Breast Cancer Gene Research and Medical Practices

The discovery of the two 'inherited susceptibility' genes BRCA1 and BRCA2 in the mid-1990s created the possibility of predictive genetic testing and led to the establishment of specific medical programmes for those at high risk of developing breast cancer in the UK, US and Europe. In the intervening fifteen years, the medical institutionalization of these knowledge-practices and accompanying medical techniques for assessing and managing risk have advanced at a rapid pace across a global and transnational terrain, whilst also themselves constituting a highly mobile and shifting terrain.

This unique edited collection brings together cross-disciplinary social science research to present a broad global comparative understanding of the implications of BRCA gene research and medical practice. With a focus on time-economies that unfold in national, transnational and global arenas (including India, UK, USA, Canada, Australia, Brazil, Germany and France) and how this facilitates a re-reading of core concepts such as prevention, kinship and heredity, this edited collection provides a unique, timely and comparative perspective on these developments.

The book provides a coherent structure for examining the diversity of practices and discourses that surround developments linked to BRCA genetics. It will be of interest to students and scholars of anthropology, sociology, history of science, STS, public health and bioethics.

Sahra Gibbon is a Lecturer in the anthropology department at University College London.

Galen Joseph is Associate Professor in the department of anthropology, history and social medicine at the University of California, San Francisco.

Jessica Mozersky is a Postdoctoral Fellow in the department of anthropology at the New School for Social Research in New York City.

Andrea zur Nieden is a sociologist and a Research Assistant at the Institute for the History of Medicine, Heinrich-Heine-Universität Düsseldorf, Germany.

Sonja Palfner is a social scientist contributing to the field of science and technology studies.

Genetics and Society

Series Editors:
Ruth Chadwick
Director of Cesagen, Cardiff University
John Dupré
Director of Egenis, Exeter University
David Wield
Director of Innogen, Edinburgh University
Steve Yearley
Director of the Genomics Forum, Edinburgh University

The books in this series, all based on original research, explore the social, economic and ethical consequences of the new genetic sciences. The series is based in the Cesagen, one of the centres forming the ESRC's Genomics Network (EGN), the largest UK investment in social-science research on the implications of these innovations. With a mix of research monographs, edited collections, textbooks and a major new handbook, the series is a valuable contribution to the social analysis of developing and emergent bio-technologies.

Series titles include:

New Genetics, New Social Formations
Peter Glasner, Paul Atkinson and Helen Greenslade

New Genetics, New Identities
Paul Atkinson, Peter Glasner and Helen Greenslade

The GM Debate
Risk, politics and public engagement
Tom Horlick-Jones, John Walls, Gene Rowe, Nick Pidgeon, Wouter Poortinga, Graham Murdock and Tim O'Riordan

Growth Cultures
Life sciences and economic development
Philip Cooke

Human Cloning in the Media
Joan Haran, Jenny Kitzinger, Maureen McNeil and Kate O'Riordan

Local Cells, Global Science
Embryonic stem cell research in India
Aditya Bharadwaj and Peter Glasner

Handbook of Genetics and Society
Paul Atkinson, Peter Glasner and Margaret Lock

The Human Genome
Chamundeeswari Kuppuswamy

Community Genetics and Genetic Alliances
Eugenics, carrier testing and networks of risk
Aviad E. Raz

Neurogenetic Diagnoses. The Power of Hope and the Limits of Today's Medicine
Carole Browner and H. Mabel Preloran

Debating Human Genetics
Contemporary issues in public policy and ethics
Alexandra Plows

Genetically Modified Crops on Trial
Opening up alternative futures of Euro-agriculture
Les Levidow

Creating Conditions
The making and remaking of a genetic condition
Katie Featherstone and Paul Atkinson

Genetic Testing
Accounts of autonomy, responsibility and blame
Michael Arribas-Allyon, Srikant Sarangi and Angus Clarke

Regulating Next Generation Agri-Food Biotechnologies
Lessons from European, North American and Asian Experiences
Edited by Michael Howlett and David Laycock

Regenerating Bodies
Tissue and cell therapies in the twenty-first century
Julie Kent

Gender and Genetics
Sociology of the prenatal
Kate Reed

Risky Genes
Genetics, breast cancer and Jewish identity
Jessica Mozersky

The Gene, the Clinic, and the Family
Diagnosing dysmorphology, reviving medical dominance
Joanna Latimer

Barcoding Nature
Shifting cultures of taxonomy in an age of biodiversity loss
Claire Waterton, Rebecca Ellis and Brian Wynne

Negotiating Bioethics
The governance of UNESCO's bioethics programme
Adèle Langlois

Breast Cancer Gene Research and Medical Practices
Transnational perspectives in the time of BRCA
Edited by Sahra Gibbon, Galen Joseph, Jessica Mozersky, Andrea zur Nieden and Sonja Palfner

Forthcoming titles include:

Scientific, Clinical and Commercial Development of the Stem Cell
From radiobiology to regenerative medicine
Alison Kraft

Breast Cancer Gene Research and Medical Practices

Transnational perspectives in the time of BRCA

Edited by Sahra Gibbon, Galen Joseph, Jessica Mozersky, Andrea zur Nieden and Sonja Palfner

Routledge
Taylor & Francis Group
LONDON AND NEW YORK

First published 2014
by Routledge
2 Park Square, Milton Park, Abingdon, Oxon OX14 4RN

and by Routledge
711 Third Avenue, New York, NY 10017

Routledge is an imprint of the Taylor & Francis Group, an informa business

British Library Cataloguing in Publication Data
A catalogue record for this book is available from the British Library

Library of Congress Cataloging-in-Publication Data
Breast cancer gene research and medical practices : transnational perspectives in the time of BRCA / edited by Sahra Gibbon [and four others].
pages cm
Includes bibliographical references and index.
1. Breast—Cancer—Genetic aspects. 2. BRCA genes. 3. Tumor markers. I. Gibbon, Sahra, editor of compilation.
RC280.B8B67223 2014
616.99'449—dc23
2013038407

ISBN: 978-0-415-82406-4 (hbk)
ISBN: 978-0-203-38551-7 (ebk)

Typeset in Times New Roman
by Apex CoVantage, LLC

Contents

Contributors

A. Lane Baldwin was a Research Aide at the Institute of Genome Sciences and Policy, Duke University from 2012–2013. She is currently pursuing an MD at the University of North Carolina.

Susanne Bauer is Associate Professor in Sociology at Goethe University Frankfurt. Her current research interests include the sociology of infrastructure, databases and biobanks in biomedicine and environmental sciences, the history of risk assessment and population sciences. Having moved to the social studies of science from environmental sciences and epidemiology, she worked as a research scholar at the Max-Planck Institute for the History of Science, at the Institute of European Ethnology, Humboldt University Berlin, and at Medicinsk Museion, University of Copenhagen.

Pascale Bourret is an Associate Professor of Sociology at Aix-Marseille Université, and a researcher at the SESSTIM (Sciences économiques et sociales de la santé et traitement de l'information médicale) research unit in Marseille. She has published several articles on the reconfiguration of medical practices in cancer genetics. Her present work centers on the emergence of personalized cancer medicine in relation to genomics.

Alberto Cambrosio is a Professor in the Department of Social Studies of Medicine at McGill University in Montreal (Canada). His present work focuses on the sociology of innovation at the cancer/genomics interface. His most recent book is *Cancer on Trial: Oncology as a New Style of Practice* (University of Chicago Press, 2012), co-authored with Peter Keating, with whom he has also co-authored *Biomedical Platforms: Realigning the Normal and the Pathological in Late-Twentieth-Century Medicine* (MIT Press, 2003), and *Exquisite Specificity: The Monoclonal Antibody Revolution* (Oxford University Press, 1995).

Julia Carbone is currently completing her SJD at Duke University, examining the relationship between formal intellectual property laws and informal community norms surrounding innovation. She holds degrees in philosophy and law from McGill University as well as a Master of Laws from Duke University. She was a researcher at both McGill's Centre for Intellectual Property Policy and Duke University's Centre for Genome, Ethics, Law and Policy. She is co-author on a project examining the political context and implications of Myriad Genetics' patenting of human genes related to breast and ovarian cancer. She is currently a law clerk to the Honourable Marc Noël, Judge of the Federal Court of Appeal.

Subhashini (Shubha) Chandrasekharan, PhD, is currently a Research Assistant Professor in the Institute for Genome Sciences and Policy at Duke University. Her research involves studying the effects of intellectual property (IP) on innovation and access to biomedical technologies, particularly emerging genetic and genomic diagnostics.

Robert Cook-Deegan is Research Professor of Public Policy, Biology and Medicine at the Institute for Genome Sciences and Policy, Duke University. He joined Duke's faculty after twenty years in public policy positions in Washington, DC, where worked at the congressional Office of Technology Assessment (1982–1988), National Center for Human Genome Research (NIH, 1989–1990) and The National Academies (1991–2002). He is the author *of The Gene Wars: Science, Politics, and the Human Genome* and an author on over two-hundred articles.

Sahra Gibbon is a Lecturer in the Anthropology Department at University College London. She has carried out ethnographic research in the UK, Cuba and Brazil examining developments in cancer genetics and public health. She is author of *Breast Cancer Genes and the Gendering of Knowledge* published by Palgrave Macmillan (2007) and *Biosocialities, Genetics and the Social Sciences. Making Biologies and Identities* published by Routledge (2008).

Richard Gold is a James McGill Professor at McGill University's Faculty of Law where he was the founding director of the Centre for Intellectual Property Policy. He teaches in the area of intellectual property and innovation. His research centers on the nexus between innovation, development and commerce, particularly with respect to biotechnology.

Deborah R. Gordon is a medical anthropologist and affiliated faculty at the Department of Anthropology, History and Social Medicine at the University of California, San Francisco. She has conducted ethnographic research on a range of topics in the US, Israel and Italy. She worked eighteen years at the Center for the Study and Prevention in Florence, Italy, during which she followed new developments around the genetics of breast cancer in Italy, Europe and the US, and later headed a project on the International Haplotype Map in Tuscany. She is co-editor of *Biomedicine Examined* (Springer 1988) and *Unhealthy Work* (Baywood Publishing 2009) and co-author of *Narrative and the End of Life* (2000, in Italian).

Nina Hallowell currently works as an applied medical sociologist and holds an honorary position in the Medical School at Melbourne and Cambridge Universities. She formerly held teaching posts at De Montfort University, The

University of Edinburgh and Newcastle University. For the past twenty years she has undertaken research on cancer genetics, and is particularly interested in the impact of risk management on identity.

Galen Joseph, PhD, is Associate Professor in the Department of Anthropology, History and Social Medicine at the University of California, San Francisco, where she is also a member of the Helen Diller Family Comprehensive Cancer Center. Her research, at the intersection of medical anthropology and public health, investigates the socio-cultural and institutional dimensions of inequities in cancer care in the US. She has published in numerous journals in the social sciences, medicine and public health. She received her PhD in Cultural Anthropology from the University of California, Santa Cruz.

Peter Keating is a member of the Centre Interuniversitaire de la Recherche sur la Science la Technologie at the Université du Québec à Montréal where he works on the history of contemporary biomedicine. He is the co-author (with Alberto Cambrosio) of *Biomedical Platforms: The Realignment of the Normal and the Pathological in 20th Century Biomedicine* (MIT Press, 2003) and *Cancer on Trial: Oncology as a New Style of Practice* (University of Chicago Press, 2013).

Sandra Soo-Jin Lee, PhD, is a medical anthropologist who studies socio-cultural dimensions and the ethical implications of emerging genomic technologies and their translation into biomedical practice. Dr. Lee is co-editor of *Revisiting Race in a Genomic Age* (Rutgers University Press, 2008) and is currently working on a project entitled Social Networking and Personal Genomics: Implications for Health Research. She received her undergraduate degree in Human Biology from Stanford University and her doctorate in Medical Anthropology from the University of California, Berkeley and San Francisco Joint Program. Dr. Lee is a Senior Research Scholar at the Center for Biomedical Ethics and faculty in the Program in Science, Technology and Society at Stanford University.

Dianne Nicol is a Professor at the Law Faculty at the University of Tasmania and one of the Deputy Directors of the Centre for Law and Genetics (CLG). Dianne's research particularly focuses on the legal issues associated with the commercialization of genetic knowledge and patenting of genetic inventions. She is currently the lead chief investigator on two Australian Research Council funded projects, one on patenting of biotechnology inventions and the other on the role of law in the era of personalized medicine. In October 2012 Dianne was appointed by the Australian government to examine pharmaceutical patents as part of a three-member expert panel.

Alison Macdonald completed her PhD in the department of anthropology, University College London. She has carried out ethnographic research in India examining the proliferation of breast cancer activism. Her research interests include the anthropology of South Asia, personhood, gender, kinship, religion and medical anthropology.

Inmaculada de Melo-Martin, PhD, MS, is Professor of Public Health in the Division of Medical Ethics, Weill Cornell Medical College. She holds a PhD in Philosophy and a MS in Molecular Biology. Her research interests include Bioethics and Philosophy of Science. Most of her work has been on ethical and epistemological issues related to reprogenetics and the biomedical sciences. She is the author of *Making Babies* (Kluwer, 1998) and *Taking Biology Seriously* (Rowman and Littlefield, 2005).

Jessica Mozersky, PhD, is a postdoctoral fellow in the Department of Anthropology at the New School for Social Research in New York City. She is the author of *Risky Genes: Genetics, Breast Cancer and Jewish Identity* (Routledge, 2013). She received her PhD in cultural anthropology from University College London, UK.

Andrea zur Nieden, PhD, is a sociologist and a Research Assistant at the Institute for the History of Medicine, Heinrich-Heine-Universität, Düsseldorf, Germany. She carried out anthropological research in German breast cancer genetic centers and received her PhD from Albert-Ludwigs-University in Freiburg. She is author of *Zum Subjekt der Gene werden. Subjektivierungsweisen im Zeichen der Genetisierung von Brustkrebs* [Becoming a Subject of the Genes. Ways of Subjectification in the Era of Genetification of Breast Cancer], published by Transcript (2013). Another current focus of her work is the history of German psychiatry since 1945.

Sonja Palfner, PhD, is a social scientist contributing to the field of science and technology studies. Currently she examines scientific infrastructures– especially the role of computing centers – and their impact on current transformations in the social order of the sciences (E-Science, Digital Humanities). Previously, she has conducted fieldwork on BRCA research and medical practices in Germany. She is author of *Gen-Passagen. Molekularbiologische und medizinische Praktiken im Umgang mit Brustkrebs-Genen. Wissen – Technologie – Diagnostik* [Gene-passages. Molecularbiological and Medical Practices Related to Breast Cancer Genes]. Knowledge – Technology – Diagnosis, published by Transcript (2009).

Britta Pelters is a teacher at the Department of Neurobiology, Care Sciences and Society and a research coordinator at the Department of Public Health Sciences, Karolinska Institute, Stockholm. She has done qualitative research on relational health and health norms and is the author of *Doing Health in der Gemeinschaft. Brustkrebsgene zwischen gesellschaftlicher, familiärer und individueller Gesundheitsnorm* [Doing Health in the Community: Breast Cancer Genes Between Societal, Familial and Individual Health Norms], published by transcript (2012).

Lisa R. Rubin, PhD, is an Associate Professor of Psychology at the New School for Social Research in New York City. Her scholarship examines the intersecting processes of gender, objectification and biomedicalization, particularly in the contexts of cancer (and cancer risk), infertility, and body weight and shape. Her work has been supported by the NIH Human Genome Project's

ELSI program, and has been published in journals spanning the disciplines of psychology, medicine and anthropology.

Martina Schlünder is a historian of medicine and science and a medical doctor. She is currently affiliated with the Ludwik Fleck Center at ETH-Zurich and a visiting scholar at the Max Planck Institute for the History of Science in Berlin. Her interdisciplinary research at the intersection with feminist science studies, anthropology and science and technology studies explores the history of reproduction in the long twentieth century, the history of biomedicine, and human-animal relationships in biomedicine.

Rayna Rapp is professor and associate chair in the Anthropology Department, New York University. She has published the award-winning *Testing Women, Testing the Fetus: the Social Impact of Amniocentesis in America* and many articles on the subject of gender and health, genetic testing, disability and the politics of reproduction. Some can be downloaded here: http://anthropology.as.nyu.edu/object/raynarapp.html.

Esther van Zimmeren (LLM, PhD) is Research Professor of Globalization, Multilevel Governance and Federalism at the Law Faculty of the University of Antwerp (Belgium), Assistant Professor in intellectual property (IP) law in the LLM program in European Competition and IP law at the University of Liège (Belgium) and senior research fellow at the Centre for Intellectual Property Rights of the University of Leuven (Belgium). Before joining academia in 2004, she was a legal assistant for Judge A.W.H. Meij at the General Court of the EU in Luxembourg in the area of European trademark and competition law (2002–2004). She has been a visiting professor at Hanken Business School and Aalto University (Helsinki), a visiting scholar at Gakushuin University (Tokyo), the Institute of Intellectual Property (IIP) in Tokyo, the University of California, Berkeley and Duke University and a research fellow at the Brocher Foundation (Geneva). Her research focuses on IP law, in particular patent and trademark law, competition law, international trade law and governance issues. Most of her work includes an important comparative (US, Europe and Japan) and interdisciplinary (i.e. biotechnology, genetics, economics and political sciences) component.

Foreword

Rayna Rapp

We live in genetically-entangled times. In North America and Western Europe, reports of genetic technologies, whether for prenatal or late-onset testing or surveillance databases, appear daily in our media. Broad swaths of the public, we could easily argue, are being tutored to anticipate positive outcomes from such interventions. Yet, as the fascinating and thought-provoking chapters you are about to read make clear, the moving target of breast cancer genetics continually remakes the local as well as international conditions under which it is deployed. We cannot assume that the meanings of the technology itself or its means of use are everywhere the same. Networks of research, as well as medical and activist practice, are highly heterogeneous, enacted differently with sundry consequences and implications in various countries and regions. This is surely true of all the emergent genetic tests, screens and therapeutic technologies.

There are real-time consequences of diverse and heterogeneous national and international networks of practice. As the protocols of genetic testing for breast cancer susceptibility spread unevenly (or don't spread!) from richer to developing nations, they leave in their wake traces that are signposts of historical, moral as well as political economies. In the conference at which many of these chapters were first presented, case studies drawn from India, Israel, Greece, Brazil and Uruguay as well as the US, UK, Italy and Germany illustrated startlingly different dilemmas raised by the presence or absence (or absent presence) of BRCA networks of testing and knowledge production. In India, for example, all technologies for the early detection of breast cancer are tragically absent. Families worry about transmission through 'the blood': the discourse of genetics and genetic testing plays no role, and 'blood' connotes far older, enduring notions of lineage and affiliation. This longstanding polysemic meaning to blood is deeply entangled with the hereditary cancers and plays out in a context where the biggest public health issue concerning breast cancer (and virtually every other cancer) concerns the lack of early diagnosis through which (some) lives could be saved. Yet as an echo of India's fast-paced contemporary modernization, mothers now frequently express worry about the 'life style' of their daughters: will they marry and have babies young enough to protect themselves from what is widely viewed as a modernist death sentence carried by this particular diagnosis? In India, earlier detection and access to treatment rather than genetic testing are clear paths to the reduction of both the fear and ravages of this disease.

In Cuba, where Sahra Gibbon, one of this book's editors, conducted fieldwork, resources for genetic testing are likewise absent (Gibbon 2009, 2011). But a lengthy and robust tradition of 'community genetics' makes mobilization and cooperation in the collection of family-at-risk pedigrees a welcomed public benefit: Cuban public health workers are not likely to gain access to BRCA testing anytime soon. But their educational mission in discussing this disease within families and communities is highly valued, even (or perhaps especially) by those who live with heightened consciousness of the hereditary influences on breast cancer in their own intimate networks. In Germany, genetic counselors never ask about ethnicity – widely used in North America and in some parts of Europe as a low-level screening device for deciding who is at heightened risk, and might be offered additional testing. The subject is haunted by Germany's Nazi past: healthcare professionals cannot comfortably query Jewish ancestry, but recent immigrant histories are widely viewed as clues to hapless health behavior. These, rather than the 'racialized roots' understood to be borne by Ashkenazi Jews, a population on which early BRCA testing was developed, can be more comfortably discussed, and services that might help in immigrant assimilation process can be offered. Yet in Israel, home to a large population of Ashkenazi Jews whose initial BRCA mutations have been well-researched, whole population testing is now being piloted under the assumption that BRCA risks are far higher for many families than they currently know. As Shiri Shkedi Rafid informed us in her conference paper (not included in this volume), a complex historic consciousness of both the massive premature deaths owed to the Holocaust and the dramatic decline in completed contemporary family size both enter into the scientific imaginary as new cases of BRCA 'carriers' as well as breast cancer become the objects of cutting-edge genetic epidemiological research.

These fascinating examples of differential testing ethics play out not only in terms of face-to-face interaction between counselors, nurses, physicians and women with or without 'informative' family histories. They also bear the marks of different national regulatory apparatuses, medical education, and laboratory practices, all of which are shaped by their specific local context. Thus even the networks of BRCA knowledge production are highly heterogeneous, and this situation is likely to become more complex now that the US patent held by Myriad Genetics on BRCA testing (honored in its home country, but not necessarily throughout the world) has been set aside by the US Supreme Court (see van Zimmeren *et al.*, this volume). This moment reinforces American investigators' and clinicians' participation in increasingly dense international networks of breast cancer research, part of the continual transformation of the research/clinical interface. How might methodologies, technologies, and databases be understood and harmonized to create larger-and-larger bodies of evidence on which experimental knowledge might in turn be developed? How is this new knowledge incorporated quite literally by business corporations? Or made available for public health usage? And where are the overlaps across those domains?

An examination of BRCA networks might metaphorically be viewed as a technology which is at once a telescope and a microscope: viewed through the end of extreme magnification of the microscopic, BRCA (and other instances of haplotype differences) potentially reveals histories of migration, marriage and mating across the *longue durée* of varied and mobile regional populations. When angled outward toward metaphorical magnification, a focus on BRCA leads us to query national and international institutions, connections, barriers and aspirations for preventive and clinical care for diseases like this one, in which a frank genetic connection has been identified but its significance is far from clear. We do not currently understand the impact of research, testing and the benefits and limits of clinical treatment in the many multiple stratified populations that carry BRCA and other genomic variants that increase breast cancer risk. This complexity serves as both a warning of the limits of biomedical knowledge, and as a promissory note of what the intersection of public health and genomic medicine might someday accomplish. Genetic entanglements, indeed. And these are rapidly changing before our very eyes: the time of BRCA is gaining velocity.

Of course, the connections wrought by BRCA are the subject of much activism and advocacy as some carriers form themselves into 'imagined communities' to militate for research and clinical resources in North America and parts of Europe. A genealogy of 'biological citizenship', in which those affected by specific health damages or challenges use their differences to make claims on state resources, surely owes much to the concept as enunciated by Adriana Petryna (2013). Investigating responses to the Chernobyl disaster and its aftermath in the Ukraine, Petryna analyzed the devastating marketability of exposure, radiation illness and injury, producing 'biological citizenship' as a concept to connote the specificity of an individual claim which, escalated in its collective implications, mounted on biological damage. She surely was working in the tradition of her teacher, anthropologist Paul Rabinow; his earlier publication on 'biosociality' as a form of social relations that took shape in late modernity was at once highly influential and circumscribed in ways that Sahra Gibbon and Carlos Novas explored in their edited collection (Gibbon and Novas 2008). This scholarly conversation was in turn richly indebted to notions of self-surveillance developed in the influential work of Michel Foucault, as Nikolas Rose and Carlos Novas pointed out (Rose and Novas 2005).

Much of the literature on patient and family support groups emerges from studies conducted in the US and Northern Europe (cf. Gibbon and Novas 2008); other parts of the world seem far less prone to collectivizing a biologized notion of 'fate' (see Gordon's article in this volume). The idea of organizing around one's genomic identity ('pastoral communities', as Paul Rabinow first described them (Rabinow 1992), of those seeking common meaning in their ambiguously, potentially shared fate, indeed, of organizing around a biological trait or potential health problem, sets the stage not only for biological citizenship but also for a range of concepts that were more-or-less independently invented to describe related identities and praxes: somatic citizenship (Novas and Rose 2000), genetic citizenship (Heath, Rapp, and Taussig 2004) and corporeal citizenship (Lock 2013), each deployed with considerable subtlety and under limited conditions. In a broader sense, an argument can be made that all these labels constitute useful but provisional attempts to understand new bases for claims on public resources for biologically based problems that entail both irreducibly person-centered health risks and vulnerabilities, and critiques of medical research and limited access. All these genetically sensitized forms of activism shape evolving notions of personhood, as many of the social scientists cited above have pointed out. Additionally, these conceptual umbrellas were and are in some profound sense a response to the intrusion of neoliberal market ideology into the realm of healthcare.

On a tide of rising expectations in Western countries, the market-based promissory note of rapid-response research leading to idealized, efficient and utopian therapeutic intervention has differentially taken hold of an activized health imaginary. This world-view and praxis loops right back into fund-raising as well as advocacy and public education. All this action is aimed at 'the race for the cure'. These 'Western' new-ish formations of advocacy have been strongly marked by the profusion and diffusion of medical technologies and chemotherapeutics as both a highly profitable source of investment and a site of hype/hope (Hoeyer and Lynöe 2006; Hoeyer 2007; Hoeyer 2009; Gibbon 2007; Mozersky 2013; Lee, this volume). This volatile and explosive staging of medicine-as-market coincides with and encourages the desire to publicize what had formerly been experienced as a private dilemma or tragedy for individuals and their families. Before the present era of activism, much of the personal devastation of relatively early onset hereditary illness played out in the intimacy of family life. Now, activists sensitized to hereditary breast cancer organize not only for public recognition and material support; many also search for a language that legitimates their concerns: Are they breast cancer survivors? Pre-symptomatic persons/patients? Previvors? All are relatively recent attempts to underline the lifelong dilemmas of living under a geneticized gaze (Chilibeck, Lock, and Sehdev 2011; Lippman 1993; Lock 2005). Whether viewed as biological or wounded citizens (Brown 1995), such groups are in the process of forging new collective identities dedicated to the utopian goal of 'curing breast cancer in our lifetime'.

Yet such social movements dwell on a deeply fractured landscape of breast cancer activism that is highly unstable and 'changing in front of our eyes', as Kristen McHenry pointed out in her conference paper (not included in this volume). The US, for example, is home to a powerful yet cantankerous and divided breast cancer movement; increasingly, other rich countries also manifest similar splits. Strategies may be 'pink' or 'green', depending on whether they emphasize public education and life-style changes that may well affect women's individual risk, or the consequences of carcinogenic environmental factors. Of course, there is overlap in the analysis and practice of many groups and projects, and there is change, too. For example some groups initially and quite successfully dedicated themselves to fund-raising for research. Over time, they also evolved plans to fund more mammograms, genetic testing and preventative strategies for low-income women, constituting a critique of the US healthcare system not initially in their business plan. Yet not all groups have agreed to ban carcinogens in their give-aways, or signed up to partner with the American Civil Liberties Union in the suit against Myriad, or focus on individual 'life style' (what an obfuscating word! Is it a life style choice to marry and/or have a first child late or nurse only briefly if at all or to be exposed to potential carcinogens in your backyard, your office or your supermarket? These are hardly matters of individual decision-making! Yet they are construed that way too often, at least in the US.) If breast cancer is a heterogeneous disease, so, too, is the activism that surrounds it in some rather selective national settings.

The science of breast cancer genetics is heterogeneous, as well. It includes genetic epidemiology which follows the public health implications of, for example, steady changes in reproduction borne through the shifting upward age of marriage in many countries, and therefore the elevated age for first births as well as duration of nursing. All these factors impact rising breast cancer rates. In molecular genomics, for example, the focus has increasingly turned to the building of molecular tumor signature databases that may reveal multiple pathways toward mechanisms of mutational breakdown of tumor repair capacity. These in turn may implicate 'new pharmaceuticals in search of a disease' in the felicitous words of Bourret, Cambrosio and Keating in this volume. Of course, the numerous endocrine disrupters found in industrial products have long been the object of environmental scientific scrutiny; increasingly, these are given a molecular upgrade in epigenetics, the currently popular scientific study of environmental cell-based mechanisms that turn on and off gene action. In this case, 'environment' is operationalized to include factors ranging from the cellular-biochemical to common-sense understandings of toxicity. In other words, a coterie of interested groups including advocacy organizations, clinicians, national and international policy makers and interdisciplinary bench scientists all hold stakes in the complexity of research into breast cancer, and where its battle lines are drawn. This science is located on an expansive horizon: for example the human microbiome project now much in the media will surely raise new modalities of diagnosing risk and protection.[1]

The 'Time of BRCA' is thus non-synchronous and fast-paced in some scientific, public health, advocacy and investment environments while not even ticking in others. Activists and their researcher-allies regularly encounter the heterogeneity of heredity, of cell culture and biotic synchronies and of individual and genealogical life spans in trying to map both this complex disease and potential interventions into it, some of which flow from BRCA testing. At the same time, our authors note the gendering of responsibility to the time of the future by dwelling in the past, all illuminated by how mothers and others understand and respond to stretches of their received DNA as it is potentially passed down to their daughters (and sons, although this is less well-known).

Writers and readers of this book are thus perched on a biopolitical horizon, trying to discern the events and entities that brought us here, and their implications for multiple potential futures we only partially can imagine and little control. From our diverse positions, we are of course implicated in 'the time of BRCA', as well: the production schedules of researchers, clinicians and activists located at the volatile intersection where deeply gendered embodiment, biomedical testing and clinical care, national aspirations and regulations, fatalism and hope all meet on the ground of breast cancer and its reverberations. As part of that hybrid international network of knowledge production, the book you are about to read is thought-provoking, indeed. I invite you to share 'the time of BRCA' at whatever pace prevails in the work you do and the understandings you bring to it.

Note

1. The Human Microbiome project aims to characterize the microbes found at different sites on the human body (such as nasal passages, oral cavities, skin and gastrointestinal tract) and to analyze the role of these microbes in human health and disease.

References

Brown, W. (1995) *States of Injury: Power and Freedom in Late Modernity,* Princeton, NJ: Princeton University Press.

Chilibeck, G., Lock, M. and Sehdev, M. (2011) 'Postgenomics, uncertain futures, and the familiarization of susceptibility genes', *Social Science and Medicine*, 72 (11): 1768–1775.

Gibbon, S. (2007) *Breast Cancer Genes and the Gendering of Knowledge: Science and Citizenship in the Cultural Context of the "New" Genetics*. Basingstoke, Hampstead: Palgrave Macmillan.

Gibbon, S. (2009) 'Genomics as public health? Community genetics and the challenge of personalised medicine in Cuba', *Anthropology and Medicine*, 16 (2): 131–146.

Gibbon, S. (2011) 'Family Medicine, "La Herencia" and breast cancer: Understanding the (dis)continuities of predictive genetics in Cuba', *Social Science and Medicine*, 72 (11): 1784–1792.

Gibbon, S. and Novas, C. (eds) (2008) *Biosocialities, Genetics, and the Social Sciences: Making Biologies and Identities*. London: Routledge.

Heath, D., Rapp, R. and Taussig, K.S. (2004) 'Genetic citizenship', in D. Nugent and J. Vincent (eds) *A Companion to the Anthropology of Politics*, Oxford: Blackwell.

Hoeyer, K. (2007) 'Person, patent and property: A critique of the commodification hypothesis', *BioSocieties*, 2 (3): 327–348.

———. (2009) 'Donors perceptions of consent to and feedback from biobank research: Time to acknowledge diversity?', *Public Health Genomics*, 13 (6): 345–352.

Hoeyer, K. and Lynöe, N. (2006) 'Motivating donors to genetic research? Anthropological reasons to rethink the role of informed consent', *Medicine, Health Care and Philosophy*, 9 (1): 13–23.

Lippman, A. (1993) 'Prenatal genetic testing and geneticization: Mother matters for all', *Fetal Diagnosis and Therapy*, 8: 175–188.

Lock, M. (2005) 'Alzheimer's disease: A tangled concept', in S. McKinnon and S. Silverman (eds) *Complexities: Beyond Nature and Nurture*, New York: Routledge.

Lock, M. (2013) *The Alzheimer Conundrum: Entanglements of Dementia and Aging*, Princeton University Press.

Mozersky, J. (2013) *Risky Genes: Genetics, Breast Cancer and Jewish Identity,* London: Routledge.

Novas, C. and Rose, N. (2000) 'Genetic risk and the birth of the somatic individual', *Economy and Society*, 29 (4): 485–513.

Petryna, A. (2013) *Life Exposed: Biological Citizens After Chernobyl*. Princeton, NJ: Princeton University Press.

Rabinow, P. (1992) 'Artificiality and Enlightenment: From Sociobiology to Biosociality', in Jonathan Crary and Sanford Kwinter (eds) *Incorporations*, New York: Zone; reprinted in *Essays on the Anthropology of Reason* (1996), Princeton, NJ: Princeton University Press.

Rose, N. and Novas, C. (2005) 'Biological citizenship', in A. Ong and S. Collier (eds) *Global Assemblages: Technology, Politics, and Ethics as Anthropological Problems*, Malden, MA: Blackwell. Accessed 20 July 2013. http://webfirstlive.lse.ac.uk/sociology/pdf/RoseandNovasBiologicalCitizenship2002.pdf

Preface

This book has its origins in the 'BRCA Network', an international group of social science researchers from various disciplines who began to examine BRCA practices collectively in 2009. Noting that many social science research initiatives proceed in parallel with little multi-disciplinary or cross-cultural discussion, Sonja Palfner initiated a plan to bring together social science scholars to share and discuss their research in this field. Together, Palfner and Sahra Gibbon planned a workshop, held in March 2009 at the Environmental Policy Research Centre of the Freie Universität Berlin and funded by the Fritz Thyssen Foundation. The workshop aimed to explore how micro or ethnographic research approaches can illuminate developments surrounding the BRCA genes. Workshop participants represented the fields of Science and Technology Studies (STS), sociology, political science and anthropology with expertise in the social science analysis of 'BRCA' breast cancer gene research and medical practices.[1] A follow-up workshop funded by the Wellcome Trust was held in March 2010 at University College London with more participants, and focused on the scope and meaning of 'comparative' approaches to BRCA gene research and medical practices and their socio-cultural consequences. Together, these two workshops led to the publication of a special section in BioSocieties (Gibbon *et al.* 2010), and to the organization of a larger conference at the Brocher Foundation in Geneva in December 2011, which culminated in this edited volume.

Co-funded by the Wellcome Trust and the Fritz Thyssen Foundation, the aim of the three-day conference at the Brocher Foundation was to extend and deepen research by bringing together an established network of cross-disciplinary social scientists, and specifically to broaden the discussion and understanding of these developments beyond Euro-American societies (where much attention has focused) by including those working in developing countries. The conference brought together twenty-one researchers working in the field of breast cancer gene research to compare international perspectives on these developments. The research presented addressed BRCA-related practices in Australia, Brazil, Canada, Cuba, France, Germany, Greece, India, Israel, the UK, Uruguay and the US, and included researchers in sociology, anthropology, STS, history of science, history of medicine, public health and political science. Participants' work addressed questions of patient subjectivity and female identity, family/kin relationships in the context of genetic testing, population genetics, ethnicity and race and public health and the dynamic relationship between BRCA gene research, laboratory practices, medical research and the health care professions.

While this collection brings together the work of researchers examining a variety of locations and national contexts, including some who did not participate in the Brocher Workshop, we acknowledge that many countries and contexts are not represented here. The initial workshops and subsequent conference highlighted the enormous range of socio-political issues that come up in the context of BRCA-related research, including the impact of biotechnological developments on contemporary medical practices; the interrelation of subjectivities, medical practices and socio-political rationalities; the local connections between genetics, medicine and women's health; research developments in the field of BRCA; the challenges of collaboration and interdisciplinary research and the ontological and epistemological 'being' of the breast cancer genes. This collection represents the ongoing discussions, research and comparative nature of the BRCA Network.

The authors are grateful to the Brocher Foundation (www.brocher.ch), the Fritz Thyssen Foundation and the Wellcome Trust (grant number WT095798MF) for their support. We would like to thank all of the staff at the Brocher Foundation where we were fortunate enough to be granted a three-day stay on the shores of Lake Geneva. We would also like to thank Richard Tutton for his helpful comments; Michelle Miles for proofreading; Helen Greenslade, editorial manager at the EGN Book Series; and Emily Briggs, editorial assistant at Routledge for their help throughout.

Note

1. Our first BRCA Network meeting in 2009 was composed of Sonja Palfner, Andrea zur Nieden, Jessica Mozersky, Eirini Kampriani, Galen Joseph, Sahra Gibbon and Pascale Bourret.

Reference

Gibbon, S., Palfner, S., Kalender, U., Joseph, G., Mozersky, J., Kampriani, E. and zur Nieden, A. (2010) 'Introduction to special section: perspectives on globalizing genomics: the case of "BRCA" breast cancer research and medical practice'. *BioSocieties* 5: 407–414.

Introduction

We finalize this book on the 'time of BRCA' at a pivotal moment in the history of breast cancer genetics. The BRCA genes are configured amidst dynamically interacting medical, scientific, cultural, socio-political and economic parameters, which are essential to understanding this continually evolving terrain.

Using BRCA as a case study, this book sheds light on transformations that are occurring in the wider field of genomic science and medicine as a result of new technological possibilities, transnational research collaborations and ever-widening parameters and definitions of risk. Our focus on time-economies illustrates how temporal notions of past, present and future are built into genomic developments, and as such facilitates a re-reading of core concepts like risk, prevention, kinship and heredity. We begin, however, by highlighting some key recent developments in the field of BRCA genetics that illustrate this shifting terrain.

The first and perhaps most highly anticipated development is the recent US Supreme Court decision regarding the patentability of genes. The two breast cancer genes BRCA1 and 2 were sequenced in the mid 1990s through the efforts of multiple international research teams, and shortly thereafter patented by one of the US teams managed by Mark H. Skolnick, co-founder of Myriad Genetics Inc. (Salt Lake City, US). Since then, debates about the commercialization of biological knowledge and the proliferation of the ownership of genes have continued to be highly controversial. In June 2013, the US Supreme Court announced their decision to outlaw patents on naturally occurring genes (but not on cDNA) putting an end to Myriad Genetics' long-held and contentious monopoly on BRCA testing in the US (see van Zimmeren *et al.*, this volume).[1] Significantly, several companies that were already providing genetic testing of other genes associated with breast cancer were ready to launch their own BRCA tests the day after the decision was announced (e.g. see the Ambry press release the day of the Supreme Court Announcement, www.ambrygen.com/press). The defeat of Myriad's patent monopoly could make genetic testing without threat of litigation more financially feasible and therefore a more widespread option, or lead to an increase in research by groups previously hindered by concerns about patent infringement. Of course, the ramifications of the court's decision both inside and outside the US remain to be seen, and may take years to fully unfold while also having repercussions in global arenas.[2]

Second, the emergence of Next Generation panel tests (e.g. Ambry Genetics' BreastNext panel and the University of Washington's BROCA panel), and the increasing turn towards whole genome/exome sequencing, signals another change in the landscape of genetic testing. Next Generation panel tests, which became commercially available in 2011, examine numerous genetic changes associated with elevated breast cancer risk, including those that confer moderate and relatively low risk. As Next Generation testing becomes more widely available and financially feasible (some of the panel tests cost approximately the same as or less than Myriad's BRCA test), the criteria for testing related to hereditary breast cancer syndromes will likely widen. At the same time, the decreasing cost of whole exome/genome sequencing will likely have even broader implications, as in the future individuals may have their entire genomes sequenced rather than portions of it (such as the BRCA genes only). One potential consequence is that many more individuals will learn they carry a BRCA mutation (and many other disease-associated mutations) as a result of sequencing carried out for some other purpose – a scenario that is directly explored by Sandra Lee in this volume, in the context of BRCA testing in the direct-to-consumer setting. While Next Generation panel tests and advanced sequencing technologies predate the recent Supreme Court decision on gene patents, they will likely be informed by this decision in complex ways, thereby paving the way for expanded and broader BRCA testing. This constantly changing technological landscape which now includes whole genome sequencing has exponentially increased the initial concerns raised by BRCA testing, such as those regarding privacy, incidental findings, variants of unknown significance and return of results (Green *et al.* 2013; Kohane, Masys, and Altman 2006, Pyeritz 2011).

Third, BRCA genetics has been and continues to be a test case in the field of genomic medicine (Gibbon *et al.* 2010b; Palfner 2009): a symbol of 'success' whilst also being at the forefront of challenging the new genetics. Nevertheless, in thinking about BRCA as a barometer for the shifting space and evolving trajectory of predictive medicine, it is important to stress the gendered and gendering nature of these medical interventions that are aimed primarily at women (such as the prophylactic removal of breasts and ovaries; also see Pelters, this volume). Thus as BRCA evolves and spreads into new medical arenas, women continue to find themselves the subjects of increasing medical and scientific practices. These dynamics coexist with well-established medical practices aimed at women such as annual gynecological exams and mammographic screening programmes, and are entangled with deeply gendered life-worlds in which women function as 'genetic housekeepers' (Richards 1996: 261). Furthermore, if we consider BRCA genetics to be a test case in the field of genomic medicine, then women are the experimental field on which such endeavors are taking place (Gibbon 2013b; Happe 2006, 2013; Palfner 2009).

We can see the intersection of gender and genomics with the recent high-profile announcement by Hollywood star Angelina Jolie in a New York Times op-ed that she had undergone a preventive double mastectomy due to a 'faulty' BRCA1 gene, bringing BRCA genetics to international attention. Jolie's decision was particularly striking given her status as an international sex symbol, and contributed to increased interest in testing among many women around the world. Indeed, those of us based in cancer centres can attest to 'the Angelina effect': the increased volume in calls and inquiries from members of the public following the announcement. On the other hand, media debate, and the comments from readers of the *New York Times* and many other news outlets took up questions about access to the test and the recommended screening and prevention practices (Jolie's announcement arrived just weeks prior to the Supreme Court's decision on Myriad's patents), and about the appropriateness of 'proactive' measures like the preventive double mastectomy surgery that Jolie had. Jolie's announcement about her decision thus provoked polemical discussion about prevention and risk reduction, access to testing, gene patents the options available to women identified at risk in this way, and in some cases, the right 'not to know' about genetic risk. Her announcement serves to both highlight the way that gendered idioms of female nurturance and empowerment continue to be central to this domain, and the ongoing impact of BRCA on women.

These developments and the recent intense media attention to BRCA that has resulted provide an opportune moment for us as social scientists to engage and explore the shape-shifting present and future terrain of BRCA genetics. The confluence of events, while each of a different scale and magnitude, has heightened interest and attention to genetic testing for hereditary cancer and related matters. This book thus provides a timely contribution which reflects on the diverse socio-cultural spaces as well as the scientific and medical practices that constitute genomics in the era of BRCA.

BRCA histories

The identification of the BRCA genes in the mid 1990s was accompanied by an enormous amount of expectation, hype and hope, and swiftly led to the establishment of predictive genetic testing and specific medical programmes for those at high risk of developing breast cancer in many countries, particularly the US, Canada and Europe. Carriers of mutations in the BRCA genes are thought to have a higher risk of breast and ovarian cancer, although risk estimates vary from 45–80 per cent for breast (compared to 10 per cent for an average woman) and 10 to 60 per cent for ovarian cancer (compared to 1.8 per cent for an average woman). While they do not account for the majority of breast cancers, BRCA mutations are thought to be responsible for 5 to 10 per cent of breast cancers. Although BRCA1 and 2 have been primarily discussed in the context of familial breast and ovarian cancer, since their initial identification there has been a concurrent hope that the knowledge gained from BRCA research would have relevance for, and be transferable to, the treatment of sporadic breast cancers, which affect many more women than the rare instances of familial breast cancer (Palfner 2009). However the establishment of a robust connection between the clinical utility of BRCA and the sporadic cancer domain emerged only recently, in 2004–2005, when the concept of 'BRCAness' took hold, as discussed by Bourret and co-authors in this collection.

Since their discovery, the medical institutionalization of BRCA knowledge-practices and accompanying techniques for assessing risk have advanced at a rapid pace, involving different scientific or medical specialties, routinizing programmes of genetic testing, developing risk assessment for breast cancer and increasing health management options for those identified at increased cancer risk. The availability of BRCA samples obtained through programmes of genetic testing and risk assessment has facilitated further research (Gibbon *et al.* 2010b; Mozersky 2013; Palfner 2009), illustrating the mutually constitutive interactions between BRCA research and clinical practices. The emergence and use of BRCA genetic knowledge in clinical settings has raised questions about the social consequences of genomic information for 'patients', family and their kin as well as the scientific and clinical utility of novel knowledge of genetic risk for breast cancer. Social scientists have studied these developments in different countries from diverse perspectives, which include: examining the historical dimensions of genetic research and the related medical practices or the laboratory life that surrounds novel techniques linked to BRCA genetics (Bourret, 2005; Löwy, 2010; Palfner, 2009; Parthasarathy, 2007); analyzing the social consequences for health, identity and perceptions of risk for women undergoing assessment in cancer genetic clinics (Gibbon, 2007; Hallowell, 1999; zur Nieden, 2010, 2013) or comparing the cultural and institutional specificity of these developments, demonstrating the unevenness of the complex global intersections that are forming across a diverse field of genomic knowledge and technology (Gibbon *et al.* 2010a, Gibbon 2013b; Mozersky and Joseph 2010; Shkedi-Rafid *et al.* 2012).

While the medical and laboratory practices surrounding the BRCA genes expand, their scientific and medical bases, on the other hand, continue to raise questions. In fact, very shortly after the sequencing of BRCA1 and 2, predictive genetic testing made it apparent that very few people actually carry the BRCA1 or BRCA2 mutations (5–10 per cent as previously mentioned), and many mutations were found in families without increased incidences of breast cancer. This variability in risk and penetrance estimates reflects gaps in medical knowledge about the BRCA genes which are based on databases of known mutations and previously identified 'at risk' families and/or populations. This variability has become increasingly apparent particularly in national contexts outside the US, Canada and Europe (see Mozersky and Gibbon, this volume), and highlights the role of nongenetic and epigenetic factors in determining risk.

At the same time, the BRCA genes have led to new avenues of medical research, particularly in the use of genetic technologies for the diagnosis and treatment of breast cancer (e.g. clinical trials of targeted drug therapies for BRCA mutation carriers; see also Section 3 in this volume) and raised questions concerning the medical management of female mutation carriers and women at high risk, such as the effectiveness of mammography, the benefits of tamoxifen in chemoprevention and prophylactic mastectomy. Thus this field of medical practice and scientific engagement continues to evolve, in part as a response to the *limitations* of BRCA genetic testing. In this sense, breast cancer genetics provides a vital arena for examining how scientific stability or transition is achieved in different contexts, for example from lab to clinic or from BRCA genetics to other research arenas (e.g. epigenetics, 'Next Generation' panel testing and whole genome/exome sequencing). In other words, BRCA shifts and spreads in various directions far beyond the very limited medical programmes for familial breast and ovarian cancer.

Time-economies

As the title of this book and the chapters within indicate, we are living in the time of BRCA. In this sense, BRCA not only stimulates enormous research and pushes it in various directions; it also reconfigures the life-worlds of many women (and men), enhances specific medical programmes and puts economic, legal and ethical issues on the agenda of many health care systems. However, BRCA genes do not hold innate agency or power; rather as Palfner (2009), drawing on Haraway (1997) and Latour (2004) suggests, we should understand BRCA as an assemblage. For Haraway (1997: 142), 'a gene is not a thing, much less a "master molecule" or a self-contained code but rather the term gene signifies a node of durable action where many actors, human and nonhuman, meet'. Latour (2004: 233) underlines that the word *thing* also means 'assembly': 'A thing is, in one sense, an object out there and, in another sense, an issue very much in there, at any rate, a gathering'. In terming the breast cancer gene an assemblage, we aim to heighten awareness of how it orchestrates and performs biomedical practices, stimulates socio-political discourses and connects various medical and research arenas through times and spaces, as the essays throughout this volume demonstrate.

Temporality is a theme that weaves through all three sections of the collection, from looking back at history and genealogy (Section I), to the ways in which risk is embodied and lived in the present (Section II), to the changing landscape and future developments of BRCA testing (Section III). While the principal aim of this book is to give an overview of BRCA research and medical practices in different countries, the contributing authors also analyze the theme of temporality as it emerges in the varied contexts they explore. The political scientist Wolf-Dieter Narr reminds us that time is a social product and intersects with relations of power: 'Ruling power is always characterized by its own calendar, its own hierarchy, its own assignment of time and its own quality of this assigned time, regardless of whether every ruling power, such as the brief rule of the Jacobins during the French Revolution, literally had their own calendar' (2003: 239; author's [SP] own translation). In other words, time itself is heterogeneous and performative, and we suggest that living in the time of BRCA should encourage us to take into account time itself and recognize that understanding time is a precondition for better understanding the ongoing research and multiple medical practices related to BRCA. Thus, we think it is appropriate to speak about BRCA 'time-economies', seeing these as social matters and hence infused with power in different ways and making it vital to understand more deeply the interplay of various temporalities.

In the context of biomedicine, the matter of time materializes clearly in the notion of disease prevention. In her commentary (this volume), Martina Schlünder argues that the most important epistemic change from medicine to biomedicine is the reconfiguration of the relation between the normal and the pathological with an increasing emphasis on health instead of disease (Clarke *et al.* 2010; Keating and Cambrosio 2003). The prevention of diseases is now seen as one of the most urgent tasks in medicine as opposed to limiting actions to the treatment of pathological events that have already happened (in an unalterable past) or are still ongoing in the present. According to Adams *et al.* (2009: 248), disease prevention and predictive medicine are practices that occur in a mode of anticipation and the attempt to envision, control and manage the future and its risk of possible pathological events: 'Crucially, the future increasingly not only defines the present but also creates material trajectories of life that unfold as anticipated by those speculative processes. Anticipation is rapidly reconfiguring technoscientific and biomedical practices as a totalizing orientation.' Following this, we begin to understand the discursive power to name genes 'breast cancer genes'. On the one hand, BRCA1 and 2 are understood as tumor suppressor genes, with a single germ line mutation increasing the risk for developing breast and/or ovarian cancer; such genes thus protect cells from one step on the path to cancer. On the other hand, to call a gene a 'breast cancer gene' implies the opposite, namely that this gene is responsible for the cancer and carrying the gene means having cancer. In other words, this overlap of the pathological and the normal rolls out through the anticipation of breast cancer in the gene.

This unfolding in the identification of 'risk' for breast and ovarian cancer via BRCA testing has resulted in the normalization of preventive procedures (Robson *et al.* 2010) such as prophylactic mastectomy and prophylactic oophorectomy (see Pelters and Gordon, for discussions of prophylactic mastectomy), chemoprevention as well as Preimplantation Genetic Diagnosis (PGD) to screen embryos at risk of carrying a BRCA mutation (Rubin and de Melo-Martin, this volume). Although the acceptance and use of these preventive measures varies significantly within and across national contexts, these practices must be situated within this biomedical maelstrom in which prospective diseases are pushed into the present and thereby have a major impact on present life-worlds including the meaning of patienthood and cancer survivorship (Bell 2013).

The increasing focus on prevention in biomedicine shows up in BRCA-related practices in other ways too. In some instances, the shift toward prevention is constituted by a move toward wider screening for deleterious BRCA mutations in particular populations. For example, a recent study of African American women with breast cancer which found high rates of deleterious mutations in BRCA and other 'breast cancer genes' (e.g. CHEK2, PALB, PTEN) suggested screening for all these genes in women of African descent with breast cancer diagnosed at a young age, with a family history, or with triple negative breast cancer (Churpek *et al.* 2013). In both Israel and Canada, population-wide screening of all Ashkenazi Jews (regardless of family history) has been proposed as a viable method to identify BRCA carriers who might not otherwise come to clinical attention (Levy-Lahad *et al.* 2011; Metcalfe *et al.* 2009). On another track, public health scientists and practitioners in the US are making efforts to identify potential BRCA carriers prior to a diagnosis by screening – in both clinical and community settings – for family history and appropriate referrals to genetic counseling (rather than genetic testing) for a full assessment of BRCA risk (e.g. Bellcross *et al.* 2009; Joseph 2012 and this volume). Thus the categories of who is at risk continue to encompass more and more people, in the name of prevention, as does the notion of being at risk for breast cancer itself.[3] In other words, the enormous potential for BRCA research to be applied to a wide range of arenas of medical research and treatment and to incorporate different clinical disciplines has made and continues to make BRCA genetics significant.

The shift toward prevention also reflects breast cancer activists' and researchers' increasing attention to the causes of breast cancer rather than only treatment and survivorship. While some argue that treatment for breast cancer has improved over recent decades in terms of the survivorship rates, others suggest this is due to overdiagnosis (e.g. Esserman *et al.* 2013). Most agree, however, that the treatments themselves remain terribly damaging with enormous side effects. As a result, the goal of preventing breast cancer in the first place has become more prominent in certain national contexts. In addition, the failure to identify the causes of breast cancer to date, particularly the environmental factors that contribute and may intersect with hereditary susceptibility, is recognized as a huge barrier to reducing morbidity and mortality due to breast cancer – and as a failure of the research community. The politics of environmental pollution and the lack of regulation of polluters has also become a target for activists, particularly in the US, who have shifted their focus to prevention as discussed by Kirsten McHenry in her paper at the Brocher Conference where this volume originated (see also BreastCancerAction.org).[4] While epigenetic research holds out the promise that the parameters of research related to prevention of breast cancer may eventually encompass a more biopolitical framework that addresses collective responsibilities for disease and health, this is unlikely to mean the disappearance of individualized framings of risk. As Landecker and Panofsky (2013) point out, this may in fact paradoxically entail an intensification of the moral framing of gendered health responsibilities given that the 'critical windows' at stake in epigenetic research often relate to nutrition in early childhood and maternal-fetal health exposures (see also Mansfield 2012).

Transnational perspectives

By offering perspectives on the transnational arenas in which BRCA genetics is now evolving, this collection directly responds to the vital need for social science to engage with genomics in the context of globalizing health care agendas *and* local moral worlds of practice. Some of the chapters directly take up the task of providing a comparative perspective with reflections on the way that for instance the so called 'Ashkenazi mutations' associated with the BRCA genes are being configured differently in Brazil and the UK (Mozersky and Gibbon) and in Germany (zur Nieden). The varying ways that questions of race and ethnicity are being drawn into the developments surrounding breast cancer genetics are also highlighted in the contrasting perspective on these issues provided by papers reflecting how different national histories concerning the politics of inclusion and discrimination play out in Germany (zur Nieden) and the US (Joseph). For example, in Germany, the history of racial hygiene and the Holocaust as well as a specific tradition of perceiving the nation as 'ethnically homogenous' continue to have an effect on contemporary medical discourse. In the US, historical and ongoing discrimination experienced by African Americans affect how risk of genetic breast cancer and interventions may be viewed. Other chapters in this volume provide a reflection on the space which BRCA occupies, or rather does *not* occupy in contexts such as India (Macdonald) and Italy (Gordon), providing an important reminder of the 'absent spaces' that BRCA also constitutes. In Alison Macdonald's discussion, we see how this absence relates to overwhelming socio-economic challenges and lack of resources in treating those with breast cancer, but also very specific beliefs about disease risk and its transmission between gendered bodies, as well as 'biomoral' concerns around family relations. Deborah Gordon similarly reminds us of the way a comparative perspective can illuminate the diverse routes through which BRCA has emerged. Gordon highlights how discourses of disease risk related to BRCA genetics and the temporal anxieties they have provoked elsewhere (especially the US) have not resonated in Italy where different cultural logics of 'risk' are at play. This is reflected, for example, in the limited institutionalization of some BRCA medical practices such as prophylactic mastectomy in the Italian context.

At our Brocher workshop, we were fortunate to have participants who offered further contrasting reflections on the way that BRCA research and medical practices were evolving in Greece, Israel and Uruguay, providing additional illuminating and invaluable perspectives not present in this volume. Eirini Kampriani's work in Greece has been and continues to be central to discussions in the BRCA group (see Kampriani 2009). Her presentation at the Brocher meeting showed the complex ways that religious philanthropy and gendered ideologies have been a key dimension of BRCA medicine in Greece against a backdrop of limited and finite public health resources – an issue that is also addressed in a number of papers in the collection concerning BRCA genetics in India (Macdonald) and Brazil (Mozersky and Gibbon). Shiri Shkedi-Rafid provided fascinating perspectives on the field of BRCA in Israel where the prospect of identifying BRCA carriers through population screening of Ashkenazi Jewish individuals without a family history is emerging as a viable avenue of intervention. Her work on the meaning of 'carrierness' for those identified in this way has important implications, particularly given the expanded possibilities of Next Generation sequencing for identifying individuals with BRCA mutations without a significant family history (Shkedi-Rafid *et al.* 2012). Finally, Ana Egana's work as part of a transnational collaborative initiative in Uruguay examined the relationship between ancestry and breast cancer. She highlighted the extent to which, for participants and also local researchers in Uruguay, socio-economic factors rather than ancestry per se were as important if not sometimes more relevant in perceptions of disease risk, raising important challenges to the homogenizing potential of global research paradigms, an issue that is also discussed by Mozersky and Gibbon.

Challenges of being engaged/positioned/situated in our research fields

In the course of our discussions at Brocher, one of the themes that recurred was our own embeddedness in the medical and scientific field of BRCA genetics. As social scientists analyzing, engaging and sometimes even collaborating with what has become a multi-million-dollar industry that is now expanding across a global terrain of medical practice and scientific research, there is an awareness (for some uncomfortably so) that our own research trajectories have been informed (and in many cases funded) because of the high public profile that BRCA genetics continues to garner. As Haraway (1988: 581) pointed out, there is of course no view 'from nowhere' and we are all necessarily 'situated' by working in the domain of BRCA genetics, whether we carry out research at the clinical interface, in the laboratory or with patient or activist populations. Entering and acknowledging the complexity of our situatedness in the context of interdisciplinarity or collaborative research is part of the challenging task of social scientists examining developments in the life and medical sciences, and one that others have begun to address. Prainsack and colleagues (2010) note the ever-present ambiguity of conducting social science research in such settings, highlighting the challenges of creating the space for critical social science perspectives and negotiating differences in authority and the legitimacy of contrasting methodological approaches. Barry *et al.* (2008) suggest the need for a more complex understanding of interdisciplinarity and stress that interdisciplinarity has diverse histories and can take a multiplicity of forms. They interrogate how different modes of interdisciplinarity come into play and intersect, and raise valuable questions about the conditions under which particular styles of interdisciplinary practices appear and the ways they inform the outcomes of scientific knowledge production.[5] Drawing on their approaches and reflecting on our own embeddedness as social science researchers in the field of BRCA genetics the following questions emerge: When – or even – is it possible to reach a synthesis of natural scientific and social scientific knowledge? Under which conditions does our own social science research function in a 'service-mode' to facilitate the research goals of the life and medical sciences? And how can the existing disciplinary epistemological and ontological assumptions be contested in such interdisciplinary collaborations? While these issues are implicit in many of the chapters presented, the questions raised about the ethics and politics of doing social science research at the interface with BRCA genetic research remain ongoing challenges that are of central interest to a number of the book's contributors, and which we suggest are crucial to social science research more generally in the field of genomic science and medicine, beyond BRCA.

* * *

The book is organized across three sections interspersed with a foreword from Rayna Rapp, commentaries from Nina Hallowell and Martina Schlünder and an afterword from Susanne Bauer, all of whom we were fortunate to have in attendance at the Brocher workshop. The first section, 'Practices of population politics and history in the production of BRCA', brings together three papers that place concerns with temporal pasts and presents centre stage. Collectively these papers tease out some of the complex questions concerning genetic research and categories of race/ethnicity and populations in the context of BRCA genetic research and medical interventions in different national contexts and/or for various 'under-served' populations. The second section, entitled 'Risk, personhood and subjectivity', provides the framework for three papers that consider core issues of politics, gender and identity in the way that BRCA research and medical practice is enacted, whilst also importantly revealing the spaces where it is absent or resisted. The third section of the book, 'Shifting terrains of BRCA knowledge and practices', brings into view the emerging horizons of this dynamic domain of genetic research as it becomes incorporated into direct to consumer testing, translational research and pre-implantation diagnosis and is informed and potentially transformed by the recent decision in the US on the patentability of genes.

Notes

1. cDNA is complementary DNA and refers to a form of DNA that is artificially synthesized.
2. Within weeks of the Supreme Court decision, Myriad sued two competitors (Ambry Genetics and Gene by Gene), who began offering BRCA testing claiming violation of some of their remaining patents not invalidated by the Supreme Court (*New York Times*, July 10, 2013, www.nytimes.com/2013/07/11/business/2-competitors-sued-by-genetics-company-for-patent-infringement.html). At the same time, Myriad has pledged that it 'will not impede non-commercial, academic research that uses patented technology licensed or owned by us'. (www.myriad.com/responsibility/myriads-pledge/)
3. See for instance the new UK NICE guidance on the preventative use of Tamoxifen or raloxifene for those with a family history of breast cancer as part of a strategy of chemoprevention. The same guidelines have suggested reducing the threshold for BRCA genetic testing for women from 20 per cent chance of having a BRCA gene mutation to 10 per cent, greatly widening the number of women eligible for genetic testing in the UK (www.nice.org.uk/newsroom/news/MoreTreatmentOptions WomenRiskBreastCancer.jsp)
4. See Preface.
5. Barry *et al.* 2008 suggest three difference interdisciplinary modes – *integrative-synthesis* mode, *subordination-service* mode and *agonistic-antagonistic* mode.

References

Adams, V., Murphy, M. and Clarke, A. (2009) 'Anticipation: technoscience, life, affect, temporality'. *Subjectivity* 28: 246–65.

Barry, A., Born, G. and Weszkalnys, G. (2008) 'Logics of interdisciplinarity'. *Economy and Society* 37 (1): 20–49.

Bell, K. (2013) 'Biomarkers, the molecular gaze and the transformation of cancer survivorship'. *BioSocieties* 8 (2): 124–43.

Bellcross, C. A., Lemke, A. A., Pape, L. S., Tess, A. L. and Meisner, L. T. (2009) 'Evaluation of a breast/ovarian cancer genetics referral screening tool in a mammography population'. *Genetics in Medicine* 11 (11): 783–9. doi:10.1097/GIM.0b013e3181b9b04a.

Bourret, P. (2005) 'BRCA patients and clinical collectives: new configurations of action in cancer genetics practices'. *Social Studies of Science* 35 (1): 41–68.

Churpek, J. E., Walsh T., Zheng Y., et al. (2013) 'Inherited mutations in breast cancer genes in African American breast cancer patients revealed by targeted genomic capture and next-generation sequencing', *Journal of Clinical Oncology* 31 (suppl; abstr CRA1501).

Clarke, A. E., Mamo, L., Fosket, J. R., Fishman, J. R. and Shim, J. K. (eds) (2010) *Biomedicalization: Technoscience, Health, and Illness in the U.S.,* Durham: Duke University Press.

Esserman, L. J., Thompson, I. M., Jr. and Reid, B. (2013) 'Overdiagnosis and overtreatment in cancer: an opportunity for improvement'. *JAMA*. 310 (8): 797-798. doi:10.1001/jama.2013.108415.

Gibbon, S. (2007) *Breast Cancer Genes and the Gendering of Knowledge: Science and Citizenship in the Cultural Context of the 'New' Genetics.* London: Palgrave Macmillan.

———. (2013a) 'Ancestry, temporality and potentiality: engaging cancer genetics in Southern Brazil'. In Taussig, K-S., Hoeyer, K. and Helmreich, S. (eds), Special Issue of *Current Anthropology* 54 (7) 'Potentiality and humanness: revisiting the anthropological object in contemporary biomedicine' S107-S117.

———. (2013b) 'BRCA genes and the "pluripotency" of gender'. In Horstman, K. and Huijer, M. (eds), *Special Edition Year Book of Women's History.* Amsterdam: Amsterdam University Press.

Gibbon, S., Kampriani, E. and zur Nieden, A. (2010) 'BRCA patients in Cuba, Greece and Germany: comparative perspectives on public health, the state and the partial reproduction of "neoliberal" subjects', *BioSocieties* 5: 440–66.

Gibbon, S. and Novas, C. (eds) (2008) *Biosocialities, Genetics and the Social Sciences: Making Biologies and Identities.* London: Routledge.

Gibbon, S., Palfner, S., Kalender, U., Joseph, G., Mozersky, J., Kampriani, E. and zur Nieden, A. (2010b) 'Introduction to special section: perspectives on globalizing genomics: the case of "BRCA" breast cancer research and medical practice'. *BioSocieties* 5: 407–14.

Green, R. C., Berg, J. S., Grody, W. W., et al. (2013) 'ACMG recommendations for reporting of incidental findings in clinical exome and genome sequencing'. *Genetics in Medicine* 15 (7): 565–74. doi:10.1038/gim.2013.73.

Hallowell, N. (1999) 'Doing the right thing: genetic risk and responsibility'. *Sociology of Health and Illness* 21: 597–621.

Happe, K. E. (2006) 'Heredity, gender and the discourse of ovarian cancer'. *New Genetics and Society* 25 (2): 171–96.

———. (2013) *The Material Gene: Gender, Race and Heredity After the Human Genome Project.* New York: New York University Press.

Haraway, D. (1988) Situated knowledges: the science question in feminism and the privilege of partial perspective *Feminist Studies.* 14: 575–99.

Haraway, D.J. (1997) *Modest_witness@ Second_Millennium. FemaleMan©_Meets_OncoMouse ™: Feminism and Technoscience.* New York: Routledge.

Joseph G. and Dohan D. (2012) 'Recruitment practices and the politics of inclusion in cancer clinical trials'. *Medical Anthropology Quarterly* 26 (3): 338–60.

Joseph, G., Kaplan, C., Luce, J., Lee, R., Stewart, S., Guerra, C. and Pasick, R. (2012) Efficient identification and referral of low-income women at high risk for hereditary breast cancer: a practice-based approach. *Public Health Genomics* 15:172–80.

Kampriani, E. (2009) 'Between religious philanthropy and individualized medicine: situating inherited breast cancer in Greece. Biomedical technology and health inequities in the global north and south'. *Anthropology and Medicine Special Issue* 16: 165–78.

Keating, P. and Cambrosio, A. (2003) *Biomedical Platforms: Realigning the Normal and the Pathological in Late-Twentieth-Century Medicine.* Cambridge, MA and London: MIT Press.

Kohane, I. S., Masys, D. R. and Altman, R. B. (2006) The incidentalome: a threat to genomic medicine'. *JAMA,* 296 (2): 212–15. doi:10.1001/jama.296.2.212.

Landecker, H. and Panofsky, A. (2013) 'From social structure to gene regulation and back: a critical introduction to environmental epigenetics for sociology'. *Annual Review of Sociology* 39: 333–57.

Latour, Bruno (2004) 'Why has critique run out of steam? From matters of fact to matters of concern'. *Critical Inquiry* 30: 225–48.

Levy-Lahad, E., Gabai-Kapara, E., Kaufman, B., Catane, C., Regev, S., Renbaum, P., Beller, U., King, M.-C. and Lahad, A. (2011) 'Evidence for population-based screening of BRCA1 and BRCA' (Program Number 1191T) Presented at the 12th International Congress of Human Genetics/61st Annual Meeting of The American Society of Human Genetics 13 October, 2011, Montreal, Canada.

Löwy, I. (2010) *Preventive Strikes: Women, Precancer and Prophylactic Surgery.* Baltimore, MD: The John Hopkins University Press.

Mansfield, B. (2012) 'Race and the new epigenetic biopolitics of environmental health'. *Biosocieties* 7: 352–72.

Metcalfe, K. A., Poll, A., Royer, R., Llacuachaqui, M., Tulman, A., Sun, P. and Narod, S. A. (2009) 'Screening for founder mutations in BRCA1 and BRCA2 in unselected Jewish women', *Journal of Clinical Oncology,* 28: 387–91.

Mozersky, J. (2013) *Risky Genes: Genetics, Breast Cancer and Jewish Identity.* London UK: Routledge.

Mozersky, J. and Joseph, G. (2010) 'Case studies in the co-production of populations and genetics: the making of "at risk" populations in BRCA genetics'. *BioSocieties* 5 (4): 415–39.

Narr, W. D. (2003*)* 'Zeit der Politik, Politik der Zeit: Zu Zeiten ihrer globalen Verkürzung und Verlängerung'. In *Jussi Kurunmäki and Kari Palonen: Zeit, Geschichte und Politik.* [Time, History and Politics.] Zum achtzigsten Geburtstag von Reinhard Koselleck, Jyväskylä, 235–61.

zur Nieden, Andrea (2010) 'The embodiment of genetic risk. Women's experiences of genetic testing for breast cancer susceptibility mutations'. In Arno Bammé, Guenter Getzinger and Bernhard Wieser: *Yearbook 2009 of the Institute for Advanced Studies on Science Technology and Society.* München und Wien: Profil.

———. (2013): *Zum Subjekt der Gene werden. Subjektivierungsweisen im Zeichen der Genetisierung von Brustkrebs.* [Becoming Subject of the Genes. Ways of Subjectification in the Era of Genetification of Breast Cancer]. Bielefeld, Germany: Transcript (in German).

Palfner, S. (2009) *Gen-Passagen. Molekularbiologische und medizinische Praktiken im Umgang mit Brustkrebs-Genen. Wissen – Technologie – Diagnostik* [Gene-passages. Molecularbiological and Medical Practices Related to Breast Cancer Genes. Knowledge – Technology – Diagnostic]. Bielefeld, Germany: Transcript (in German).

Parthasarathy, S. (2007) *Building Genetic Medicine: Breast Cancer, Technology and the Comparative Politics of Health Care.* Cambridge: MIT Press.

Prainsack, B., Svendsen, M. N., Koch, L. and Ehrich, K. (2010) 'How do we collaborate? Social science researchers' experience of multidisciplinarity in biomedical settings'. *Biosocieties* 5: 278–86.

Pyeritz R. E. (2011) 'The coming explosion in genetic testing – is there a duty to recontact?' *New England Journal of Medicine* 365 (15): 1367–9. doi:10.1056/NEJMp1107564.

Richards, M. (1996) 'Families, kinship and genetics'. In Marteau, T. and Richards, M. (eds) *The Troubled Helix: Social and Psychological Implications of the New Human Genetics,* 249–73. Cambridge: Cambridge University Press.

Richards, M.P.M. (1996) 'Genetics and health: a family affair'. *Biological Sciences Review* 9: 26–30.

Robson, M. E., Storm, C. D., Weitzel, J., et al. (2010) 'American Society of Clinical Oncology policy statement update: genetic and genomic testing for cancer susceptibility'. *Journal of Clinical Oncology* 28 (5): 893–901.

Shkedi-Rafid, S., Gabai-Kapara, E., Grinshpun-Cohen, J. and Levy-Lahad, E. 'BRCA genetic testing of individuals from families with low prevalence of cancer: experiences of carriers and implications for population screening'. *Genetics in Medicine* 14 (7): 688–94. doi:10.1038/gim.2012.31.

Section I

Practices of population, politics and history in the production of BRCA

1 The presence of the past

‘Ashkenazi BRCA mutations’ and transnational differences in categories of ‘race’ and ‘ethnicity’: the German case[1]

Andrea zur Nieden

I cannot ask a woman if she is Jewish!

(Genetic counsellor)

Introduction

In this chapter, I will address how ‘populations’ as well as ancestral or migratory pasts are related to issues such as health disparities in German public health debates. I will begin with the example of the striking *absence* of ‘Ashkenazi BRCA mutations’ from clinical discussions in comparison to other countries such as the US and UK. While the German past, in particular Nazi history, can partly help explain this absence, I will outline some characteristics of the more general German public health discourse and its political implications, which also account for this phenomenon.

In some countries, especially in the US, it has become common practice in medicine and public health to differentiate between ‘races’ and ‘ethnicities’ inside the country’s own population due to supposed biological or genetic differences. Despite the wide-spread notion that race and ethnicity are socially constructed categories, searching for biological differences along the lines of populations has experienced a recent renaissance in the age of genetics, as patterns of genetic variations are analysed in their relation to health. Initially, genetics research focused on rare genetic conditions, like sickle cell anaemia and its relatively greater rate of occurrence in tropical Africa and among people of African descent, or Tay-Sachs and Gaucher diseases as being more common among Ashkenazi Jews. Since then, research has begun to concentrate more and more on common diseases like cancer, diabetes and heart failure and how these relate to genetic variations in order to better explain racial/ethnic differences in susceptibilities. Often, the initial intent of this research was to address social causes of disparities in health between race or ethnic groups, but the claim of social justice has increasingly intermingled with the realm of biological and/or genetic difference (Bauer 2003; see also Joseph in this volume). Especially well researched are Ashkenazi Jews and, for example, their higher risk of carrying mutations (1/40) in the so-called BRCA or breast cancer genes, which are associated with a higher risk of breast and ovarian cancer (Mozersky and Joseph 2010). These mutations are even commonly named the 'Ashkenazi mutations'.[2] The use of 'population' categories in genetic research are also discussed with regard to different local contexts in other chapters in this book section – for example, public health genomics and health disparities as related to the African American population in the US (Joseph) and research on Ashkenazi mutations in the UK and Brazil (Mozersky and Gibbon). These case studies point to the fact that, although genetics can be seen as a highly globalized field of science and medicine, there are still national differences relating to health care systems and local/national histories as well as cultural practices relating to categories of race and ethnicity. In Germany, especially, the term *Rasse* ('race') is generally considered taboo when used to refer to humans. It is also extremely politically controversial to speak of ethnicities in biological terms, mainly due to Germany's Nazi history. As I will demonstrate, population categories are rarely used in German scientific and medical discourses, while more apparently politically correct terms like *Migrationshintergrund* ('immigrant background') or *Migrant* ('immigrant'/'migrant') are often used instead.

In this respect, the *past* is very *present* in today's public health discourse on genes in many different ways. Not only is each individual's family history important – as is always the case when it comes to genetic 'dispositions' – but so is Germany's political past. What is also present, on the other hand, is a particular tradition in Germany of seeing its own population as relatively ethnically homogeneous. In this chapter I present some exploratory findings taken from an ongoing research project on categories of race and ethnicity in genetic medicine and the public health discourse in Germany. In the following sections, I will start with impressions from my fieldwork on BRCA mutations (zur Nieden 2010, 2013), during which I observed that Ashkenazi mutations demonstrated an interesting 'absent presence'. In an attempt to find deeper reasons for this phenomenon, I analyse the usage of the categories of race and/or ethnicity in other fields of health as well as in debates on health disparities while attempting to situate them in a broader political context. This context is characterized not only by the taboo of talking about race or ethnicities in biological terms for historical reasons, but also by a specific way of dealing with ethnic diversity and immigration. Ultimately, I want to suggest that, in contrast to an 'inclusion-and-difference paradigm', as Steven Epstein (2007: 7) has proposed for medicine in the US, biopolitical citizenship in Germany can rather be characterized as following an 'integration paradigm'. Thus, health disparities are not so much seen as being due to biological differences, but due to a lack of proper 'integration', and even the grandchildren of immigrants are still addressed as 'immigrants' who must work toward integration.

According to Epstein, medicine in the US is characterized by 'the assumption that social identities correspond to relatively distinct kinds of bodies – female bodies, Asian bodies, elderly Hispanic male bodies, and so on – and that these various embodied states are medically incommensurable' (2007: 2). As a consequence, one way to address health disparities among different groups is thought to be the inclusion of all ethnic, racial, gender and age groups in medical research. This was significantly formalized in the National Institute of Health Revitalization Act from 1993 for all NIH-sponsored clinical trials. A widely discussed controversial consequence of such efforts was BiDil, the first race-based prescription drug to be approved by the Food and Drug Administration in 2005 for use only by African Americans for the treatment of congestive heart failure.

There has been much debate both inside[3] and outside science about the problematic aspects of using racial/ethnic categories in research, such as their often vague and unclear meaning (e.g. Hunt and Megyesi 2008), indicating that populations are 'neither natural nor essential but are matters of practice' (M'charek 2005: 48–49). Others have critiqued the intermingling of cultural or social differences with supposed 'genetic' differences (e.g. Bauer 2003; Fujimura and Rajagopalan 2011) and the danger of a reification of social differences by presuming that they are biological (e.g. Duster 2005). Instead of summarizing this debate here again, I want to clarify the perspective that informs this chapter: race and ethnicity are primarily *social* and not innately genetic categories, although they may have biological consequences (e.g. through discrimination or cultural practices that affect one's health). Concerning genetic variations originating from a common ancestry, it has been a scientific commonplace since the 1950s to agree with the geneticists Leslie Dunn and Theodosius Dobzhansky (1946) that there is more variation within racial groups than between them (Weingart *et al.* 1988: 615–18). Another commonplace is to consider populations only as statistical entities without clear-cut boundaries (Livingstone 1962). With this in mind, my research project looks more closely at how individuals and samples are 'racialized' and 'ethnicized' in medical discourse, how boundaries are actually drawn between races/ethnicities and how *national differences* that relate to different political situations may manifest in the usage of these categories. This chapter offers a discussion on the medical and public health discourse in Germany, based primarily on a literature review of selected German journals. It sets the stage for a future study, in which I will also look at practical research routines in Germany. As Epstein has outlined, 'formal policies concerning inclusion and difference in biomedicine are mostly restricted to the United States – at least so far.' The inclusion-and-difference paradigm relates to the prominence of identity politics in the United States, while other countries 'seek instead to subsume difference under a broader conception of national citizenship' (Epstein 2007: 7–8). My goal is to shed more light on this assumption, thereby relying on political sociology in an attempt to outline what might inform these national differences.

The absent presence of Ashkenazi mutations

In Germany, the term *Rasse* ('race') is taboo when used to refer to humans, mainly due to Germany's Nazi history. Nonetheless, there has been a continuum of racially defined research in some departments of anthropology and human genetics after 1945 (Palm 2009; Plümecke 2010; Weingart *et al.* 1988). In the field of biology in Germany, the concept of population based on statistics as proposed by

Dunn and Dobzhansky replaced the typological concept of race much later than was the case in Great Britain and North America (Palm 2009: 249). In addition, in 1971 an edition of the prestigious *Brockhaus Encyclopedia*[4] still defined the term *Menschenrassen* ('human races') by referring to race categories from the works of the *Rassenkunde* (Race Studies) from the 1930s (E. von Eickstedt and H. Weinert) and by including illustrations of 'typical race' faces (*Brockhaus* 1971: 406–10). However, perhaps also due to a new postwar generation of scholars, it has been common at least since the 1980s not to use the term *Rasse* ('race') in Germany. In recent social science discourse on discrimination, the English term 'race' has been used instead of the German word *Rasse* for indicating a social category, as the German word is thought to have a historical bias toward biology. Furthermore, linking ethnic and cultural groups of people to certain biological characteristics is also considered problematic. Thus, it is interesting to examine German responses to the increasing importance of racial and ethnic differences in the international health debates. Prime examples of this are the so-called Ashkenazi mutations in the BRCA genes. In the US, Canada, Israel and the UK, the increased risk of carrying one of these mutations for Ashkenazi women is explicitly addressed in the structures of BRCA clinical and research practices (e.g. in clinical guidelines and testing recommendations). In their comparison of the application of BRCA testing in the US, France and the UK, Löwy and Gaudillière (2008) demonstrate the following:

> In the United States, experts, cancer nonprofit organizations, patient groups, and Jewish women leagues have widely discussed the Ashkenazi mutations. (. . .) Myriad's offer to test for Ashkenazi mutations at a very reduced price and the marketing strategies of this company might also account for this population's increased use of these tests and thus to a greater visibility of these mutations in it. As a consequence, breast cancer, a pathology with high prevalence in the general population, has been partly turned into a 'Jewish disease' – all this despite the fact that the presence of the Ashkenazi mutations increases but slightly the overall risk that women from Ashkenazi origins will develop breast cancer in their lifetime,[5] as compared with other Western women of similar socioeconomic strata.
>
> (Löwy and Gaudillière 2008: 312–13)

Löwy and Gaudillière state that, in spite of a tradition in the UK to analyse the correlation of class rather than ethnic origins with health and disease, the 'British do, however, pay more attention than the French to differences between communities, and genetic counselors are trained to be aware of their patients' ethnic origins to provide culturally sensitive counseling' in general (313).

This attention can best be demonstrated in the leaflet 'Are you worried about breast cancer?' by the British cancer charity CancerBACUP (which has since merged with MacMillan Cancer Support) from 2004 about familial breast cancer in which, after the number of family members with breast cancer is mentioned as a hereditary risk, it says:

> If your family is like this and you are worried about developing breast cancer yourself, you might want to talk to your GP. If you have a family history of any unusual cancers/childhood cancers or you have Jewish or other ethnic background (where a faulty gene is more common), you should mention that to your GP.[6]

Having a 'Jewish or other ethnic background' is thus depicted as a risk that can be just as threatening as having a family with several cases of breast cancer. (The formulation 'other ethnic background' is also problematic in and of itself in that 'ethnic' seems to be reserved for ethnic minorities, while the majority apparently has no ethnicity.)

Since 2005 the British National Institute for Clinical Excellence (NICE) has included Ashkenazi Jewish ancestry as a risk factor for assessing genetic risk and making referrals for genetic testing in their guidelines (Mozersky and Joseph 2010: 424): 'Family history questionnaires to assess women's risk when they are first referred to a clinic contain a question about Ashkenazi ancestry. For patients with an Ashkenazi background, testing can be offered when only one relative had breast cancer.'

This testing is thus free of charge through the British National Health Service (NHS), as is the case for other patients with many relatives with breast cancer. Some countries, including the UK and Canada, even offer population-wide screenings for BRCA mutations among Ashkenazi Jews as pilot projects with support of Jewish organizations (Mozersky and Joseph 2010: 424).

Despite the annihilation of the majority of German Jews during the Nazi regime, the number of Jews living in Germany has increased again over the last decades due mainly to immigration from Eastern European countries. The percentage of the population is approaching that of the UK (around 0.24 per cent of the German population, compared to roughly 0.5 per cent of the British population).[7] And yet, specific Ashkenazi mutations are practically invisible in the medical discourse in Germany. When looking at *Deutsches Ärzteblatt,* the most widespread German medical journal, this specific population risk is only mentioned in five of the eighty-five articles on BRCA since 1996. Two of the five papers are from 1997 (Beckmann *et al.* 1997; Meyer 1997) and one is from 1998 (Holinski-Feder *et al.* 1998), when there was no accepted general test for BRCA mutations available. Ashkenazi Jews thus serve as an example in these texts because a test for Ashkenazi mutations already existed at this time. In contrast, papers published after this time make no mention of Ashkenazi mutations at all, except for two short news reports about testing in the UK for genetic cancer in individuals without a family history: 'Gentests in Großbritannien auch für Menschen ohne Erbkrankheit' ('Gene tests in Great Britain include people without family history') (2009) and about Preimplantation Genetic Diagnosis (PGD): 'Präimplantationsdiagnostik: Erstes Baby ohne Brustkrebsgen geboren' ('Preimplantation genetic diagnostics: first baby born without breast cancer gene') (2009). While there is a well-organized infrastructure for BRCA genetic testing and special care for familial breast and ovarian cancer (covered by health insurance) with twelve specialized clinics in Germany, ethnic aspects of the disease are not addressed either in the programme's structure or in its information material for patients. Furthermore, the BRCA-Netzwerk, an organization by and for people affected by BRCA, does not mention specific risks for certain population groups either on its website or in its informative literature.[8] When I interviewed genetic counsellors and asked them whether they acknowledged differences between populations in their clinical practice, they tended to react in the following way, as this specific example from my field research illustrates:[9]

Q: Are there actually different tests for different population groups?

A: Well, within this programme, not really, no. (. . .) But, you know, it depends on which population group someone comes from. You can cover a large part [of the population] with certain mutations already. This means that if you test two BRCA1 mutations and one BRCA2 mutation in the Jewish-born population, specifically Ashkenazi Jews, then you're already going to exclude or detect a very large number of the mutations existing in this population group – this ethnic group.

But we don't test for specific mutations. In this programme we practically sequence the entire gene.

Q: Because otherwise you'd have to, you know, ask someone if they have a Jewish background, right?

A: We do ask that sometimes, actually. I tell the person that certain mutations actually occur with varying frequency . . . and, well, we also have several families of Jewish ancestry in this programme. (. . .)

Q: So, it's a standard question?

A: Well, you know, we ask about their family tree, for example, and what their ethnic background is. Unless it's clear – sometimes we don't even have to ask because it's obvious from the names in the family tree or so. Then you can conclude it more or less indirectly. We ask about the ethnic backgrounds that are relevant – you know, so whether someone has a Jewish background. I don't necessarily ask every time if someone is Jewish or not, but I'll explain to the person that there are these mutations and that it [Jewish ancestry] plays an essential role in this case.

If we take this to be representative, it would appear that there is no standard procedure for addressing ethnic differences during a clinical encounter. Although the counsellor states that they do not look for specific mutations and instead sequencing the whole gene (that is, this is done for the so-called 'index patient' in the family, who already has breast cancer – after a mutation is found in this case, other family members will only be tested for that mutation), he later says that they *do* ask about ethnic background. (Procedures also vary from clinic to clinic: In an interview with a counsellor from another clinic I was told that, if they know of Jewish or Dutch relatives,[10] they test specific population mutations first.) Probing his response further, it seems that Ashkenazi background is rather assumed than asked about. This compares to my analysis of twenty recordings of genetic counselling sessions at the same clinic in which, in contrast to what the counsellor said, I never encountered a question on ethnic background. The counsellor's hesitant choice of words in the above passage also reflects a sense of uneasiness when asking about Jewish ancestry.

Thus, in the German BRCA discourse and clinical practice, Ashkenazi mutations seem to have an 'absent presence': every counsellor knows about them, but no one addresses them. Another human geneticist addressed this issue directly by saying: 'I cannot ask a woman if she's Jewish!' This is very typical of the situation in Germany, where the memory of medicine's involvement in Nazi racial hygiene and in the Holocaust continues to have an effect today.

According to Löwy and Gaudillière (2008: 312), the situation is similar in France. In French BRCA health care, patients are not actively asked about a possible Ashkenazi Jewish origin. As in Germany, genealogy or the patient's record usually does not contain ethnic information, which can only be drawn indirectly from names or when patients themselves address the issue. This happens very rarely, however, because unlike in the US (but similar to the situation in Germany), the issue of ethnic differences is not very present in the public mind. The authors argue that this is due to the universalist conception of citizenship in France, which does not favour focusing on ethnic issues in general.

As for Jewish communities, there are a few international organizations working to raise the awareness of genetic breast cancer, such as Jews Against Cancer of the Breast (JACOB).[11] However, in the German context, in the most widespread German-language Jewish journal, the *Jüdische Allgemeine,* only two articles have dealt with familial breast cancer since 2006, and in both cases it was only a side issue.

Race, ethnicity and immigrants

Against the backdrop of the conspicuously missing Ashkenazi mutations in the German BRCA discourse and the uneasiness around this issue, I became interested in whether this 'absence' is specific to the topic of Jewish ancestry. I thus looked more generally for the prominence of ethnic or racial differences in the German medical discourse. When searching the database of the *Deutsches Ärzteblatt,* the term *Rasse* ('race'), similar to the term *Juden* ('Jews'),[12] is only used in historical articles about racial hygiene.[13] The term 'ethnic' does, however, appear in a number of articles addressing ethnic differences relating to different diseases, but mostly only as a side issue. Most of these articles are summaries of studies done in the US. However, when they do refer to research results relating to ethnic differences, these categories seem to be taken for granted and not questioned, and no consideration is given as to how these differences have come about (for example, through cultural or social conditions or genetic discrepancies) (e.g. Gerste 2012, '1000-Genom-Projekt: Gesunde Menschen haben viele Genfehler' ['1000 Genomes project: healthy people have many genetic errors']). The latter is typical for scientific articles in other countries as well (Hunt and Megyesi 2008;

Sankar *et al.* 2007), but in the German case it is interesting that, although the categories are rarely used for their own research, they are still accepted when found in other studies.

In many articles, it is clear that the German word *ethnisch* is used not only for the English word 'ethnic', but for 'racial' as well. For example, one article in the *Deutsches Ärzteblatt* summarizes several studies found in the journal *Diabetes Care,* which detected differences in the rate of occurrence and degree of severity of diabetes in Asians compared to other populations ('Diabetes bei Asiaten erfordert besonderes Augenmerk' ['Diabetes in Asians requires special attention'], 2012). The differences are argued as being based on genetic as well as environmental factors. The studies in the US (Hsu *et al.* 2012; King *et al.* 2012) referred to here in the German article distinguish between different 'race groups' (Asian and Pacific Islanders [PIs]) as well as 'ethnicities' in terms of subgroups or 'populations'. In the German translation, this is has been transformed merely to 'Asians' (or 'people in Asia or of Asian descent') as a particular 'ethnic' group – thus illustrating how the taboo of using the word 'race' leads to interesting translations or transformations of categories.

Very few of these articles discuss *German* medical studies in which a distinction has been made between ethnic differences (e.g. Frädrich 2010; Gissendanner *et al.* 2012). The only *genetic* disease[14] occasionally discussed with respect to ethnic differences (in four articles: Ernst 1998; Schönland 2006; Sudeck and Horstmann 1999; Timman *et al.* 2004) is Familial Mediterranean fever, as can be seen in the following quote from the English abstract of one: 'FMF is predominantly found in Jewish, Armenian or Turkish families whose ancestors originate from the Mediterranean basin. (. . .) With immigrants, FMF came to Germany, and for differential diagnosis, it is now of considerable importance' (Sudeck and Horstmann 1999).

This indicates another striking aspect of the German debate: not only is there uneasiness with ethnic or racial categories for historical reasons, but the population is also generally perceived as ethnically homogeneous, and differences are related to (recent) immigration. The largest group of immigrants in Germany in the postwar period comes from Turkey. Fifty years ago Germany and Turkey signed a labour recruitment agreement when West German industry desperately needed workers. The standard term for this group of immigrants used to be 'guest workers' (*Gastarbeiter*), indicating that they were not considered part of German society, but were only 'guests' for a certain time. Many of them decided to stay and they acquired different statuses of legal or illegal residence, and they now constitute part of the population living in Germany. Still, until very recently, the political mainstream continued to state that 'Germany is not a country of immigration' (see, for example, Özdemir 2006). Furthermore, at the time proponents of positions that welcomed diversity as an enrichment of society were rather marginal, and 'multiculturalism' also often tended to essentialize cultural differences. This has shifted somewhat since the late 1990s and is now moving toward the acceptance of (very restricted) immigration policies and the possibility of gaining German citizenship with a very heavy emphasis on *integration.*

Recent political struggles mostly revolve around the extent to which immigrants are able, or are willing, to *integrate* into German society with, at times, strong rhetoric used against so-called *Integrationsverweigerer,* or 'those who refuse to integrate'.[15] In this rhetoric, integration is seen as the effort or obligation of the individual immigrant, and not as a general social process. Furthermore, positions within the debate differ along the lines of the relevance they attribute to cultural and religious differences (especially regarding the Muslim religion). These differences are sometimes treated as 'essential' in their 'otherness', and they thus fulfil the same role that race used to. This has been called the 'culturalization' of racism (Çinar 1999). The 'resistance' to integration is therefore sometimes explained by referring to this essential otherness. Another specific characteristic of the German situation in contrast to, for example, the US or UK, is that the forms of identity politics of ethnically defined groups are rather marginal, and a law to abolish discrimination[16] – including discrimination based on 'race' or ethnicity – was passed only as recently as 2006 to accommodate European Union legislation.

It appears that a similar emphasis on integration is also reflected in the medical discourse in Germany. While there is almost no health disparities debate that focuses on different ethnicities as part of the German population, there is an emerging debate on health disparities with regard to 'immigrants' (called *Migranten,* or 'migrants' in German) or 'people with immigrant backgrounds' (*Migrantionshintergrund*) as they are often called, including those who are second or third generation citizens or residents. Thus, instead of searching for the terms 'race' or 'ethnicity' to find this debate in, for example, the *Deutsches Ärzteblatt* database, it can be found when performing a wildcard search of 'Migra*'. The term 'immigrant background' (*Migrantionshintergrund*) has thus replaced *Ausländer* ('foreigner') in many statistical surveys, especially since the opportunities to acquire German citizenship have been expanded, and many immigrants and their children can therefore no longer be considered *Ausländer.* While this categorization can be understood as being based on the anti-discriminatory intention of discovering more about health disparities among descendants of immigrants, the term 'immigrant background' also indicates a non-inclusive model. By definition, it means residents who either do not have German citizenship or citizens who were born in a 'typical country of emigration', or it can mean people whose parents (or grandparents) fit this description.[17] In statistics or surveys, this entire concept is often condensed into the category of *Migrant,* which is understood in opposition to the categories 'German' and 'non-(im)migrants'. This means that people in the third generation (the grandchildren), who did not immigrate to Germany themselves, are still defined as 'immigrants'.[18] This stands in contrast, for example, to the US, where the nation is regarded as consisting of different ethnicities,[19] and it also stands in contrast to the universalist conception of French citizenship. While France has a tradition of *jus soli,* in which every person born in France can principally achieve citizenship, the German tradition goes back to the tradition of *jus sanguinis,* meaning only those with German 'blood' were considered part of the German people.[20]

Interestingly, in the medical debate about health disparities in Germany among people with an 'immigrant background', *biological* or *genetic* differences are virtually not mentioned. Topics which are discussed in several papers include problems of people accessing the health care system because of social status or language difficulties (e.g. 'Kinder- und Jugendärzte: Für eine bessere Versorgung von Migrantenkindern' ['Paediatricians: better provision for immigrant children'], 2010; 'Präventionsprojekt "Mit Migranten für Migranten" erfolgreich' ['Preventative project "With Immigrants for Immigrants" successful'], 2010). Other articles note higher levels of depression in the immigrant population, with the reasons noted being either immigration in and of itself or refugee trauma (e.g. 'Psychotherapeutische Versorgung von Migranten mangelhaft' ['Poor psyotherapeutical provision for immigrants'], 2010; Hillienhof 2011). There are also studies on different relationships to childbirth and contraception (e.g. Rieser 2010) or complaints about the lack of parental support of young children in immigrant families that has to be compensated by day care (e.g. 'Kinderärzte kritisieren schleppenden Ausbau der Krippenplätze' ['Paediatricians criticize slow expansion of day care services'], 2011). Some papers propose addressing these health disparities by offering adjusted medical services, such as native-language information or cultural mediators (for example, 'Kinder- und Jugendärzte: Für eine bessere Versorgung von Migrantenkindern' ['Paediatricians: better provision for immigrant children'], 2010; 'Präventionsprojekt "Mit Migranten für Migranten" erfolgreich' ['Preventative project "With Immigrants for Immigrants" successful'], 2010; 'Patientenberatung auf Türkisch und Russisch' ['Patient consultation in Turkish and Russian'], 2011).

The groups of immigrants most discussed in these cases are those from Turkey or Russia. And although, as already mentioned, Jewish immigration from different Eastern European countries has recently increased, they are not mentioned as a particular group in these papers. Instead they appear to be subsumed under the general immigration from these countries.

While all these topics relate to *cultural* or *social* aspects where immigrants differ from the supposed 'standard German patient', one of the few topics in which *biology* is regarded as a reason for health disparities is vitamin D deficiency, because darker skin is thought to reduce the impact of sunlight. But even here, biology is combined with culture and/or religion, and the religious dogma of wearing clothing that covers most of the body is put forth as another reason for the same phenomenon (Zeeb and Greinert 2010).

One of the few examples of a larger German survey that systematically differentiates between immigrants and non-immigrants is KiGGs, an ongoing survey of children's and young people's health in Germany that was launched in 2003 by the Robert Koch Institute. The survey currently includes 17,641 boys and girls and their parents. The reason given by KiGGs as to why immigrants are systematically taken into account is the assumed disparity in health due to their lower social status and because immigration itself is said to cause health risks (Schenk 2012: 2). Again, *genetic* reasons are not mentioned. Within this survey, health disparities in immigrant children and young people have been found in different fields of health (e.g. Kamtsiuris *et al.* 2007; Thiersfelder *et al.* 2007), but the explanation given for these is again mostly a cultural or social one. For example, the fact that certain infections are found more often in the immigrant population, while others are found less frequently, is explained by their different levels of awareness of disease or different levels of access to the health care system (Kamtsiuris *et al.* 2007: 696). A very interesting finding that has since been referred to occasionally in the political debate on immigration has been the 'low quality of oral hygiene' – measured by the frequency of brushing of one's teeth and visits to the dentist – as a risk factor for disease (Beauftragte der Bundesregierung für Migration, Flüchtlinge und Integration 2011: 129).

We can clearly see an emphasis in the German health disparities debate on different behaviour and compliance, which does not conform to the standard preventative strategies, including brushing one's teeth regularly. These are seen as part of the cultural practices that differ from the ideal German patient and thus point to non-integration rather than biology or genetics.

For the sake of further illustrating the political background and specific situation also reflected in the medical discourse in Germany, I will outline a discussion that has been called the 'Sarrazin debate'. In the summer of 2010, Thilo Sarrazin, the chairman of the German National Bank and a member of the Social Democratic Party, published the book *Germany Is Abolishing Itself* (*Deutschland schafft sich ab,* Sarrazin 2010). It became the best-selling political book of the last decade, but it was also severely criticized. His line of argument was clearly a racist mixture of biologistic and culturalist rhetoric.[21] On the one hand, by drawing on theories of 'intelligence genes' and so forth, Sarrazin predicted that Germany would abolish itself biologically due to the 'inferior' genetic material from 'too many immigrants'; on the other hand, he specifically held Muslim culture responsible for individuals refusing to integrate and exert themselves economically. The arguments varied between genetic determinism and appeals toward immigrants to strive to achieve more.

Interestingly, the publishing company refused to leave the term *Rasse* ('race') in the book, although Sarrazin had originally used it, and replaced it with *Ethnie* ('ethnic group').[22] What is also significant for the German discussion is the reaction to Sarrazin's statements. Prior to the book's publication, Sarrazin stated in an interview – as an example of the genetic identity of populations – that all Jews share a common gene. This was rejected by many people as racist and defamatory, including the secretary general of the German Jewish Council, Stephan Kramer, and Chancellor Angela Merkel. The critics stated, for instance, that defining Jews by their genetic heritage is part of a racial fanaticism in which Judaism does not share (Kramer, quoted in Deutsche Presse-Agentur 2010). Sarrazin later apologized and resigned from his post at the German National Bank (which by that time was in the process of dismissing him anyway). Despite all this, after the first wave of criticism, many people applauded Sarrazin for having stood up against those who refuse to integrate and are thus a burden to German society. In the end, the debate resulted in a shift in the domain of what is 'sayable' (Foucault 1974: 45) toward the right.[23] The position that multiculturalism has failed and that immigrants should adapt to the German culture thus became mainstream. Newspapers featured portraits of 'well-integrated' immigrants in contrast to those unwilling to integrate. Thus, while on the face of it, this discourse seems less prone to racism because biological categories of race or ethnicity are rejected, speaking of 'cultural differences' can be as exclusionary for those who are described as being too 'alien' to integrate and very normative and disciplining for those who are obligated to integrate.

In addition, the media took up a debate about genetic differences, which had not been prominent in the public before. All of a sudden, there were articles that explained, with reference to the Sarrazin debate, that there is no such thing as a Jewish gene, or a gene for intelligence, while on the other hand, Jews were said to share many genetic features and also have a higher probability for certain diseases, like Gaucher or Tay-Sachs (see, for example, the left-leaning German newspaper *Frankfurter Rundschau* on 3 September, 2010). Even prominent Social Democrats like Klaus von Donanyi challenged this specifically German taboo and argued that it should be acceptable to say the words *Rasse* ('race'), 'Jews' and 'Muslims' (Friedrich 2011: 21).

Conclusion

Based on these explorative findings, it appears that, in contrast to an inclusion-and-difference paradigm (Epstein), the political and medical discourse in Germany could be characterized more as following an integration paradigm of political citizenship. Starting with the observation that BRCA 'Ashkenazi mutations' are practically invisible in Germany and based on an examination of more general categories of 'race' and 'ethnicity', it seems that health disparities are seen less as being due to biological differences neglected by science so far and more as being due to a lack of the integration of immigrants in Germany. There is much more attention paid to this behavioural aspect of integration, which also includes a certain set of preventative strategies (like brushing one's teeth regularly) than to (biological) differences. This contrasts with a 'bio-multiculturalism' (Epstein) that includes all members of a population and their supposed differences in research, which characterizes certain sections of public health in the US. While Epstein built his argument on the analysis of this inclusion in clinical research, he also claims a more general extension of this new 'biopolitical paradigm' in the debate on health disparities. Others have also noticed the spread of biologically or genetically defined research as compared to the traditional calls for social justice – for instance, by improving access to health care – that used to be the focus of these debates (e.g. Lee 2009; see also Joseph in this volume).

Similar to this tradition, the German public health discourse analysed here occasionally calls for addressing disparities by offering adjusted medical services – for example, by providing native-language information or cultural mediators. Integration is therefore not only understood as a demand made of people with an 'immigrant background', but also as a concession on the part of the social majority. In the end, however, the latter is only meant to facilitate their integration and hence their adaptation to the norms of German health care. This therefore contrasts with approaches in other countries in which cultural (or biological) diversity is more accepted as such and is actively addressed by powers like the NHS in the UK or the NIH in the US.[24] Although there are some calls to be more open to diversity and slight indications of awareness of ethnic differences, the German population is mostly perceived as homogeneous and immigrants as the ones who have to assimilate. On the one hand, this reflects Germany's refusal to accept the reality of an immigration society and its tendency to continue to try to keep huge parts of the population out of society. When differences are addressed, in the majority of cases they are not defined biologically, which on the other hand may be due to a historical taboo. Both phenomena serve as a general background for the absence of not only so-called Ashkenazi mutations, but also of general biological ethnic differences in medical discourse and practice. Especially individuals with a Muslim background – defined as having an 'immigrant background' rather than different 'ethnicities' – have been the focus of recent debates on health disparities. These debates tend to focus in turn on 'integration' or 'non-integration', which also reflects a recent, sometimes Islamophobic political discourses on immigration. In contrast, Ashkenazi Jews and BRCA Ashkenazi mutations are practically not discussed. Regardless of primarily hidden, but still prevailing, anti-Semitism in the German population, which attributes all kinds of 'alien' features to Jews, Jews remain officially perceived in terms of a religious community rather than as a different ethnic or somehow biologically defined group, as demonstrated in the Sarrazin debate. Linking Jews with specific genetic features and diseases, as is common in the international medical discourses on Ashkenazi mutations, causes uneasiness and is rather ignored in clinical encounters.[25] In the health disparities debates involving immigrants, Jews who have recently immigrated to Germany from Eastern Europe also do not receive specific attention but seem to be subsumed under the general immigration to Germany from these countries.

An interesting question will thus be whether or not, and how, the discursive changes in the context of the Sarrazin debate will lead to a renaissance in discussions about biologically defined differences in different fields, including medicine, with all the ambivalent aspects I have pointed out in the beginning of this chapter. The number of papers quoting ethnic differences in studies from the US demonstrates that there is no general resistance toward this category. While in this chapter I concentrate on the medical discourse in Germany, it will be a very interesting question for further research to follow what happens in practical research routines – for example, in international studies or studies in which international data are reviewed for Germany. Given that it is currently still not common to differentiate between racial or ethnic categories in German studies, it would therefore be challenging to see how the categories used in international studies are applied or transformed in Germany.

Notes

1. I want to thank my fellow editors of this book and Tino Plümecke and Birgit zur Nieden for their very helpful comments on earlier versions of this chapter, and also Michelle Miles for her help with the English version.

2. For a detailed explanation of the history of these 'founder mutations', see Mozersky and Gibbon in this volume.
3. See, for example, the 2004 special 'Genetics for the human race' issue of *Nature Genetics* (November 2004, volume 36, no. 11).
4. The German equivalent of the *Encyclopaedia Britannica.*
5. The authors are referring to the overall population risk of Ashkenazi women here, not the risk of mutation carriers. The prevalence of these mutations among Ashkenazi women is approximately 2.5 per cent (one in forty). A mutation carrier has a 50 to 60 per cent cumulative lifetime risk of breast cancer.
6. CancerBACUP is a charity that merged with Macmillan Cancer Support in 2008 and changed its name to CancerBACKUP. The cited leaflet was printed with funding from the Department of Health and has been reprinted in several editions. On its website, it states that patient information is accredited by the NHS. Interestingly, the wording of the leaflet has been slightly changed. In 2011, it was more precise concerning the 'ethnic background': 'and have Jewish ancestry or come from another ethnic background (Icelandic, Dutch or Norwegian) where BRCA gene changes are more common' (Macmillan Cancer Support 2011).
7. Figures from 2011 and 2007. See REMID's webpage: www.remid.de/index.php?text=Info_Zahlen.
8. www.brca-netzwerk.de/startseite0.html.
9. This passage from the interview has been translated from German into English by the author.
10. She was referring to known mutations that are particularly common to the Dutch population.
11. See Mozersky and Joseph (2010: 424) for more on the rhetoric used by this organization, who understands its mission to inform people about BRCA as contributing to the survival of the Jewish people.
12. Except for very few articles that *do* address differences in some diseases among Ashkenazi Jews – such as breast cancer or Crohn's disease – the only other topic is the reflection in medical discourse of a wide public debate in the summer of 2012 about religious (Muslim and Jewish) male circumcision after a surprising judicial decision that considered doctors' circumcision of boys a criminal act. Similar to the discourse outlined later on health disparities among immigrants, medical 'problems' discussed in this debate refer to religion or culture, and not genetics.
13. Except for one very recent article that critically discusses categories of race and ethnicity referring to international developments, which he calls 'racial pharmacotherapy' (Müller *et al.* 2013).
14. Another genetic disease mentioned several times is sickle cell anaemia, which has been found more frequently in Germany lately 'because of increasing immigration'('Sichelzellanämie: Hydroxycarbamid wirkt auch bei Kleinkindern' ('Sickle cell anaemia: Hydroxycarbamide also works in infants') 2011). Concerning sickle cell anaemia and thalassaemia, one doctor even complained in a letter about the insufficient treatment of patients because of the low awareness of these diseases that only affect immigrants in Germany (Dickerhoff 2013).
15. This is only a very brief overview of the development in this debate. What can be said is that the discourse frequently fluctuates between more inclusive forms, in which immigration is defended as a 'demographic necessity', and debates about a 'German *Leitkultur*' and the willingness or (in)ability of immigrants to integrate. For more detailed descriptions, see e.g. the contributions in S. Friedrich's *Rassismus in der Leistungsgesellschaft* (2011).
16. Called *Allgemeines Gleichbehandlungsgesetz.*
17. See, for example, in the survey by Schenk (2012) 'Studie zur Gesundheit von Kindern und Jugendlichen in Deutschland (KiGGs): Migrantenbericht': 6–7.

18. In most surveys, participants do not classify themselves, but are classified by others.
19. I do not intend to say that US society does not also at times exclude and discriminate against immigrants or other specific populations, but the official concept of society is multi-ethnic.
20. Nations of course have never followed these models to their full extent, and they are becoming more and more diffused today, but the general attitude still informs many political institutions and practices.
21. See Shooman's chapter 'Keine Frage des Glaubens. Zur Rassifizierung von "Kultur" und "Religion" im antimuslimischen Rassismus' (Shooman 2011) for more on how culture and religion gained the same function in Sarrazin's rhetoric that race had before (similar to what Çinar [1999] said about the 'culturalization' of racism. See D. Çinar [1999]).
22. Quoted in 'Es war ein langer und lauter Furz'. Henryk M. Broder interviewt Thilo Sarrazin ['It was a long and loud fart.' Henryk M. Broder interviews Thilo Sarrazin] (2010) *Taz,* 7 December, www.taz.de/!62422/.
23. See Friedrich's introduction 'Rassismus in der Leistungsgesellschaft. Einleitung' in Friedrich (2011) for a detailed discursive analysis.
24. Although sometimes these efforts also include propagating a normative (proactive) patient subjectivity, as has been noted by Joseph in this volume, for the case of breast cancer prevention among African Americans.
25. This uneasiness around topics of Jewish ancestry parallels with that in Brazil, where geneticists tend not to inform patients about found Ashkenazi mutations in their families, as described by Gibbon (Mozersky and Gibbon) in this volume. However, it certainly has a different historical background in Germany, given the history of the Holocaust.

References

'1000-Genom-Projekt: Gesunde Menschen haben viele Genfehler' (2012) *Deutsches Ärzteblatt,* 1 November. Accessed 26 July, 2013. www.aerzteblatt.de/nachrichten/52254

Bauer, Susanne (2003) 'Krankheit im Raster des Umweltgenomprojekts – Koordinaten, Lokalisationen, Fakten auf der Flucht'. In Nusser, T. (ed.) *Rasterfahndungen. Darstellungstechniken – Normierungsverfahren – Wahrnehmungskonstitution.* Bielefeld: Transcript.

Beauftragte der Bundesregierung für Migration, Flüchtlinge und Integration (2011) *Zweiter Integrationsindikatorenbericht. Erstellt für die Beauftragte der Bundesregierung für Migration, Flüchtlinge und Integration.* Cologne/Berlin.

Beckmann, M. W., Niederacher, D., Goecke, T. O., Bodden-Heidrich, R., Schnürch, H. G. and Bender, H. G. (1997) 'Hochrisikofamilien mit Mamma- und Ovarialkarzinomen: Möglichkeiten der Beratung, genetischen Analyse und Früherkennung', *Deutsches Ärzteblatt* 94 (4): A–161.

Brockhaus Enzyklopädie in zwanzig Bänden. Siebzehnte völlig überarbeitete Auflage des großen Brockhaus (1971) vol. 12. Wiesbaden: F.A. Brockhaus.

CancerBACUP (2004) 'Are you worried about breast cancer?' 6-page leaflet.

Çinar, D. (1999) 'Alter Rassismus im neuen Europa? Anmerkungen zur Novität des Neo-Rassismus'. In Kossek, B. (ed) *Gegen-Rassismen: Konstruktionen – Interaktion – Interventionen.* Hamburg: Argument.

Deutsche Presse-Agentur (2010) 'Sarrazins Provokationen: "Alle Juden teilen ein bestimmtes Gen"', *Die Zeit,* 28 August. Accessed 25 July, 2013. www.zeit.de/gesellschaft/zeitgeschehen/2010–08/sarrazin-juden-gene-migration

'Diabetes bei Asiaten erfordert besonderes Augenmerk' (2012) *Deutsches Ärzteblatt,* 1 May. Accessed 25 July, 2013. www.aerzteblatt.de/nachrichten/50231

Dickerhoff, R. (2013) 'Gesundheitschancen: Thalassämien Nur Bei Migranten', *Deutsches Ärzteblatt,* 18 January. Accessed 26 July, 2013. www.aerzteblatt.de/archiv/134105/Gesundheitschancen-Thalassaemien-nur-bei-Migranten

Dunn, L. C. and Dobzhansky, T. (1946) *Heredity, Race, and Society.* New York: The New American Library of World Literature.

Duster, T. (2005) 'Race and reification in science', *Science* 307 (5712): 1050–1.

Epstein, S. (2007) *Inclusion: The Politics of Difference in Medical Research.* Chicago: University of Chicago Press.

Ernst, J., Saeger, W., Linke, R.P., et al. (1998) 'Praktische Hinweise zur Diagnose und Therapie generalisierter Amyloidosen', *Deutsches Ärzteblatt* 95 (42): A–2626.

Foucault, M. (2001) *Die Ordnung des Diskurses,* 6th ed. Frankfurt: Fischer. (Original work published 1974.)

Frädrich, A. (2010) 'Teilnahme an Klinischen Prüfungen: Spezielle Art des Geldverdienens', *Deutsches Ärzteblatt* 107, 44: A-2162.

Friedrich, S. (2011) *Rassismus in der Leistungsgesellschaft: Analysen und kritische Perspektiven zu den rassistischen Normalisierungsprozessen der 'Sarrazindebatte',* Münster: Assemblage.

Fujimura, J.H. and Rajagopalan, R. (2011) 'Different differences: the use of "genetic ancestry" versus race in biomedical human genetic research', *Social Studies of Science* 41 (1): 5–30.

'Gentests in Großbritannien auch für Menschen ohne Erbkrankheit' (2009) *Deutsches Ärzteblatt,* 2 January. Accessed 24 July, 2013. www.aerzteblatt.de/nachrichten/34999

Gerste, R.D. (2012) 'Kurzsichtigkeit: Kinder werden meist im Alter von 9 bis 13 Jahren myop', *Deutsches Ärzteblatt* 109 (47): A-2361.

Gissendanner, S.S., Ngassa Djomo, K. and Schmid-Ott, G. (2012) 'Ethnisch-kulturelle Vielfalt und psychosomatische Rehabilitation: Transkulturelle Kompetenz', *Deutsches Ärzteblatt* 108 (50): A 2709–12.

Hillienhof, A. (2011) 'Baden-Württemberg: Traumatisierte Migranten besser versorgen', *Deutsches Ärzteblatt* 10: 488.

Holinski-Feder, E., Brandau, O., Nestle-Krämling, C. et al. (1998) 'Genetik des erblichen Mammakarzinoms: Grundlagen – Forschung – Diagnostik', *Deutsches Ärzteblatt* 95 (11): A–600.

Hsu, W.C., Boyko, E.J., Fujimoto, W.Y. et al. (2012) 'Pathophysiologic differences among Asians, Native Hawaiians, and Other Pacific Islanders and treatment implications', *Diabetes Care* 35 (5): 1189–98.

Hunt, L.M. and Megyesi, M.S. (2008) 'The ambiguous meanings of the racial/ethnic categories routinely used in human genetics research', *Social Science and Medicine* 66: 349–61.

Kamtsiuris, P., Atzpodien, K., Ellert, U., Schlack, R. and Schlaud, M. (2007) 'Prävalenz von somatischen Erkrankungen bei Kindern und Jugendlichen in Deutschland: Ergebnisse des Kinder- und Jugendgesundheitssurveys (KiGGS)', *Bundesgesundheitsblatt – Gesundheitsforschung – Gesundheitsschutz,* 50: 686–700.

'Kinder- und Jugendärzte: Für eine bessere Versorgung von Migrantenkindern' (2010) *Deutsches Ärzteblatt* 107 (50): 83. Accessed 26 July, 2013. www.aerzteblatt.de/archiv/79784

'Kinderärzte kritisieren schleppenden Ausbau der Krippenplätze' (2011) *Deutsches Ärzteblatt,* 9 November. Accessed 26 July, 2013. www.aerzteblatt.de/nachrichten/47983

King, G.L., McNeely, M.J., Thorpe, L.E. et al. (2012) 'Understanding and addressing unique needs of diabetes in Asian Americans, Native Hawaiians, and Pacific Islanders', *Diabetes Care* 35 (5): 1181–88.

Lee, S.S. (2009) 'Pharmacogenomics and the challenge of health disparities', *Public Health Genomics* 12 (3): 170–9.

Livingstone, Frank B. (1962) 'On the non-existence of human races', *Current Anthropology* 3 (3): 279–81.

Löwy, I. and Gaudillière, J.P.P. (2008) 'Localizing the global: testing for hereditary risks of breast cancer', *Science, Technology and Human Values* 33 (3): 299–325.

Macmillan Cancer Support (2011): 'Are you worried about breast cancer?' Accessed 26 July, 2013. http://be.macmillan.org.uk/Downloads/CancerInformation/CancerTypes/MAC12153Worriedaboutbreastcancer.pdf

M'Charek, A. (2005) *The Human Genome Diversity Project: An Ethnography of Scientific Practise*. Cambridge, UK: Cambridge University Press.

Meyer, Rüdiger (1997) 'BRCA-Gentest: Entscheidungshilfe oder Wahrsagerei?' *Deutsches Ärzteblatt* 94 (24): A–1600.

Mozersky, J. and Joseph, G. (2010) 'Case studies in the co-production of populations and genetics: the making of "at risk populations" in BRCA genetics', *BioSocieties* 5 (4): 415–39.

Müller, D.J., Kluge, U. and Heinz, A. (2013) 'Genetische Varianz: Haben die Ostfriesen andere Gene?' *Deutsches Ärzteblatt* 110 (8): A-314.

zur Nieden, A. (2010) 'The embodiment of genetic risk: Women's experiences of genetic testing for breast cancer susceptibility mutations'. In Bammé, A., Getzinger, G. and Wieser, B. (eds) *Yearbook 2009 of the Institute for Advanced Studies on Science Technology and Society*. München und Wien: Profil.

———. (2013) *Zum Subjekt der Gene werden. Subjektivierungsweisen im Zeichen der Genetisierung von Brustkrebs.* [*Becoming Subject of the Genes. Ways of Subjectification in the Ara of Genetification of Breast Cancer.*] Bielefeld: Transcript (in German).

Özdemir, C. (2006) 'PERSPECTIVE: Germany's integration challenge'. Accessed 22 July, 2013. https://litigation-essentials.lexisnexis.com/webcd/app?action=DocumentDisplay&crawlid=1&doctype=cite&docid=30+Fletcher+F.+World+Aff.+221&srctype=smi&srcid=3B15&key=d4a7d45fa640fc68b69a393ff459583a

Palm, K. (2009) 'Der "Rasse"-Begriff in der Biologie nach 1945', AG gegen Rassismus in den Lebenswissenschaften (ed) *Gemachte Differenz: Kontinuitäten biologischer 'Rasse'-Konzepte.* Münster: Unrast.

'Patientenberatung auf Türkisch und Russisch' (2011) *Deutsches Ärzteblatt,* 17 October. Accessed 26 July, 2013. www.aerzteblatt.de/nachrichten/47719/Patientenberatung-auf-Tuerkisch-und-Russisch

Plümecke, T. (2010) 'Die neuen Differenzen der Lebenswissenschaften. "Rasse", Genetik und die ungenutzten Potentiale der Soziologie'. In Müller, M. und Zifonun, D. (eds) *Ethnowissen: Soziologische Beiträge zu ethnischer Differenzierung und Migration.* Wiesbaden: VS Verlag.

'Präimplantationsdiagnostik: Erstes Baby ohne Brustkrebsgen geboren' (2009) *Deutsches Ärzteblatt,* 14 January. Accessed 25 July, 2013. www.aerzteblatt.de/nachrichten/34985

'Präventionsprojekt "Mit Migranten für Migranten" erfolgreich' (2010) *Deutsches Ärzteblatt,* 30 December. Accessed 26 July, 2013. www.aerzteblatt.de/nachrichten/44085

'Psychotherapeutische Versorgung von Migranten mangelhaft' (2010) *Deutsches Ärzteblatt,* 6 October. Accessed 26 July, 2013. www.aerzteblatt.de/nachrichten/42992.

Rieser, S. (2010) 'Migrantinnen: Studie zu Verhütung und Mutterschaft', *Deutsches Ärzteblatt* 107 (45): A–2202.

Sankar, P., Cho, M. K. and Mountain, J. (2007) 'Race and ethnicity in genetic research', *American Journal of Medical Genetics Part A* 143A (9): 961–70.

Sarrazin, T. (2010) *Deutschland schafft sich ab: Wie wir unser Land aufs Spiel setzen.* Munich: Deutsche Verlags-Anstalt.

Schenk, Liane (2012) 'Studie zur Gesundheit von Kindern und Jugendlichen in Deutschland (KiGGS): Migrantenbericht'. Accessed 25 July, 2013. www.rki.de/DE/Content/Gesundheitsmonitoring/Studien/Kiggs/Basiserhebung/Fachartikel/kiggs-migrantenbericht.pdf?__blob=publicationFile

Schönland, S. O. (2006) 'Fortschritte in der Diagnostik und Therapie der Amyloidosen', *Deutsches Ärzteblatt* 103 (34–35): A–2237.

Shooman, Y. (2011) 'Keine Frage des Glaubens. Zur Rassifizierung von "Kultur" und "Religion" im antimuslimischen Rassismus'. In Friedrich, S. (ed) *Rassismus in der Leistungsgesellschaft: Analysen und kritische Perspektiven zu den rassistischen Normalisierungsprozessen der 'Sarrazindebatte'*. Münster: Assemblage.

'Sichelzellanämie: Hydroxycarbamid wirkt auch bei Kleinkindern' (2011) *Deutsches Ärzteblatt,* 13 May. Online. Accessed 26 July, 2013. www.aerzteblatt.de/nachrichten/45848/Sichelzellanaemie-Hydroxycarbamid-wirkt-auch-bei-Kleinkindern

Sudeck, H. and Horstmann, R. (1999) 'Gentest ermöglicht Diagnose des Familiären Mittelmeerfiebers', *Deutsches Ärzteblatt* 96 (21): A–1418.

Thierfelder, W., Dortschy, R., Hintzpeter, B., Kahl, H. and Scheidt-Nave, C. (2007) 'Biochemische Messparameter im Kinder- und Jugendgesundheitssurvey (KiGGS)', *Bundesgesundheitsblatt – Gesundheitsforsch – Gesundheitsschutz* 50: 757–770.

Timmann, C., Schumacher, J., Lamprecht, P., Sudeck, H. and Horstmann, R. (1999) 'Genetisch bedingte Fiebersyndrome: Klinik, Genetik, Diagnose und Therapie', *Deutsches Ärzteblatt* 101 (48): A–3262.

Weingart, P., Kroll, J. and Bayertz, K. (1988) *Rasse, Blut und Gene – Geschichte der Eugenik und Rassenhygiene in Deutschland.* Frankfurt: Suhrkamp.

Zeeb, H. and Greinert, R. (2010) 'Bedeutung von Vitamin D in der Krebsprävention: Konflikt zwischen UV-Schutz und Anhebung niedriger Vitamin-D-Spiegel?' *Deutsches Ärzteblatt International* 107 (37): 638–43.

2 Mapping Jewish identities

Migratory histories and the transnational re-framing of 'Ashkenazi BRCA mutations' in the UK and Brazil

Jessica Mozersky and Sahra Gibbon

Much social science attention has been paid to the notion of 'genomic futures' and the implications of *medical* genetics for health, identity and how we conceptualize risk and prevention of disease for self and family (Finkler 2000; Gibbon 2007; Hallowell 1999; Mozersky 2013). More recently, others are directing us to the ways in which *population* genetics can reconfigure the past (El Haj 2007; Nelson 2008; Palmié 2007). Moreover, there is an increasingly complex intertwining of medical and population genetic research, with the former exploring what genetic variation may reveal about health, disease and drug response and the latter focusing on ancestral and migratory histories. It has also been suggested that genomic knowledge acts as a 'telescope' to the past (and future) in the ways that narratives of migration, colonization and origin have become part of the temporal logic of the medical, scientific and social discourse surrounding BRCA mutations (cf. Adams *et al.* 2009; El-Haj 2007; Gibbon 2013; M'Charek 2013; Schlünder, this volume). This is particularly evident, as new technologies such as high-throughput sequencing are impacting the scope and reach of genomic interventions and as the marketing of direct-to-consumer (DTC) testing (particularly in the US) is combining a so-called 'recreational' interest in genetic genealogy with medical genetic testing and the promise of preventative health (Koenig *et al.* 2008; Lee 2013).

This chapter builds on studies at the emerging intersection of medical and population genetics by examining the different ways in which narratives of ancestry and migratory history have been, and are becoming, linked to mutations in the high-risk breast cancer genes BRCA1 and BRCA2. In particular, it examines how these historical narratives – initially associated with Ashkenazi Jewish communities and subsequently with diverse regions and populations – have become variously incorporated into different domains of transnational medical research and clinical practices. Drawing on ethnographic research in the UK and Brazil, this article compares the ways in which health professionals (research scientists and clinicians) communicate, understand and situate narratives of history and migration associated with Ashkenazi Jewish populations and the varied consequences this has for the way patients engage with and incorporate this knowledge into understandings of risk and identity.[1] In this way, we aim to highlight several contrasting dynamics surrounding the transnational re-framing of 'Ashkenazi BRCA mutations'.

Before turning to our ethnographic data, we begin with a discussion of the 'Ashkenazi' BRCA founder mutations and their relationship to migratory and demographic history of both Jewish and, more recently, non-Jewish populations.

Founder mutations as links to the past

The increased incidence of genetic disease among populations can be the result of processes known as the founder effect and genetic drift. A founder event occurs when a population has a small number of founding ancestors who are separated from the larger parent population and who goes on to found a new population (Stone *et al.* 2007). Alternatively, a founder event can be the result of an extreme reduction of a population, by over 50 per cent, due to famine, war, epidemic or some other event that causes a significant number of a population's members to die. In both of these situations, the new founding population carries only a fraction of the original population's genetic variation and is not representative of the entire diverse population from which it was derived (Stone *et al.* 2007). A founder effect occurs when one of the members of the new founding population carries a genetic mutation, which is then passed on to future generations, and the concept of genetic drift refers to this happening purely by chance. The mutation may substantially increase in frequency if the population remains reproductively closed – for example, due to geographic isolation or cultural/religious practices, such as endogamy (Janavicius 2010). Founder mutations can sometimes be traced to a single common ancestor or 'founder', and as such can create temporal links to a group's ancestral past.[2]

The Ashkenazi BRCA founder mutations

The increased risk of BRCA breast cancer among Ashkenazi Jews is the most well-known and established population risk that has been identified to date, having emerged shortly after the cloning of the BRCA genes over 15 years ago. Ashkenazi Jews have the highest known population risk of carrying three specific founder mutations in the BRCA1 and 2 genes. The three 'Ashkenazi mutations', as they initially came to be known in medical and scientific literature, are illustrative examples of the ways in which founder mutations create temporal links to the past.[3] Population geneticists have dated the Ashkenazi founder mutations, and each has been correlated with a specific event and time point in Jewish history when the population was suddenly reduced and then re-expanded (Neuhausen *et al.* 1998; Risch *et al.* 2003; Slatkin 2004). For instance the oldest mutation (185delAG on BRCA1) was originally estimated to be between 2,000 and 2,500 years old and believed to have originated in the Middle East prior to the first important founder event in Ashkenazi Jewish history when Jews left the Middle East and settled in Europe following the destruction of the Second Temple around 70 CE (Slatkin 2004). The second mutation (6174delT on BRCA2) was estimated to be about 700 years old and to have arisen in Eastern Europe, as most Jews settled there at this time. It is associated with a second important founder event – the severe persecution of the Jews during the Crusades and the Black Death, both of which led to an extreme population reduction (Slatkin 2004).[4]

While other populations are also the subject of genetic research, Ashkenazi Jews are considered to be ideal genetic research subjects because they are descended from a small number of founding ancestors who were confined to one particular geographical area (primarily Eastern Europe) and who practised endogamy. Furthermore, the Ashkenazi Jewish population was often extremely reduced as a result of famine, war or epidemic. At the same time, Jewish history is fairly well documented over the past 4,000 years in terms of migration, location and population events, making them a particularly attractive study population. Without such historical knowledge, it would be much more difficult to make conclusive genetic statements. When individuals are stripped of all prior information about their ancestry, geographical origins or ethnic group and are then assigned to groups *a posteriori,* racial categories or geographical origins based on genetic data become much less reliable (Bamshad *et al.* 2004). Without external information such as texts, oral history or archaeology, it is difficult, if not impossible, to tell a coherent story about a population based on genetic information alone (Goldstein 2008). Genetic differentiation and mutations are therefore a reflection of the particular geographic, migratory, reproductive and socio-cultural histories of populations.

In addition to the reasons stated above, much is known about genetic diseases among the Ashkenazi Jewish population because they have historically been active participants in research and screening programmes, and they are over-represented in genetic literature (Birenbaum Carmeli 2004).[5] For example, the identification of the first Ashkenazi founder mutation on BRCA1 was derived from a set of approximately 700 samples screened for Tay-Sachs disease that had been stored since the 1970s.[6] Tay-Sachs screening brought thousands of Ashkenazi Jews into clinics, where their blood samples were not only screened for Tay-Sachs, but often stored for future genetic research. The 'unexpected research payoff' (Kahn 2005: 8) was the availability of stored blood samples that were subsequently used for other research studies. One consequence of the prevalence of the Ashkenazi Jewish population in research is that, when researchers find a particular mutation or disease risk among this group, the results are often labelled as 'Jewish' (as in the case of 'Ashkenazi BRCA mutations'), even though the existence of these mutations in other populations who are studied less is entirely possible (cf. Azoulay 2003). Perhaps unsurprisingly, as researchers have broadened their pool of subjects, Ashkenazi and other founder mutations are increasingly being identified in populations who do not identify themselves as Ashkenazi Jewish (cf. Hamel *et al.* 2011; Janavicius 2010; Weitzel *et al.* 2013).

Beyond Ashkenazi Jews

Despite increasing discoveries of the Ashkenazi mutations in other populations, these are often situated and discussed in scientific or popular discourse in ways that suggest that the presence of these mutations are diagnostic of 'hidden' or 'original'

Jewish identity. For instance, in 2005 a scientific study by Weitzel *et al.* to determine the frequency of BRCA mutations among Hispanic American women living in Los Angeles found a high number of one of the Ashkenazi founder mutations in the sample. This led the authors to conclude that these 'apparently non-Jewish' families likely descended from the Spanish Jews known as *conversos* who hid their identities by converting to Christianity during periods of anti-Semitism in Spain from the twelfth to sixteenth centuries (Weitzel *et al.* 2005: 1669). Building on this study, Laitman *et al.* (2013) led an international genetic study that found the presence of this same 'Ashkenazi founder mutation' among a population of Indians living in the state of Colorado who had immigrated from Mexico, which was considered evidence that this mutation originated among the same group of *conversos* who had immigrated from Spain. This research gained international interest not only in scientific publications, but also in popular media in the US and abroad. For example, the Israeli newspaper *Haaretz* ran the headline: 'Group of Colorado Indians have genetic Jewish roots' (Even 2012). According to this article, the study 'proves' that this group of Indians has 'genetic roots going back to the expulsion of Jews from Spain' (Even 2012), showing how such information is not just diagnostic of risk, but in this case indicative of migratory history and previously unknown Jewish identity. According to another article in the *Smithsonian* magazine, when one US oncologist was alerted to the discovery of this mutation among Hispanic Catholics, she reportedly said, 'Those people are Jewish' (Wheelwright 2008). Rather than raising doubts about whether the mutations are specific to Ashkenazi Jews, the researchers' focus on the migratory history of Jewish populations, and their conclusion about the mutations' origin have reinforced the notion of 'Jewish genes' and common ancestry to all of those who carry them.[7]

According to Neulander's (2006) research in New Mexico with non-Jewish individuals who were found to carry supposedly 'Jewish' genetic diseases or mutations, genetic disease may be used to infer 'secret' or 'crypto-Jewish' descent from ancestral Jews. These claims often serve a broader purpose of asserting an overvalued line of white ancestral descent and restoring 'prestige lineage'. Neulander (2006) argues that the use of the label 'Jewish' to determine who is at risk of genetic disease has paved the way for the popular use of heritable diseases to determine who is a Jew. This 'disease-based Judaism' (Neulander 2006: 389) is in fact a failure to differentiate between heritable characteristics acquired through DNA and cultural characteristics widely attributed to Jews, which are only acquired through learning. Neulander (2006) argues strongly against genetically labelling faith-based communities, and instead proposes that diseases be identified in terms of geographical origins, such as Eastern Europe, rather than Ashkenazi Jewish, since every heritable disease will have a founder who can be located in time and place. As our chapter suggests, in the context of transnational research and medical practices associated with the Ashkenazi BRCA founder mutations, there are signs that processes of reframing and renaming the Ashkenazi founder mutations are taking place, while Jewish origins are simultaneously still being inferred for those who carry them.

This chapter contributes to these recent developments by exploring the diverse social, cultural and scientific implications involved when researchers find Ashkenazi BRCA mutations in apparently non-Jewish populations. The existence of Ashkenazi founder mutations among self-identified Ashkenazi Jews, Hispanic Californians, Brazilians and Mexican Indians is thought to be evidence of a common ancestor among all of them. How might this knowledge of a supposedly shared Jewish ancestry affect the ways genetic risk information is understood by health professionals and/or communicated at the clinical interface? How do individuals (self-identified as Jewish or not) conceive of themselves and the groups to which they belong? Some social scientists suggest that renewed attention in scientific and medical research to genetic ancestry raises profound questions for the configuration of identity (El Haj 2008; Palmié 2007). The discovery of genetic mutations or markers, including those not related to disease, has the potential to strengthen or threaten a group's communal narrative, religious, cultural and even ethnic identity (Davis 2004).[8] As a result, examining how new knowledge about the origin of the BRCA mutations intersects with pre-existing narratives of identity and history is central to understanding these developments. A key issue is the potential role of newly geneticized historical narratives of migration and origin for the 'naturalization' of pre-existing identities as well as their partial or unexpected transformation

In the section below, we compare developments and scientific findings regarding the 'Ashkenazi BRCA mutations' in both the UK and Brazil, drawing on ethnographic fieldwork in each location. In the UK, research and clinical interventions regarding the Ashkenazi mutations have primarily been aimed at those who already identify themselves as Ashkenazi Jews. One result is that, in such a context, Ashkenazi mutations can have the effect of reiterating pre-existing or known Jewish identity and understandings of collective history. In Brazil, the discovery of Ashkenazi mutations among those who do not consider themselves to be Jewish can have diverse ramifications. For some, it might reveal previously unknown or hitherto hidden aspects of identity and history – the consequences of which can serve to both reaffirm pre-existing notions of being of 'European' origin and/or having mixed ancestry and as a result offering a confirmation of being 'Brazilian'. At the same time, an inferred Jewish origin can also be an uncomfortable scenario for Brazilian patients and practitioners, despite the positive symbolic value in Brazil of *mesticagem* – having mixed-race ancestry. These contrasting comparisons therefore reveal the multiple, context-specific ways in which genetic knowledge can affect notions of individual and group identity as well as the boundaries, moral frameworks and affective alignments through which genes, risk and identity are variously co-configured.

The UK context: reiterating Jewish identity

In the UK, genetic testing is available free of charge through the National Health Service to any individual who meets the risk criteria set by the National Institute for Health and Care Excellence (NICE). In 2005, NICE published revised guidelines for the management of familial breast cancer, including the addition of Ashkenazi Jewish ancestry as an important risk factor to be taken into account by physicians when considering whether to refer a woman to genetic counselling services.

It is standard clinical practice to send women who are referred to genetic counselling a family history questionnaire in advance of their appointment. This questionnaire includes a question about Jewish ancestry for the purposes of determining an individual's risk. Women who self-identify as Ashkenazi and opt to undergo genetic testing are initially only tested for the three Ashkenazi BRCA founder mutations (as opposed to sequencing the entire large BRCA1 and 2 genes). Screening only for specific founder mutations is a cheaper, faster way to carry out genetic testing, as most Ashkenazi Jews who are tested will be found to carry one of the three founder mutations. Sequencing the entire BRCA1 and 2 genes (a more expensive and time-consuming process) only occurs if no mutation is found after this initial round of targeted testing. There is thus a very practical benefit for clinicians and scientists to be had from knowing whether particular founder mutations exist within a given population (Janavicius 2010).

In the UK, such clinical practices, alongside national guidelines and a large body of scientific research about this population, have had the effect of routinizing the clinical association of Ashkenazi ancestry with genetic breast cancer risk.[9] In fact, genetic counsellors have reported a lower threshold for offering genetic testing to Ashkenazi patients (for example, one first-degree relative with breast/ovarian cancer) as opposed to the more stringent criteria used with other patients. This clinical practice reflects both the fact that testing for founder mutations is faster and more economical and the perception that being Ashkenazi Jewish is strongly associated with an increased risk of genetic breast cancer.

Mozersky (2013) has shown elsewhere how genomic knowledge about breast cancer risk can reiterate pre-existing ways of how Ashkenazi Jews understand their group belonging and collective history. For instance, the existence of Ashkenazi BRCA mutations is interpreted by some individuals as evidence of the interrelatedness of all Jews, their common ancestors or a collective history (including suffering) in the ghettos of Eastern Europe. The examples below illustrate this reiteration from the perspective of patient advocacy organizations, clinicians/researchers and patients.

Patient advocacy

Jews Against Cancer of the Breast (JACOB) International is an international breast cancer advocacy organization dedicated to helping Ashkenazi Jewish women learn more about their increased risk of genetic breast cancer. Their goal is not only to educate Ashkenazi women, but to encourage all women (not just those at high risk) to seek genetic testing in order to fulfil their mission of breaking the cycle of hereditary breast and ovarian cancer. JACOB's website explains the Ashkenazi mutations as follows:

> It is believed that these mutations can be traced back hundreds of years to their common ancestors, or founders. As the result of numerous intermarriages among Jews, all of today's Ashkenazi Jews are descended from a very small group of Jews who lived in Eastern Europe 500 years ago. These 'founding Ashkenazis' carried the particular BRCA1 and BRCA2 gene mutations which were subsequently passed on to their descendants.
>
> (JACOB International 2013)

JACOB explicitly relates these mutations to the common history of Ashkenazi Jews in Eastern Europe. The US Jewish advocacy organization Sharsheret (Hebrew for 'chain') supports young Jewish women and their families who are facing breast cancer and acknowledges the 'unique concerns' of Jewish women, particularly by putting them in contact with one another and offering various support programmes. The cover of their education booklet about genetic breast cancer, entitled 'Your Jewish Genes', has a photo of four women of all different ages and generations and contains an explanation of '*what's Jewish* about hereditary breast and ovarian cancer' (Sharsheret website 2013, italics added). This further demonstrates how genetic breast cancer is framed as a Jewish disease caused by supposedly Jewish genes.

Donelle *et al.* (2005) have compared the portrayal of breast cancer risk in Jewish newspapers as opposed to newspapers intended for the general population and found that genetic breast cancer is especially associated with being a Jewish woman. They found a significantly higher proportion of articles that identified genetics as the main risk factor for breast cancer in Jewish newspapers as compared to non-Jewish newspapers (75 per cent of the articles in Jewish newspapers versus 12 per cent in general newspapers). Despite the fact that a very small proportion of breast cancer is genetic, even among Ashkenazi Jews, the Jewish newspaper articles 'insinuate that the identity of Jewish women, in part, entails the genetic risk of breast cancer' (Donelle *et al.* 2005: 191).

Clinical and research context

In the UK and several other national contexts, population-wide screening programmes are being piloted with the aim of screening all Ashkenazi Jews, regardless of family history, for the three BRCA founder mutations (Levy-Lahad *et al.* 2012; Metcalfe *et al.* 2009). In the UK, a pilot population screening programme began in October 2008. It aims to recruit 10,000 Ashkenazi Jews and 'to develop a strategy for prediction and prevention of genetic cancer. Over the long term it is hoped this will reduce cancers in the community.'[10] The study is supported by a major Jewish charity in the UK, the liberal and reform Jewish movements, rabbis, other Jewish organizations and a major high street chemist. Similar to the UK, it was announced in May 2008 that Jewish women in Ontario, Canada, would be offered a free genetic test for BRCA mutations as part of a research study. Within 10 days after a national Canadian newspaper began advertising the study, over

2,100 women volunteered, illustrating 'considerable interest for genetic testing among Jewish women' (Metcalfe *et al.* 2009: 1). This study found that 45 per cent of the mutations identified were in women who did not meet the local genetic testing criteria, leading the study authors to conclude that genetic testing should be extended to women who do not meet the current criteria (Metcalfe *et al.* 2009). One female Canadian rabbi claimed that BRCA mutation screening will one day be offered in a similar way to Tay-Sachs screening because the 'rate of this gene is so high' (Priest 2008). In Israel, a general population screening study found mutations in 63 per cent of families that would not have otherwise been considered high risk due to minimal or no family history of breast or ovarian cancer, leading to the suggestion that population-wide screening of the Ashkenazi population is feasible, cost-effective and justified (Levy-Lahad *et al.* 2012).

These studies demonstrate how researchers stratify samples based on notions of a discrete Ashkenazi population with a unique risk of BRCA mutations, which in turn justifies population-wide screening. At the same time, self-identified Ashkenazi Jews actively participate in research, which has the effect of reinforcing notions of specific 'Ashkenazi' mutations and genetic diseases.

BRCA mutations are also portrayed as indicative of a collective Jewish history and identity because they have been dated and correlated to particular historical events. In addition to the two founder mutations described earlier, the third mutation (5382insC on BRCA1) is estimated to be approximately 1,800 years old but to have entered the Ashkenazi population about 400–500 years ago (Hamel *et al.* 2011). According to Hamel *et al.*, the mutation may have spread due to the rapid expansion of Jews in Poland beginning in the sixteenth century, which 'significantly improved the odds of admixture' (2011: 305) between Jews and non-Jews, even for an otherwise relatively genetically isolated group (admixture refers to reproduction across groups). In contrast, the origins of this mutation have also been associated with another Jewish founder event: the Cossack massacres in 1648, which resulted in the 'total destruction of many Jewish communities' and the death of at least 25 per cent of the population (Risch *et al.* 1995: 157). According to one British Jewish breast surgeon, this mutation may have spread as a result of rapes during pogroms, leading him to describe it as 'another tragic event in Jewish history' and a 'component in the repertoire of humiliations experienced in the Jewish ghettos of the Pale of Settlement between the 13th and 19th centuries' (report of the Anglo-Israeli Workshop on the Genetic Risk of Breast Cancer 2006: 4). Of course, rape is not the only mechanism by which genetic mutations can be transferred across groups, as Hamel *et al.*'s (2011) more neutral suggestion of admixture suggests. The surgeon's comment rather demonstrates how specific aspects of the historical suffering of Ashkenazi Jews are invoked to explain hereditary disease-causing mutations.

Inferring Jewish origins from genetic BRCA mutations has also been reflected in clinical practice, as when one genetic counsellor reported that occasionally an 'Ashkenazi mutation' is found in families who do not identify as Jewish. When asked whether this actually indicates that a family is really Jewish, given that some of these mutations are present in non-Jewish Eastern European individuals, she explained that it just shows how 'somewhere back there genes got mixed in' and that she usually has chosen not to inform the family that the mutation was specifically a Jewish one, presumably to avoid altering how this family/individual already conceives of themselves.

Women

Although most high-risk Ashkenazi women in the study were not aware of the specific Ashkenazi founder mutations and the endeavour of population geneticists to date each of them, they did attribute the origins of genetic disease and mutations to the collective endogamous history, and suffering, of Ashkenazi Jews in the shtetls of Eastern Europe. For instance, Jennifer was a British woman in her 40s who had a very strong family history of breast cancer. She was awaiting her genetics appointment and explained her understanding of the increased risk as follows:

> I know the history, you know, was that we were in tiny shtetls so I guess it makes sense, um, and it's just one of those things . . . we've all seen *Fiddler On The Roof,* so I guess you know it does make sense, they don't marry that far out really do they? It's different today I suppose there's a lot more, well for a start we're not living in tiny little shtetls. We live in big cities and we're just sort of out there much more, and everything has changed beyond measure what our great grandparents would have imagined, um, so I suppose it's probably reducing as well now, maybe . . . even if you were still marrying a Jewish person, it wouldn't necessarily be from your village, it could be from Birmingham or you know whatever, so that the kind of risk, that kind of intermarriage, is probably reducing now.

For Jennifer, life in the shtetls of Eastern Europe and the intermarriage between Jews helps explain the risk of genetic breast cancer. While this history 'makes sense' and is consistent with her understanding of Jewish history, she relegates such practices to the past. Jennifer's first cousin Anna was in her mid-40s and had lost her mother (Jennifer's aunt) to breast cancer when she was in her twenties. She was awaiting the results of her BRCA mutation test. Anna also related the increased risk to historical reproductive patterns:

> But it's interesting to understand this background because . . . presumably it's all through intermarriage. It's sort of fascinating . . . well it must be cousins, I presume it's coming through cousins, I suppose we have no idea of what background, I mean what sort of communities they lived in and one assumes it was an acceptable way of life in being introduced to what must be your first or your second cousin.

The existence of genetic breast cancer among Ashkenazi Jews has the potential to reiterate a collective historical narrative of Jews living in Eastern Europe, isolated in small shtetls and ghettos and practising endogamy. In this context, genomic knowledge does not transform or alter understandings of the past; rather, it serves to naturalize a social/cultural narrative about a shared past.

The passages from interviews below demonstrate how genetic disease can reiterate a sense of group belonging and boundaries based on blood, genes and biology. Lori was an American graduate student living and studying in London. She was in her mid-twenties and had lost her mother to breast cancer as a teenager. Although Lori was too young for genetic testing at the time of the interview, she was advised that it was something she might consider in future. Although Lori was not raised in a religious home – she described herself as secular and her Judaism as a 'cultural background' – she also said: 'I think that these potential genetic mutations, Tay-Sachs disease, breast and ovarian cancer mutations, I mean that's what brings it back to a biological level obviously.'

For Daniel, an unmarried, successful, retired businessman in his late 40s, genetic disease among Ashkenazi Jews helped to define them as a distinct group:

> I would have thought that if there are distinctive Jewish diseases then there must be distinctive Jewish genetic components. Now it may not be enough to found a whole identity, but . . . it makes it quite difficult to resist the conclusion that if one was trying to define a group, meaning draw boundaries between it and another group, even if they weren't clear boundaries . . . still it's an indicator!

Despite Daniel's acknowledgement that the boundaries would be unclear and porous when trying to define the group, it is hard for him to resist the conclusion that genetic mutations are an indicator that there are genetic aspects to being Jewish, and that this serves to reinforce the boundaries between Jews and non-Jews. For Lori and Daniel, disease-causing mutations, or 'genetic components', demarcate Jews in a certain way and reiterate a boundary between Jews and non-Jews. This 'disease-based Judaism' (Neulander 2006) demonstrates that the existence of supposedly Jewish genetic diseases reinforces the pre-existing boundaries and ways in which individual 'Jewish' identity has been understood. Thus, this way of thinking about Jewish belonging did not challenge or conflict with the other social and cultural ways in which individuals also experienced being Jewish.

The Brazilian Context

The field of BRCA research in Brazil has been active since the early 2000s, when the 'unknown' contribution of BRCA genes to breast cancer incidence in the country became a source and site of inquiry and transnational research, contributing to the emergence of Brazilian *oncogenetica* as a clinical specialty (Gibbon 2013). From an early stage, there has been an explicit focus on identifying the frequency of possible founder mutations in the Brazilian population.

Initially, this included mutations identified in populations outside of Brazil, including those associated with the Ashkenazi Jewish population. The focus on these specific mutations was initially directly tied to the possibility of developing 'rapid inexpensive genetic tests' in the Brazilian context (Gomes *et al.* 2007) – an issue of considerable importance in developing cancer genetics in low-income country settings (Narod 2011).[11] A number of Brazilian studies have subsequently identified these mutations at variable but 'significant' frequencies in different regions of the country (Da Costa *et al.* 2008; Dufloth *et al.* 2005; Esteves *et al.* 2009; Ewald *et al.* 2011; Lourenco *et al.* 2004). Initially, this research suggested that 'a small number of founder mutations may be predominant' and called for 'screening for all Brazilian women with breast cancer' (Gomes *et al.* 2007).

The focus on these mutations in Brazil reflects an international research agenda for the BRCA genes in which the Ashkenazi mutations are some of the most common identified worldwide. Nonetheless, given that nearly all of the Brazilian studies have been undertaken, entirely or in part, with individuals who do not identify themselves as Jewish, there has unsurprisingly been significant speculation in these published papers about the reason for finding these mutations in the Brazilian population. Common narrative explanations in published papers include the reference to the large Jewish population who used to live in Portugal and or Spain but who were deported during the Inquisition known as *conversos* (Ewald *et al.* 2011; Gomes *et al.* 2007). By contrast a study by Da Costa *et al.* in 2008 of the 'origin' and 'diffusion' of one so-called Ashkenazi mutation (5382insC) highlights the potential for a 'significant Eastern European contribution to the present day genetic background of the Brazilian population, contrary to an alternative hypothesis of a contribution from new Christians emigrating in the 16th century' (2008: 65). It is argued that this reflects the specificity of Brazilian migratory history, especially as this concerns German immigration to the region in the late nineteenth and early twentieth centuries.[12]

In a more recent article, Ewald *et al.* (2011) also turn their attention to the range of different founder mutations that they have identified in non-Ashkenazi women in their publications, including historical explanations for the identification of these mutations in Brazil. While acknowledging that a more detailed understanding of their entrance and distribution in Brazil remains to be determined, the article nevertheless counters prior speculation that those who carry the mutation may be *conversos* from Portugal. Instead they suggest that the more likely explanation is that the 'mutation probably originated in Scandinavia or Northern Russia . . . and could have entered Brazil through one or more several large European immigration waves in the 18th and 19th century' (Ewald *et al.* 2011: 5).

There is thus an understanding 'that the population from the Brazilian cities studied here show trihybrid ancestries that are distinct from Central American populations' (Ewald *et al.* 2011: 6).[13] In the above publication, such an acknowledgement becomes the broader context in which a position *against* population screening for the Ashkenazi founder mutations is made, as this would mean 'more than 90% of mutation carriers would remain unidentified' (2011: 6).[14]

We can therefore see how, in contrast to previous publications, instead of attempting to associate the presence of so-called Ashkenazi mutations with a particular national origin or specific migratory histories, such research contributes to knowing and making evident the 'mixed' ancestry of the Brazil population. This (re)framing of the meaning of Ashkenazi mutations is strongly consistent with long-standing notions of Brazil as a place of mixture, or *mesticagem,* which has been historically positively associated with Brazilian national identity. As emerging social science research in Brazil suggests, an emphasis on genetic mixture is being reconstituted through different domains of genetic research, conjoined to powerful, affective and moral alignments of national identity and nationhood (Gibbon 2013; Santos and Silva 2011; Santos and Maio 2006).

A brief overview of publications in the Brazilian context therefore illustrates the ways in which scientific and medical research associated with the Ashkenazi mutations is both simultaneously shifting away from this association while it is also being incorporated into Brazilian cancer genetics. Nevertheless, observations and interviews with health practitioners in Brazil show how this continues to generate complexities at the clinical interface and ambivalence about the meaning, significance and utility of attending to certain categories of population difference through a focus on Ashkenazi mutations.

Practitioners

While the Brazilian census categories (black, brown, white, yellow and indigenous) were sometimes filled in on the family history forms used by practitioners in consultations I witnessed, questions surrounding *etnia,* or the more common term *raca,* were not commonly raised in clinical consultations as a matter of course. When they were discussed, often little or no information was given by patients beyond stating that they were 'Brazilian'. In the southern city of Porto Alegre, discussions of family origin sometimes elicited further details, especially when it was obvious from a surname or during the consultation that a person had German, Eastern European or Italian ancestry. But there was little explicit discussion or even direct questioning of whether someone had Jewish ancestry. When I commented on this with one cancer geneticist in Porto Alegre, he explained this reticence in ways that also reflected the relevance and perhaps also moral worth of emphasizing and recognizing 'mixture':

> I think there is a bit of fear about suggesting to the patient that perhaps you have a Jewish origin. I think we're a bit different in that respect because we're so mixed here we haven't got 'oh so you're only Jewish' – it's difficult to find that in Brazil. You've got your African part and your Indigenous and European, but I think that helps too to have less prejudice.

Another scientist who worked in the field of genetic epidemiology in clinical research projects associated with the BRCA genes expressed similar sentiments about the difficulties of categorizing risk in relation to unique population groups.

> We're so mixed here I think it's difficult to find a unique influence, so we really don't worry about this. We just don't have this, the first time that I heard about the studies with specific Ashkenazi models I didn't know what it was but then saw that there are lots of studies with this population so for instance

> the "Gail" models[15] with the race component if you are African or white. But it's really difficult to do that here. When we use the model here to estimate risk, we never know what to calculate. We have in various moments opted to put all the population as white, because at least we can compare one woman with another.

There was also a sense among practitioners that patients in clinics often 'didn't know' whether they had Jewish ancestry. As one researcher working with the cancer genetics team put it: 'You could ask the patient directly – do you have Jewish ancestry? Then she'd reply, "No, no, as far as I know we don't have," but then you find out that she does'. A number of clinicians and researchers talked about the rapidly changing field of identifying BRCA mutations inside and outside of Brazil, which has raised questions about the extent to which certain mutations could still be described as exclusively associated with Ashkenazi Jewish populations. This was how one practitioner put it:

> For example, that mutation that the team here found, that we thought was associated with the Ashkenazi population from the literature, now there are lots of articles that say there were possibly two entry points for the mutation. Perhaps it was a characteristic of the Ashkenazi Jewish population but perhaps it was from another that had different mutations. So imagine if you say to a patient that it was associated with Ashkenazi ancestry and two or three years later an article is published saying no it's not – it gets complicated. So in science if it's not something certain I don't think we should be saying anything, otherwise we could cause more confusion. Of course, if they are really Ashkenazi and say they are, fine but if they're not Ashkenazi then you're going to be thinking, "Is it that they have an Ashkenazi origin or just that they don't know?" You might try to speak to them to ask them to see if they can discover something but afterwards you might find that that mutation isn't associated in that way and it gets complicated.

Another professional reflecting on the 'origin' of these mutations in Brazil also underlined, as other international publications have recently suggested, that it might not be appropriate in Brazil to describe what was identified as Ashkenazi mutations or to use a stated Ashkenazi ancestry as a criteria for testing, as has been done in other countries:

> You know those families that we have here who have Ashkenazi mutations – with rare exceptions they don't recognize themselves as Jewish . . . but perhaps these mutations are very old. I think they could be Christian converts who centuries before were Jewish, and today culturally aren't . . . so I think in Brazil we can't call them "Ashkenazi mutations" and as a result I'm a little bit reluctant to use this idea as an indication to test or not.

Practitioners' comments reveal how a variety of concerns and issues emerge when considering the utility and value of Ashkenazi BRCA mutations in Brazilian cancer genetics. This includes the economic logistics of being able to undertake genetic testing in resource-poor contexts with the complex cultural histories of race, ancestry and 'mixture' in Brazil and perhaps most importantly with the inapplicability of population categories developed elsewhere for informing the significance and meaning of finding Ashkenazi mutations in non-Ashkenazi-identified persons and families in Brazil. The following sections reflect on how two Brazilian families, neither of whom identified themselves as Jewish, responded to the information given to them by practitioners that the identified BRCA mutations were associated with this population.

Elenice and Angela

Elenice and her sister Angela attended a consultation in the mixed private/public hospital in Sao Paulo. They had travelled several hundreds of miles from the neighbouring state of Parana for a follow-up clinical appointment to receive the results of the BRCA test they had (in this case) paid to have done. Both the sisters were in their mid-to-late-40s, had each been diagnosed with cancer 10 years earlier and had many cases of breast cancer in the family.

During the consultation, they were told that an initial mutation test had positively identified a specific BRCA mutation. They were in the consultation with five of their daughters, all of whom were in their 20s or late teens, to discuss the possibility of genetic testing for them.

Before discussing the result that she'd received that morning, Elenice talked about what she thought had caused her cancer, pointing out that, although genetic factors were significant, she believed that the interaction of other factors with genetic aspects were important. For Elenice, 'external factors' such as 'smoking and stress' were, she said, 'together in this'. In other words, in her view, genetic factors were necessary but not sufficient to explain the incidence of cancer in her family.

Responding to an open question at the start of the interview about how she would describe her ethnicity or race, she immediately asked if this meant 'ancestry'.[16] This being affirmed, she went on to say 'the ancestry well what we discovered in all this process is that the genetic mutation that we have amongst us came from the Jews so we discovered that we have Jewish ancestry.'

She pointed out that she had a brother who had investigated this also and discovered Jewish ancestry on both sides of the family. When asked directly if they were Jewish, Elenice immediately said, 'No, no, we're Brazilian. I might have a [Jewish] genetic characteristic but I'm Brazilian.' Probing this response further and asking what being Brazilian meant to her she added, 'I think that being Brazilian means being Indian and I'm more on that side.' Toward the end of the interview, she described in more general terms how the information that they had received today about the test result would affect how she saw her family history or the identity of the family. She was hesitant and uncertain, pointing out that this was still 'new information', but said, 'I think there will be changes, yes . . . internal . . . personal, psychological perhaps.'

Elenice's younger sister Angela also directly responded to the initial question about ethnicity at the start of the interview with information about ancestry and cancer risk, saying

> We have a little bit of Italian with Portuguese but my oncologist was saying that there is a very rare cancer that was detected in Curitiba that was discovered in 1800 linked to the Portuguese so Elenice discovered just a while ago we have Portuguese in the family . . . we never worried about this but now we have to worry about this, go back in the family.

For Angela the information they'd received in the consultation about having a mutation associated with particular ancestry seemed in this case to have been linked to other information they had been given by a different oncologist.[17] This was even more evident when Angela pointed out how their current surname 'was one of the names the Jews used to change their name that really isn't Portuguese its Jewish'. Unlike Elenice, who saw the causes of cancer in her family as a mixture of factors, for Angela genetic aspects seemed to dominate, as she said: 'It's all in the blood [*tudo esta no sangue*] – not just disease but everything, isn't it – something that you carry forever.' At the same time, when asked what this meant in relation to the ancestry she had recently discovered in the family associated with the risk of cancer, it was clear that a notion of Brazil as a place of population mixture also informed this understanding of at-risk ancestry. As she said, talking of Brazil, 'There isn't just one ethnicity or population, there are unions [*unioes*]. I think that one union of one ethnicity with another creates this [risk] . . . because [here] the mixture is very big.'

For both these sisters, the information that they'd been given in the clinic about the BRCA mutation that had been identified in the family as being associated with Jewish ancestry was contextualized in a variety of ways with differing repercussions. While for Elenice, genetic risk factors were nested in a complex mix of other causal aspects, it was clear that there might be consequences associated with knowing this risk information in terms of 'identity' (read through an idiom of 'internal' psychological factors) for the family. Yet, like Angela, she also situated information about genetic ancestry associated with the BRCA genes in the broader context of Brazil being a place of population mixture such that it was hard to think of 'just one ethnicity', even if the explanatory weight of genetic knowledge was for her a powerful one.

Yvonete and Viviane

Yvonete was in her mid-20s and worked in a pharmacy in the city of Porto Alegre in the southernmost state of Rio Grande do Sul. She had been attending the cancer genetic service of a government-funded SUS hospital there for the last few years and had recently heard that she was (like her mother who had had breast cancer a number of years before) carrying a BRCA mutation, although she herself had not developed the disease.

Initially Yvonete mentioned nothing about the information she had been given about the mutation, which had been associated with the Ashkenazi Jewish population. This emerged more directly during a discussion about how she would describe her ethnicity. She initially described herself as being 'half German and half Italian . . . and all the Brazilian outside influence as well . . . so I'm really well mixed'. When asked if she associated ethnicity or ancestry in any way with an increased risk of developing the disease, the subsequent exchange followed:

Yvonete: I think yes . . . in fact the geneticist said something to my mum about this gene that they have been studying appearing in a Jewish community that existed . . . that all the women had it . . . all of them had cancer. So it appeared initially that it was obvious, but my German grandfather nearly fainted, you know saying that it had come from the Jews!!

SG: So you are not Jewish then?

Yvonete: No! No, well, you see my grandfather is German, so we started teasing him "you know you have Jewish ancestry" . . . but it looks like it started in that Jewish community. But really I've never stopped to think about this very much . . . well I suppose it's interesting that its with us now and we don't know how . . . or we'll never know. . . . But what we have to think about at the moment is how not to pass it on right? If there existed that possibility, that's what I would like to know now.

Yvonete's mother, Viviane, later also talked about her ancestry as a 'mixture' of 'German, with Brazilian and Portuguese' while also emphasizing her German ancestry. But when asked if she associated ancestry as a risk factor for the disease, she was more hesitant, saying:

> I've never thought about this in a direct way. I've heard people speaking about this . . . but now that I'm talking I remember that the doctor mentioned this to me that some races [*racas*] have more diseases or types of cancer. I'd never heard this before, never thought about it. I guess those who have lighter skin have more skin cancer in that sense . . . but in relation to my history it could be but I wouldn't know to say for sure.

While this response suggests that she recalled something about the association with Jewish ancestry that her daughter also remembered, Viviane does not directly mention this link. More explicitly, later on when asked directly whether the test result had affected the way she thought about her ethnicity or identity, she said emphatically and explicitly, 'No, it's got nothing to do with this.'

Thus, while both mother and daughter remembered in part some of the information they had been given – that the identified mutation was associated with Jewish Ashkenazi ancestry – this was in both cases nested in a sense of having mixed European and 'Brazilian' ancestry. While Viviane explicitly rejected the relevance of that information to the family's identity, Yvonete suggested that it initially had repercussions in the family, given the family's sense of having particular 'German' origins.[18] Yvonete, nevertheless, like many others, seemed less concerned with recent or older family or ancestral origins than with making future preventative histories for herself and her children.

Conclusion

Through a comparison of ethnographic research in the UK and Brazil, this chapter has examined how changing scientific and medical understandings regarding the origin, genealogical history and patrimony of the so-called Ashkenazi mutations have been diversely taken up and put to use in clinical/research contexts. It has explored the very differing consequences this can have for the way health care practitioners, scientists, patients and their families engage with and incorporate knowledge about hereditary BRCA mutations into scientific narratives, clinical practices and understandings of clinical/familial risk and identity.

We have shown how the recently discovered presence of Ashkenazi mutations in non-self-identified Jewish individuals from diverse geographical regions reveals the complexities and fluid boundaries of categories such as population, race and ethnicity. In particular, it reveals the complexity and incommensurability of translating scientific findings and categories originating in European/North American contexts to other diverse regions.

At the same time, genomic knowledge is temporally configured by bringing narratives of migration, ancestry and colonization into view alongside the medical, scientific and social discourse surrounding the origins of the BRCA mutations (cf. Adams *et al.* 2009; Gibbon 2013; M'Charek 2013). In this sense, BRCA founder mutations have the ability to constitute not only promissory futures but also to de/re/construct or 'abduct' genomic pasts (Adams *et al.* 2009; Palmié 2007), 'telescoping' both the past and future into the lived present (see Schlünder in this volume).

While several researchers examining the turn to ancestry and history in the wider field of genomics, particularly in relation to commercial ancestry testing, have warned about the potential in these developments to lend scientific legitimacy at the molecular level to 'unscientific' constructions of the past (El Haj 2008; Palmié 2007), others point at different dynamics, where the 'strategic' selection and use of genetic genealogy and ancestry is complexly unfolding. Nelson (2008) has shown that there is considerable variance in how individuals interpret genetic ancestry information. That is, scientific data are not always accepted as definitive proof of identity, but are rather often interpreted within the context of personal experience and the historical politics of identity.

Such variation in the significance and meaning of genetic ancestry information is particularly notable in the examples discussed in this chapter that reveal the affective and moral ramifications of the transnational reframing of Ashkenazi mutations, which move far beyond a simple telescoping of past and present. In Brazil, the disjuncture in alignments between Ashkenazi mutations and being Brazilian is evident in the hesitancy and ambivalence of the cancer genetic practitioners, as they negotiate newly emerging understandings and gaps in epidemiological knowledge associated with the BRCA genes. Here, a focus on Ashkenazi mutations facilitates transnational research and a reflection on migratory histories while it can also be used to valorize and make material 'hybrid' ancestries. At the same time, we see how knowledge of the mutations associated with Jewish populations and history is diversely incorporated within an understanding of being 'Brazilian' as being of mixed ancestry by families in the cancer genetic clinics, where newly discovered specificity and solidity of family history generates discomfort or ambivalence.

In contrast, for Ashkenazi Jews in the UK, genetic information about BRCA mutations and Jewish history are consistent with the pre-existing ways in which individuals self-identify. While such knowledge may also be nested in other understandings of risk (such as diet or environment), genetic research and medical practices reiterate narratives of shared ancestry and collective belonging as Ashkenazi Jews. On the one hand, it is plausible that, for historical reasons (such as the Holocaust), genetic research and discoveries might be met with scepticism or anxiety regarding 'biological' thinking about Ashkenazi Jews. In the UK context, however, this appears not to be the case for the majority of individuals. Knowledge about genetic mutations does not necessarily lead to ambivalence or a reconfiguration of identity, but rather allows individuals to situate genetic disease within a complex sense of self and community that includes shared history, ancestry and belonging.

As BRCA testing continues to expand and to be undertaken in diverse global arenas it will become increasingly important to monitor the extent to which we may see further reclassifications of the so-called Ashkenazi and other founder mutations and/or the way that historical narratives of colonization and migration of other populations are (or are not) used in the explanatory scientific and medical discourses associated with these new understandings. As the examples in this chapter suggest, the socio-cultural consequences of inferred Jewish origins from genetic research can be highly variable. While for some, this may be unproblematic or even culturally valued, for others such information may sit uneasily with pre-existing national or regional histories, creating an unsought and sometimes undesired solidity out of what are in fact heterogeneous and fluid identities and modes of identification. Equally, we may see a more cautious approach to categorization, or a redefinition, of categories with reference to continental ancestry or geography (Neulander 2006; Fujimura and Rajagoplan 2009) that could help constitute new spaces of identity and identification. At the same time, practical issues such as cost and available resources may continue to encourage researchers to look for founder mutations, or other population-wide risk factors, that may help ease the economic burden that incorporating genomics into health care raises for many countries.

Notes

1. The two authors carried out their fieldwork separately in the UK and Brazil. In the UK, Jessica Mozersky worked in clinical research for BRCA carriers (2002–2010) and carried out participant observation of cancer genetic appointments followed by in-depth interviews with high-risk Ashkenazi women over a 24-month period.

The ethnographic research carried out by Sahra Gibbon in Brazil was based on 18 months of research in three different cancer genetic clinics in urban centres in the southern region of Brazil. This research included participant observation in cancer genetic clinics as well as interviews with patients and their families, health practitioners and scientists working in the arena of cancer genetics.

2. The same founder mutation can arise independently in different populations and is therefore not always linked to a single common ancestor.
3. Although we do not use quotation marks for Ashkenazi for aesthetic reasons here, as this article suggests, we take this term to be contingent and fluid.
4. The third founder mutation is discussed in a later section.
5. See Mozersky (2013) for a detailed discussion of the many reasons – genetic and otherwise – why Ashkenazi Jews have become such prominent subjects of research.
6. Tay-Sachs is a severe and lethal recessive disorder that usually leads to death before the age of 5.
7. It might be suggested that Israeli newspapers have a particular socio-political interest in claiming Jewish origins for other populations. However, it is also evident that these scientific discoveries are being picked up in other national contexts as well, suggesting that this research generates interest in both scientific and popular domains.
8. For example, the Lemba are a South African tribe who claim to be descendants of one of the lost tribes of Israel. They have certain traditions, such as circumcision, dietary laws and rituals related to conversion that are similar to those of Judaism. When researchers found that some of the Lemba carried the Cohen modal haplotype (a set of genetic markers found among some Jewish men who identify as Cohens), this was considered evidence that they were likely descended from Jews in ancient Israel, as their oral history suggests (Thomas et al. 2000). Cohen refers to a biblical priestly class of Jewish men who passed priesthood down from father to son. When another group in Ethiopia who also claim to be descended from Jews in ancient Israel were tested and found not to carry the haplotype, this was taken as proof that they were not Jewish (Azoulay 2003).
9. It is worth noting that even this clinical association is contextual and not prevalent in all of Europe. For example, in France the universalist conception of citizenship does not favour focusing on ethnic issues in general or in relation to breast cancer. Thus, ethnicity and Ashkenazi Jewish origin are not significantly associated with breast cancer (Lowy and Gaudilliere 2008). In Germany, clinicians avoid discussion about disease risk and Ashkenazi or 'racial/ethnic' identity as a result of the contentious German past for Ashkenazi Jews during the Holocaust (see zur Nieden in this volume).
10. www.instituteforwomenshealth.ucl.ac.uk/academic_research/gynaecological cancer/gcrc/gcapps> (accessed 20 January, 2012).
11. However, the development of NextGeneration sequencing and cheaper panel tests may, in the future, significantly change the parameters of the situation in the context of emerging and developing economy contexts such as Brazil as well as elsewhere.
12. While other South American countries have historically been associated with colonization from Spain, the southern part of Brazil, and to a large extent Argentina and Uruguay, have been associated with more recent immigration from other parts of Europe.
13. They add here 'additionally it has been demonstrated that even Mestizos from different Central and South American regions have intra-and inter-ethnic variability and admixture profile' (Ewald et al. 2011: 6).
14. The authors also note it is a situation that they suggest is exacerbated by 'lack of coverage through both private and public health based insurance of germline mutation testing' (2011: 6), showing how such research is also linked to calls for expanded public health provision for cancer genetic services.

15. The Gail model is a statistical model for calculating the risk of breast cancer that incorporates age, reproductive history, breast biopsy history and breast cancer incidence in first-degree relatives. Other models, such as BRCAPRO, incorporate Ashkenazi Jewish heritage.
16. This question forms part of the collection of more socio-demographic data collected at the start of the interviews with those attending the cancer genetic clinics.
17. There is an association in Brazilian oncogenetics with a different mutation R337h also linked to a high incidence of cancer in the southern region of Brazil and in research publications has been associated with Portuguese ancestry (see Gibbon 2013). Angela seemed to have mixed these narratives in discussing issues related to ancestry.
18. This region of the southern part of Brazil is historically associated with German populations who themselves have a complex history in Brazil. As a group, German immigrants to Brazil at the turn of the twentieth century have a history of being culturally suppressed but are also more recently celebrated as having a distinctive history within southern Brazil. In this region, there is a popular association between having German ancestry and conferring to specific phenotypic features, such as blue eyes and a 'whiter' skin tone. This is set against a contrasting broader background of 'mixture', which is valorized as being more Brazilian.

References

Adams, V., Murphy, M. and Clarke, A. (2009) 'Anticipation: technoscience, life, affect, temporality', *Subjectivity,* 28: 246–65.

Azoulay, K. G. (2003) 'Not an innocent pursuit: The politics of a "Jewish" genetic signature', *Developing World Bioethics,* 3, 2: 119–26.

Bamshad, M., Wooding, S., Salisbury, B.A. and Stephens, J. C. (2004) 'Deconstructing the relationship between genetics and race', *Nature Review Genetics,* 5, 8: 598–609.

Birenbaum Carmeli, D. (2004) 'Prevalence of Jews as subjects in genetic research: figures, explanation, and potential implications', *American Journal of Medical Genetics,* 130A: 76–83.

Da Costa, E.C.B., Vargas, F. R., Moreira, A. S. et al. (2008) 'Founder effect of the BRCA1 5382insC mutation in Brazilian patients with hereditary breast ovary cancer syndrome', *Cancer Genetics and Cytogenetics,* 184, 1: 62–66.

Davis, D. S. (2004) 'Genetic research and communal narratives', *Hastings Center Report,* 34, 4: 40–49.

Donelle, L., Hoffman-Goetz, L. and Clarke, J. N. (2005) 'Ethnicity, genetics, and breast cancer: media portrayal of disease entities', *Ethnicity and Health,* 10, 3: 185–197.

Dufloth, R. M., Carvalho, S., Heinrich, J. K. et al. (2005) 'Analysis of BRCA1 and BRCA2 mutations in Brazilian breast cancer patients with positive family history in Sao Paulo', *Sao Paulo Medical Journal,* 123, 4: 192–197.

El-Haj, N. A. (2007) The genetic reinscription of race, *Annual Review of Anthropology,* 36, 1: 283–300.

Esteves V. F., Thuler, L. C., Amendola, L. C. et al. (2009) 'Prevalence of BRCA1 and BRCA2 gene mutations in families with medium and high risk of breast and ovarian cancer in Brazil', *Brazilian Journal of Medical and Biological Research,* 42, 5: 453–7.

Even, D. (2012) 'Israeli researchers: group of Colorado Indians have genetic Jewish roots', *Haaretz.* Accessed 13 June, 2013. www.haaretz.com/jewish-world/jewish-world-news/israeli-researchers-group-of-colorado-indians-have-genetic-jewish-roots.premium-1.433227

Ewald, I., Izetti, P., Vargas, F.R., et al. (2011) 'Prevalence of the BRCA1 founder mutation c.5266dupin Brazilian individuals at-risk for the hereditary breast and ovarian cancer', *Hereditary Cancer in Clinical Practice,* 9, 11: 1–8.

Finkler, K. (2000). *Experiencing the New Genetics: Family and Kinship on the Medical Frontier,* Philadelphia: University of Pennsylvania Press.

Fujimura, J. and Rajagoplan, R. (2011) 'Different differences: the use of "genetic ancestry" versus race in biomedical human genetic research', *Social Studies of Science,* 41, 1: 5–30.

Gibbon, S. (2007) *Breast Cancer Genes and the Gendering of Knowledge. Science and Citizenship in the Context of the 'New' Genetics,* London: Palgrave Macmillan.

———. (2013) 'Ancestry, temporality and potentiality: engaging cancer genetics in Southern Brazil', *Current Anthropology,* publication pending.

Goldstein, D.B. (2008) *Jacob's Legacy: A Genetic View of Jewish History,* New Haven: Yale University Press.

Gomes, M.C., Da Costa, M.M., Borojevic, R. et al. (2007) 'Prevalence of BRCA1 and BRCA2 mutations in breast cancer patients from Brazil', *Breast Cancer Research and Treatment,* 103, 3: 349–53.

Hallowell, N. (1999) 'Doing the right thing: genetic risk and responsibility'. In Conrad, P. and Gabe, J. (eds) *Sociological Perspectives on the New Genetics,* Oxford: Blackwell.

Hamel, N., Feng, B.J., Foretova, L.et al. (2011) 'On the origin and diffusion of BRCA1 c.5266dupC (5382insC) in European populations', *European Journal of Human Genetics,* 19, 3: 300–6.

Jews Against Cancer of the Breast (JACOB). Accessed 11 June, 2013. www.jacobintl.org/

Janavicius, R. (2010) 'Founder BRCA1/2 mutations in Europe: implications for hereditary breast-ovarian cancer prevention and control', *EPMA Journal,* 1: 397–412.

Kahn, S.M. (2005) 'Are genes Jewish? Conceptual ambiguities in the new genetic age', paper presented at Jean and Samuel Center for Judaic Studies, University of Michigan, 16 March, 2005.

Koenig, B., Lee, S., Richardson, S. and Marshall M. (eds) (2008) *Revisiting Race in a Genomic Age.* Piscataway, NJ: Rutgers University Press.

Laitman, Y., Binj-Jian, F., Zamir, I.M. et al. (2013) 'Haplotype analysis of the 185delAG BRCA1 mutation in ethnically diverse populations', *European Journal of Human Genetics.* 21: 212–16.

Lee, S.S. (2013) 'American DNA: the politics of potentiality in a genomic age', *Current Anthropology,* publication pending.

Levy-Lahad, E., Gabai-Kapara, E., Kaufman, B. et al. (2012) 'Evidence for population-based screening of BRCA1 and BRCA', *International Journal of Gynecological Cancer,* 22: S43.

Lourenco, J. J, Vargas, R.F., Bines, J. et al. (2004) 'BRCA1 mutations in Brazilian patients', *Genetics and Molecular Biology,* 27, 4: 500–4.

Lowy, I. and Gaudilliere, J.P. (2008) 'Localizing the global: testing for hereditary risks of breast cancer', *Science, Technology and Human Values,* 33: 299–325.

M'Charek, A. (2013) 'Making faces, making races', paper presented at the seminar series Globalization and Biomedical Technologies: Circulation, Appropriation and Diversion, Ecole Des Hautes Etudes en Sciences Sociales, Paris, France, 8 January.

Metcalfe, K.A., Poll, A., Royer, R. et al. (2009) 'Screening for Founder Mutations in BRCA1 and BRCA2 in Unselected Jewish Women', *Journal of Clinical Oncology*, 28: 387–91.

Mozersky, J. (2013) *Risky Genes: Genetics, Breast Cancer and Jewish Identity.* London: Routledge.

Narod, S. (2011) 'BRCA1 and BRCA2 mutations and breast cancer', *Discovery Medicine,* 12, 66: 445–53.

National Institute for Health and Clinical Excellence (NICE) (2005) 'Familial breast cancer: full guideline'. Accessed 13 January, 2012. http://guidance.nice.org.uk/CG41/Guidance/pdf/English

Nelson, A. (2008) 'Bio science: genetic genealogy testing and the pursuit of African ancestry', *Social Studies of Science,* 38, 5: 759–83.

Neuhausen, S.L., Godwin, A.K., Gershoni-Baruch, R. et al. (1998) 'Haplotype and phenotype analysis of nine recurrent BRCA2 mutations in 111 families: results of an international study', *American Journal of Human Genetics,* 62, 6: 1381–88.

Neulander, J.S. (2006) 'Folk taxonomy, prejudice and the human genome: using disease as a Jewish ethnic marker', *Patterns of Prejudice,* 40: 381–98.

Palmié, S. (2007) 'Genomics, divination, "racecraft"', *American Ethnologist,* 34, 2: 205–22.

Priest, L. (2008) 'Cancer test a genetic crystal ball for women', *The Globe and Mail,* 24 May. Accessed 22 December, 2011. www.theglobeandmail.com/life/cancer-test-a-genetic-crystal-ball-for-jewish-women/article687467/

Report of the Anglo-Israeli Workshop on the Genetic Risk of Breast Cancer (2006), unpublished report of meeting held in Israel, 22–26 April, 2006.

Risch, N., de Leon, D., Ziv, E. et al. (1995) 'Genetic analysis of idiopathic torsion dystonia in Ashkenazi Jews and their recent descent from a small founder population', *Nature Genetics,* 9, 2: 152–159.

Risch, N., Tang, H., Katzenstein, H., and Ekstein, J. (2003) 'Geographic distribution of disease mutations in the Ashkenazi Jewish population supports genetic drift over selection', *American Journal of Human Genetics,* 72, 4: 812–22.

Santos, R.V. and Maio, M.C. (2006) 'Race, genomics, identities and politics in contemporary Brazil', *Critique of Anthropology,* 24, 4: 347–78.

Santos, R.V. and Silva, G. (2011) 'Pharmacogenomics, race/ancestry and admixture: a view from Brazil', paper presented at EASA Biennial Conference, Paris, France 12 July.

Sharsheret: Your Jewish community facing breast cancer. Accessed 11 June, 2013. www.sharsheret.org/

Slatkin, M. (2004) 'A population-genetic test of founder effects and implications for Ashkenazi Jewish diseases', *American Journal of Human Genetics,* 75: 282–93.

Stone, L., Lurquin, P.F., and Cavalli-Sforza, L.L. (2007) *Genes, Culture and Human Evolution: A Synthesis,* Malden, Mass: Blackwell Publishing.

Thomas, M.G., Parfitt, T., Weiss, D.A. et al. (2000) 'Chromosomes traveling south: the Cohen modal haplotype and the origins of the Lemba – The Black Jews of Southern Africa', *American Journal of Human Genetics*, 66, 2: 674–86.

Weitzel, J.N., Lagos, V.I., Blazer, K.R. et al. (2005) 'Prevalence of BRCA mutations and founder effect in high-risk Hispanic families', *Cancer Epidemiology Biomarkers Prevention,* 14, 7: 1666–71.

———. (2013) 'Prevalence and type of BRCA mutations in Hispanics undergoing genetic cancer risk assessment in the southwestern United States: a report from the Clinical Cancer Genetics Community Research Network', *Journal of Clinical Oncology,* 31, 2: 210–16.

Wheelwright, J. (2008) 'The "Secret Jews" of San Luis Valley', *Smithsonian Magazine.* Accessed 11 June, 2013. www.smithsonianmag.com/science-nature/san-luis-valley.html

3 Genetics to the people

BRCA as public health and the dissemination of cancer risk knowledge

Galen Joseph

For some time now, social scientists and other researchers have been tracking the idea of the genetically 'at-risk' subject and related technologies, medical practices and biosocialities. While the BRCA-positive woman has become emblematic of this 'at-risk' subject, the idea of being 'at risk' for breast cancer and the forms this takes are still evolving. The institutionalization of cancer genetic medicine in the US over the past 15 years has occurred within the context of the biopolitical paradigm of 'health disparities'. In this context, public health researchers have begun to assess how the dissemination of clinical and technological advances in genetics and genomics differentially reach and impact population groups identified by race/ethnic categories and, to some extent, income, education and geographic location (rural/urban). They have also begun to assess what might be done to eliminate the resulting disparities (Armstrong *et al.* 2012, Fullerton *et al.* 2012, Hall and Olopade 2006, Ponce 2007, Shields and Crown 2012).

In this chapter, I examine how two developments – BRCA research and clinical practices, and the biopolitics of health disparities – intersect in the context of the emerging field of public health genomics. To date, public health genomics, defined as the translation of discoveries in genetics and genomics for the benefit of public health, has been most advanced in the realm of newborn screening, but efforts to expand to cancer and other adult-onset conditions are growing (see Bowen *et al.* 2012). This chapter focuses on a health promotion programme in African American churches as an exemplar of this new public health genomics that is emerging within the biopolitical paradigm of health disparities.[1]

The Family History Project (FHP) is a train-the-trainer programme designed to enable health ministry leaders in African American churches to educate members of their congregations and communities about hereditary breast cancer.[2] Health ministries are lay groups within churches 'that integrate faith and health for their members and the communities they serve' (Carter-Edwards *et al.* 2006). The immediate objective of the FHP is to identify women who are at risk of hereditary breast cancer and refer them to genetic counselling; the long-term goal is to develop an 'evidence-based' intervention which ultimately could be disseminated in churches across the country. The FHP was developed in the context of an ongoing academic-community collaboration that is part of the community outreach and education required of the comprehensive cancer centres funded by the US National Institutes of Health.[3] The project is one of several programmes within this academic-community partnership that aims to foster health ministries in African American churches explicitly as a means to reduce cancer disparities. The project team is led by a senior public health researcher who specializes in cancer disparities and health education. It also includes a genetic counsellor, two outreach programme managers, four members of the Faith Committee of the academic-community partnership (two of whom also support church health ministries in their day jobs at community benefits departments of private healthcare organizations) and myself, an anthropologist. My role as a co-investigator and project director has been to help implement the programme and the evaluation study.[4] As such, over the course of the project's initial two years, I collaborated on the development of materials used in the workshop, participated in project meetings and trainings, observed workshops led by participating churches and participated in informal conversations with workshop participants and health ministry leaders.

Here, I reflect on the FHP and its implications (beyond its specific short- and long-term goals) by locating the development of this project within the broader context of the biopolitics of health disparities and BRCA-related clinical and public health practices in the US. I argue that in the FHP workshops, despite the focus on breast cancer risk, the 'disparities paradigm' – as it echoes other forms of historical inequities experienced by African Americans – resonates more strongly than the risk of breast cancer. This health promotion project represents an effort to 'biosocialize' the participants, offering an 'at-risk' subjectivity to African American women in the context of 'health disparities'. I use the term biosocialize to emphasize the processes of forming, or attempting to create, a biosociality or biological citizenship, in this case through the intertwined narratives of breast cancer risk and disparities offered in the workshops. These narratives encourage participants to 'know your family history' in order to 'know your risk' and are followed with the familiar public health directive to do the things that can be done to reduce one's risk. The workshop thus simultaneously offers a message about both the past and future: we need to know our family's history in order to address the future risk of breast cancer in ourselves or our family, especially our children. While there has been much social science analysis of the future-oriented thinking required by users of predictive technologies such as BRCA testing, much less has been said about the temporal orientation to the past that is also required in the form of individual family history (e.g. Clark *et al.* 2010, Gibbon and Novas 2008). In addition, the disparities paradigm raises a particular 'politics of temporality' (Adams *et al.* 2009) in which *collective* conditions of health inequity in the present and medical segregation, neglect and abuse in the past are highlighted. Of course in the era of BRCA, the conceptualization of breast cancer risk increasingly reflects a focus on prevention (for example, through mastectomy and chemoprevention) and a broadening scope of risk. Several tools are now being employed that broaden the range of individuals screened for breast cancer risk. These include tools that integrate multiple biological risk assessments (such as Gail, Claus and BRCAPRO at the point of mammography screening), social categories (such as race) and behavioural factors (such as tobacco use and alcohol intake) to estimate risk.[5]

Furthermore, as in the Family History Project, there are tools that screen for eligibility for genetic counselling rather than for genetic testing (Bellcross *et al.* 2009, Joseph *et al.* 2012). In the following, I will provide background for the multifaceted nature of the current health disparities paradigm (Epstein 2007) and the unsettled place of genetics within it. Through an examination of the FHP, I illustrate how these dynamics play into the emerging field of public health genomics.

The biopolitics of health disparities and public health genomics

While inequities in the US are well documented, the relationship between *health care* inequities and *health* inequities is still being debated. Disparities are tackled simultaneously as a social issue to be addressed through social means and as a biological issue to be addressed through genomic and other biological interventions. In 1990, when the US government first established an Office of Research on Minority Health, a government infrastructure documenting disparities among population groups and facilitating their elimination began to be constructed. The NIH Revitalization Act of 1993 mandated the inclusion of minorities and women in clinical research, and the National Institutes of Health (NIH) 'blueprint' from 2000 declared the explicit goal of eliminating health disparities by the year 2010 (Epstein 2007, USDHHS 2000). This blueprint defined a population as 'a health disparity population if there is a significant disparity in the overall rate of disease incidence, prevalence, morbidity, mortality or survival rates in the population as compared to the health status of the general population'.[6] With ample statistical evidence demonstrating higher incidence, morbidity and/or mortality for a range of diseases,[7] 'minority populations' such as African Americans and Hispanics were defined as 'health disparity populations'. The Office of Research on Minority Health was promoted to a *Center* in 2000, and in 2010 to the National *Institute* of Minority Health and Health Disparities at the NIH – making it comparable to other NIH institutes, such as the National Cancer Institute and the National Human Genome Research Institute.[8]

Epstein (2007) argues that the focus on health disparities reflects a broader transformation in 'the way of thinking about medical difference in the United States' and a focus on 'embodied difference' that problematically assumes a correspondence between social identities and distinct kinds of bodies, or what he calls the 'inclusion and difference paradigm' (Epstein 2007, 2010). In this context, 'communicating and thinking in a multiracial, race positive idiom has become a norm for the field' of genomic science (Bliss 2012: 135). Genomic scientists, according to Bliss, 'assert genomics as a plausible solution to racial dilemmas' through a complex process or consciousness about race that she calls 'biosocial reflexivity' (Bliss 2011, 2012). Bliss contends that this race-positive norm results in a shift away from 'sociological approaches to understanding race' toward a genomic paradigm (Bliss 2011: 1026). Although a great deal of research has been conducted to identify social causes of disparities in health outcomes (including access to health care and racial discrimination in health care), the realm of biological or genetic difference is increasingly being funded and sought out as an explanation (Bliss 2012, Sankar *et al.* 2004). For example, in her analysis of recent developments in pharmacogenomics, Sandra Soo-Jin Lee (2009) argues that requiring 'the use of racial and ethnic categories in genetic research and increasing interest in identifying untapped racial market niches by the pharmaceutical and biotechnology industries – and weak governmental oversight of race-based therapeutics converge to create an "infrastructure of racialization"'. As a result, she warns of an 'emerging discourse that tethers racial justice to notions of racial biology' (Lee 2009: 170).

In contrast to genomics researchers, public health researchers and several clinical researchers (and their funders) have focused on the goal of extending the reach of genomic science by expanding access to genetic services, such as BRCA counselling and testing, to ensure equal access to and utilization of these new scientific and medical developments across race, income, education, literacy and language. Within the context of the health disparities paradigm, this objective is a logical outgrowth of the uneven availability and use of BRCA clinical services in the US. Although the American Society of Clinical Oncology and the National Comprehensive Cancer Network (NCCN) view genetic testing as standard care for those meeting high-risk criteria for hereditary breast cancer, there is no national mandate for insurance coverage of testing or related screening and preventive practices, and equal access remains elusive (Bruinooge 2003, NCCN 2013, Robson *et al.* 2010). Myriad Genetics held patents on the BRCA genes and charged over $3,000 for full sequencing until the Supreme Court decision from June 2013 (see van Zimmeren in this volume).[9] The patchwork health insurance system combined with the issue of who is able to access health care services and where, including genetic testing and counselling for breast cancer, reflect US norms of race and class stratification (Nelson 2011, Omi and Winant 1986, Washington 2006). As a result, people of colour are over-represented among the poor and the uninsured, and they thus disproportionately seek care in public 'safety-net' hospitals and clinics (Hasnain-Wynia *et al.* 2007, Haynes and Smedley 1999) where typically two-thirds of the patients are minorities (Regenstein and Huang 2005). The provision of BRCA counselling, testing and follow-up services in such safety-net settings is uneven, limited or non-existent. Medicaid (the federally funded health insurance for the poor) covers genetic counselling and/or testing for hereditary cancer in only 26 of the 50 states,[10] and Medicare, the federal insurance for those aged 65 and older, covers genetic testing but not genetic counselling for breast cancer. A study from 2009 showed that less than 13 per cent of all women who receive BRCA testing in the US are of non-European ancestry (Hall *et al.* 2009), while people of colour make up 35 per cent of the US population.[11]

Some public health and clinical researchers who advocate for increased access to genetic counselling and testing nevertheless make the case in partially biological terms, arguing that insufficient representation of 'disparities populations' and their BRCA variants in genetics research presents a range of clinical problems, including the inability to accurately estimate risk and a lack of knowledge about the spectrum of mutations and penetrance of breast and ovarian cancer among BRCA1/BRCA2 mutation carriers (Hall and Olopade 2006, Olopade 2004, Ponce 2007). In an editorial in *JAMA* from 2007, Huo and Olopade encouraged interventions to improve genetic testing (GT) uptake in underserved populations, 'so that genetic testing can achieve full potential as a tool for effective cancer control and prevention' (Huo and Olopade 2007). These arguments extend beyond the disparate access to genetic testing and counselling to address the content of the biological databases on which the accuracy and utility of test results depend – what Fullerton has called 'the input-output problem' (2011). The underlying argument here is that social exclusion from clinical testing and research databases (which often overlap) leads to a lack of genetic diversity in the database, which in turn makes the same BRCA test less useful for the excluded populations.

Fullerton *et al.* (2012), in examining the question of how genomics might be used to reduce health disparities, suggest that

> the best way to maximize the benefits of population-based genomic investigations, and mitigate potential harms, is to direct research away from the identification of genetic *causes* of disparities [the current focus of genomics scientists interested in reducing disparities], and instead focus on applying genomic methodologies to the development of clinical and public health *tools* with the potential to ameliorate healthcare inequities, direct population-level health interventions or inform public policy. (italics in original)

Given the multifactorial nature of many diseases, the low penetrance of many genes, gene-environment interactions and internal diversity of populations, genomic causes of disease or disparity are rarely simple and straightforward (such as x mutation explains y disparity). This is why Fullerton and co-authors suggest a focus less on research striving to identify genomic causes of disparities and more on using genomic data in conjunction with social/environmental knowledge to reduce disparities. For example, they suggest using 'algorithms that integrate both genotype and local air quality data . . . to identify families, apartment buildings, neighborhoods or cities with increased asthma risk to target for home or employment-focused air quality interventions' (2012: 159).

The Family History Project, as I describe it below, is a public health education project that draws both on discourses of disparities and emerging knowledge about the genetic causes of breast cancer. It aims to reduce disparities in the awareness of and access to genetic testing for hereditary breast cancer through a community-based approach that takes into account the social context of the women it aims to reach.

The Family History Project

The Family History Project, which relies on health ministries to implement and sustain it, follows in a long tradition of African American churches of addressing the community's health. While it is tempting to view the FHP as indicative of larger neoliberal patterns of shifting the social safety net from the state to the private sector,[12] it is equally important to consider the specific role of the church in African American life and the role of health activism in African American history (Nelson 2011) and, in this context, to note the only partial influence of neoliberalism (Hackworth 2009).

The African American church is widely understood as 'the anchoring institution in the African American community' (Pattillo 1998: 769), both historically and in contemporary America (Lincoln and Mamiya 1990). Black churches were among the organizations providing 'alternative avenues for delivering healthcare services and health education to black communities' in the era preceding medical desegregation (Nelson 2011: 25). Black churches provided free health clinics as early as the 1920s (Campbell 2007: 215). In the 1980s, the Parish Nurse movement promoted a holistic approach to health, incorporating the mind, body and spirit and encouraging the active role of nurses in the church to promote the health of congregants. This movement, with support from health care organizations[13] as well as denomination hierarchies, evolved into lay health ministries. The FHP relies on health ministries to implement and sustain it and thus follows in this tradition.

The workshops, as carried out by the trained health ministry leaders, consist of an opening prayer, a videotaped testimonial by an African American woman who is BRCA positive (a member of the Faith Committee and our team), a short educational video about hereditary cancer (Joseph *et al.* 2010) and a self-assessment of hereditary risk. In the initial two years of the project (on which this chapter is based), approximately 25 health ministry leaders from 10 churches participated in several trainings. They then held approximately 15 workshops in their churches and communities. Each workshop included 6–15 people and was open to all adults, whether or not they had had breast cancer. Participants were mostly women, ranging in age from their 20s through to their 80s. The churches represent communities in low- and middle-income neighbourhoods across three counties in the San Francisco Bay Area. In what follows, I closely examine three components of the FHP and analyse how narratives of health care disparities and breast cancer risk are knit together in the workshops.

Training: 'Know your story, know your breast cancer risk'

The training to prepare health ministry leaders to conduct the workshops in their churches and communities was framed as an opportunity to address disparities faced by African American women with regard to breast cancer. Facts were provided to define the disparity: the higher mortality for African American women with breast cancer and the higher rate of young African American women who are diagnosed. 'We have taken up the challenge to change that disparity,' the principal investigator said, comparing this effort to a prior successful effort 20 years earlier to eliminate disparities in African American women's use of mammography. The workshop was described to the health ministry leaders as offering information that has not been brought to the African American community before, despite the fact that this information and cancer genetics services have been used for 10 years by 'insured and highly educated women' – i.e. most frequently white middle-class women. The concluding message was: '*There are things you can do – life saving measures you can take* – if you have a family history or a gene mutation.'

The introduction of the training, which provides the Health Ministry (HM) leaders with a framework for carrying out the workshops, intertwines a narrative about healthcare disparities and inequities in breast cancer outcomes – the younger diagnoses and higher mortality rates – which so far remain unexplained by science but are increasingly explored as the result of specific molecular/biological differences. Despite the success in promoting screening mammography to African American women, who now use it at roughly equivalent rates compared with white women, there has been no consequent drop in mortality for African Americans with breast cancer. As a result, biological, and specifically molecular, causes of particular types of breast cancer, such as triple negative breast cancer, have been the focus of increasing investigation. Although an explicit discussion of these biological issues was avoided for the sake of time and the clarity of message, the question of how to convey the risk to African American women was complicated by the trainers' awareness of the research on the potential biological and molecular particularities of breast cancer in African American women. For example, one discussion among team members centred around how to convey the idea that, although most breast cancer occurs after 50, African American women are more likely to get it before 50, and how getting breast cancer before 50 can be a 'red flag' for hereditary cancer. Confusion among participants about what age group was most likely to get breast cancer was evident in the post-training evaluation questionnaire. As social scientists and/or public health researchers, we are influenced by some of the same conditions shaping the genomics scientists' 'reflexive biosociality' (Bliss 2012). We address the social injustice of health inequities with tools of health education, but we also draw on 'facts' about potential biological or molecular difference from medical science. Thus, the disparities conveyed in the training reflected the multifaceted state of the disparities paradigm, with a primary focus on health *care* disparities, but also with reference to potential biological causes of disparate breast cancer outcomes.

On another register, the training presented a dual message of empowerment ('knowledge is power') and responsibility – 'there are things you can do to protect yourself' and to 'change that disparity' – which is familiar in this era of biomedicalization (Clark *et al.* 2010). The solutions offered were not social or collective action (despite the group educational context), but rather individual responsibility to 'know your family history' and thus 'know your risk' – and also 'to use that knowledge to monitor your risk with genetic counselling and/or testing'. This future-oriented message is paradoxically accompanied by the message that, in order to address risk for breast cancer in the future, in ourselves or our children – we need to know our family's history, we need to know our past. This message was developed to reflect prior research as well as team members' experience that cancer was not discussed in many African American families. To make the message culturally appropriate, it was considered important to first clearly acknowledge that typically there is a lack of family communication about cancer, and then to directly challenge that norm by making the case that it could save lives, that 'talking is love'.

Marion's testimonial

To reinforce the message about knowing one's family history, the workshop presents a testimonial by a BRCA-positive breast cancer survivor named Marion. In the five-minute video, Marion talks about being initially diagnosed and successfully treated at age 31, and diagnosed and treated again at age 41. Only years later did she discover that she was BRCA-positive. Her story begins with her diagnoses and her doctor's disrespect and dismissal of her initial concerns when she found a lump in her breast. As she describes it, her doctor essentially told her not to worry about the lump because she was too young to have breast cancer. After a year, he finally agreed to do a biopsy so she would stop 'bothering' him. She emphasizes that she was not taken seriously and that it was only through her persistence and her knowledge as a nurse that she was eventually diagnosed and treated.

She also reveals that she did not learn her family's history until years after her diagnoses, when she discovered that three of her paternal aunts had all had breast cancer before they turned 40. At that point, she went to her gynaecologist and then her oncologist in pursuit of the BRCA test. She said:

> At the time of my diagnosis, neither the doctor nor 'science' knew the importance of family history. But now, there is new information out there for African American women. I do have the breast cancer gene. And this is important because I have two sons and a granddaughter. Knowing my family history is vital. I want my sons to be tested – they need to test – for my granddaughter.

Marion's narrative touches on a number of issues: the need to persistently advocate for oneself, the hope a new technology offers for future generations, and her own empowerment (in the course of learning how to negotiate her care in the health care system and learning about her family history). In the discussions in the workshops following her testimonial, participants tended to focus on Marion's difficulty getting appropriate care and treatment rather than on the hereditary nature of her cancer and her belated discovery of her family's cancer history. Furthermore, the participants' reactions to her story of delayed diagnosis and treatment suggest that at least some of them have heard a familiar story of discrimination and racism. For example, in one workshop, after watching Marion's testimonial, a participant told the group a story about her own difficulty getting her doctor to be responsive to her requests. After 'asking around' about the doctor, she told us, she found out he was a 'skinhead'. In another workshop, the video led to a discussion about how to get what one needs despite discrimination in the medical system. After that, the discussion returned to the need to advocate for oneself, to take responsibility for one's own care, because doctors and others in the medical system cannot be relied on to have patients' best interests at heart. Such experiential testimonies from participants are disturbing but not surprising, as they coincide with historical and contemporary documentation of racism and discrimination in US health care. Critically, they suggest a lay understanding of disparities as a social structural issue that overlies and masks biology or individual behaviour.

Self-assessment: the family history score

The next parts of the workshop, which include a video about hereditary cancer (discussed elsewhere, see Joseph *et al.* 2010, Mozersky and Joseph 2010) and a risk-assessment questionnaire, are meant to clarify who is 'at risk' and therefore who should see a genetic counsellor. While several assessment tools have existed for many years to predict the likelihood of a BRCA mutation and thus appropriateness for genetic testing (for example, BRCAPRO, Myriad II, BOADICEA, PENN II) – referral for genetic counselling is another matter when involving screening the general population (Antoniou *et al.* 2004, Bellcross *et al.* 2009, Evans *et al.* 2004, Lindor *et al.* 2010). Determining the appropriateness of genetic testing requires a complete pedigree, including enumeration of family members who have and have not had cancer, types of cancer and age at diagnosis. Identification of those whose level of risk is such that they should be referred for counselling to obtain an in-depth family history has received far less attention.

The Family History Score Sheet is an 11-question questionnaire that assigns points for a personal and family history of breast and ovarian cancer in an algorithm intended to identify those with a high enough risk to warrant genetic counselling.[14] It was adapted and simplified from another validated screening tool designed to be administered by telephone operators at a California State referral service for free mammograms and pap tests in the context of a study intended to identify low-income women at high risk of hereditary breast cancer (Joseph *et al.* 2012).

The shift from screening for likelihood of a BRCA mutation to screening for an appropriate referral for genetic counselling reflects an attempt to broaden the scope (to any woman) and context (beyond the clinic) in which women are screened for hereditary breast cancer risk. It also reflects the tools needed for the translation of the technology for the benefit of public health. In the context of the FHP workshops, the disciplining practice of self-assessment for the risk of hereditary cancer relies on a knowledge of one's family history as well as a level of health literacy – including knowledge of biology and cancer – that is not always available. Low health literacy affects 36 per cent of all Americans and is disproportionately found among those who have less education and are living in poverty and/or are of ethnic/racial minority background (Kutner *et al.* 2006, Nielsen-Bohlman *et al.* 2004). For example, the common confusion between ovarian and cervical cancer is difficult to clarify with such a questionnaire. Nevertheless, when using this questionnaire as a self-assessment tool, approximately one-fifth of the 100 participants in the workshops scored high enough for a referral to genetic counselling. As part of the study, a genetic counsellor was tasked with calling participants identified as 'high risk' who provided a phone number, indicating their willingness to be contacted. (Several who had a high score did not provide a phone number.) In this study and in other research aiming to identify 'high risk' women who are outside the clinical setting or who do not already have cancer (Joseph *et al.* 2012), we have found that responsibility or empowerment only goes so far. Participation in the workshop and the potential 'at-risk' status, identified through the family history screener, does not motivate most women to call a genetic counsellor on their own. That is, this screener does not appear to produce a subject with a sense of embodied risk.

Among those called and reached by the genetic counsellor, only two were considered high enough at risk to be offered a BRCA test.[15] One chose to go to another medical facility, and the other declined the test, indicating concerns about health insurance discrimination. She had been under the impression that the testing, as well as the counselling, would be free and therefore not be in her medical record, and when she found out that she would have to use her insurance for the $3000 test (required for participants who have insurance that covers testing), she declined. The Genetic Information Nondiscrimination Act of 2008 (GINA), a federal law that protects people from genetic discrimination in health insurance and employment, and the broader legal protections in the state of California provided no comfort.[16] Although it is quite possible that there were other, perhaps more significant, reasons for declining to test, it was rather striking that being at risk of discrimination seemed to weigh more heavily than being at risk of breast cancer. The disparities argument, which favours receiving genetic counselling, is one about overcoming discrimination in access to care and overcoming a perhaps greater risk posed by molecular subtypes of breast cancer believed to be more common in African American women. Yet, the concern about discrimination re-emerged here in the face of the opportunity to test.

Conclusion

Karen-Sue Taussig has argued that the production of biosocial citizens is occurring in the context of a 'major historical transformation in which developments in the life sciences play a significant role' (2007: 192). Genomics is a critical arena of this transformation, and it is unfolding in different ways across the globe. One of the specificities of its development in the US is the biopolitical context of health disparities. The intersection between genomics and the biopolitics of health disparities has led to biosocialization processes such as the Family History Project as well as other public health or health promotion projects that attempt to educate people about particular genetic risks, such as hereditary breast cancer, and to identify 'at risk' individuals while also addressing inequities in health (Taussig 2007).

The Family History Project offers an opportunity to explore the intersection between, and articulation of, the biopolitics of health disparities and breast cancer risk related to BRCA in this era of expanding public health genomics. I have suggested that, for the women participating in these workshops, the disparities biopolitical paradigm resonates more strongly than the particular risk of breast cancer. The biosocialization process in which participants are offered an 'at-risk' subjectivity in the context of 'health disparities' is multi-layered and temporally complex. The workshop offers messages of both empowerment and responsibility, invoking possible futures and calling on us to know our family's past: we need to know our family's history in order to responsibly address the future risk of breast cancer for ourselves or our children. However, for the women in the workshops, the past is more than an individual's family history of cancer. In framing the risk of hereditary breast cancer in terms of disparities, the workshop raises the spectre of a long history – as well as a present and possible future – of discrimination in health care and beyond. The resonance of this larger social context was clear in the discussions following Marion's testimonial in which the issue of Marion's BRCA status and family history were virtually ignored. Instead, the testimonies offered by participants in response were about their own experiences of deeply embodied discrimination in the health care system, and the need to advocate for oneself and to learn to navigate the system effectively. Adams and colleagues have argued that 'anticipation has become a common lived affect-state of daily life, shaping regimes of self, health and spirituality' (Adams *et al.* 2009: 247). Yet, that is not clearly the case for the women in these workshops. Chanita Halbert's recent finding that low rates of BRCA counselling and testing among African American women may be due to their 'preferences and values' rather than disparities also suggests that the future-oriented, anticipatory 'habitus' is neither universal, nor is it equally valued or prioritized (Halbert 2012: 781).

Indeed, for those who lack 'cultural health capital', this lack of anticipatory habitus may contribute to disparities (Shim 2010). Shim argues that 'in the current US health care system – with its emphasis on consumerism, patient initiative, self-knowledge, self-surveillance, and self-management, particular characteristics [and skills] tend to be rewarded in clinical interactions' and their absence contributes to 'the social production of unequal treatment' (2010: 2–3). Among the characteristics of cultural health capital are 'an enterprising disposition and a proactive stance toward health, both of which presuppose a sense of mastery and self-efficacy' as well as a 'belief in the value of, and the resources to practice, self discipline' and a knowledge of medical topics (Shim 2010: 3). It also includes an orientation toward the future. Over time, the embodiment of such characteristics becomes one's 'habitus' in Bourdieu's terms. Cultural capital, and likewise cultural health capital, is 'deeply relational' (Shim 2010: 5), reflecting hierarchy and power. In essence, in the discussions following Marion's testimonial video, participants recognized their own lack of cultural health capital and provided each other with support and encouragement to counter that lack. Thus, the biosocialization processes in these workshops occur not only between the trainers and participants, but also among the participants. Despite the trainers' focus on breast cancer risk in their intertwined narratives of breast cancer risk and disparities, the participants seemed to focus on and take up the disparities paradigm. As it echoes other forms of historical inequities experienced by African Americans, the risks posed by disparities appear to resonate more strongly than the risk of a particular disease, even breast cancer.

Notes

1. A recent study suggests a higher prevalence than previously thought of deleterious mutations in BRCA and other breast cancer susceptibility genes (CHEK2, PALB2, ATM, PTEN) using the BROCA next generation sequencing panel test (Churpek *et al.* 2013).
2. This project is funded by a grant from Susan G. Komen for the Cure. I would like to thank the principal investigator of the Family History Project, and the rest of the team of researchers and community partners who have made it possible. I also acknowledge with great appreciation the comments of my co-editors on earlier drafts whose thoughtful suggestions helped me to hone my argument.
3. According to the National Cancer Institute's website:

   > An NCI-designated comprehensive cancer center must demonstrate reasonable depth and breadth of research in each of three major areas: laboratory, clinical, and population-based research, as well as substantial transdisciplinary research that bridges these scientific areas. In addition, a comprehensive center must also demonstrate professional and public education and outreach capabilities, including the dissemination of clinical and public health advances in the communities it serves.
   >
   > (www.cancer.gov/researchandfunding/extramural/cancercenters/about)

4. I was simultaneously a co-investigator for another study funded by the National Center for Minority Health and Health Disparities to evaluate the overall Abundant Life initiative. The description of the FHP here represents the first iteration of a workshop programme that remains under development in an attempt to refine its messages and feasibility, thus achieving effectiveness in identifying at-risk women and referring them to genetic counselling. Over the next year, as part of these efforts, we will conduct interviews with workshop participants and leaders.
5. For example, see http://athenacarenetwork.org/.
6. Minority Health and Health Disparities Research and Education Act United States Public Law 106–525, 2000, p. 2498, National Cancer Institute Center to Reduce Cancer Health Disparities (http://crchd.cancer.gov/disparities/defined.html, accessed 21 July, 2010).
7. For example, while the overall breast cancer incidence rate is lower for African American women than white women, the mortality rate is significantly higher. For women under the age of 40, the incidence rate is higher for African American women than all other ethnic/racial groups in the US. www.cdc.gov/cancer/breast/statistics/race.htm (accessed 16 July 2013)
8. NCMHD was re-designated the National Institute on Minority Health and Health Disparities (NIMHD) with the passing of the Patient Protection and Affordable Care Act of 2010 (President Obama's health care reform).
9. While Myriad offers a 'hardship programme' for the uninsured, the ability to access those funds varies.
10. The advocacy organization FORCE: Facing Our Risk Empowered has the most up-to-date list of state Medicaid programmes that cover BRCA testing (www.facingourrisk.org/info_research/finding-health-care/financial-help/index.php).
11. This article reports on testing via Myriad Genetics, which, up until June 2013, was the only lab in the US legally able to test the BRCA genes. Some additional BRCA testing is carried out through research that includes or focuses on minority populations (see, for example, Weitzel *et al.* 2013).
12. Faith-based initiatives became an important space for this shift in the early 1990s when President George H. W. Bush pushed for volunteerism as an alternative to government support for social services with his 'thousand points of light' campaign.

This was continued under President Clinton's Welfare Reform policy and President George W. Bush's Faith Based Initiative.

13. For example, UCSF and the organizations where Faith Committee members work are all private, not-for-profit medical centres with community benefits programmes.
14. A validation study of the screen tool is currently underway.
15. The participants in the workshop were, for the most part, not women with very strong family histories of breast and ovarian cancer, so the message of risk was less relevant to them personally. Even those whose risk score was high did not initiate calls to the genetic counsellor, and some were not responsive when the counsellor called.
16. California Genetic Information Nondiscrimination Act (CalGINA), which took effect on January 1, 2012: 'CalGINA amends anti-discrimination laws already in effect to prohibit genetic discrimination in areas, such as housing; mortgage lending; employment; education; and public accommodations' (www.duanemorris.com/alerts/california_law_prohibits_genetic_discrimination_can_result_significant_damages_if_violated_4222.html).

References

American Society of Clinical Oncology (ASCO) guidelines 2003, 2010.

Antoniou, A. C., Pharoah, P. P., Smith, P. and Easton, D. F. (2004) 'The BOADICEA model of genetic susceptibility to breast and ovarian cancer', *British Journal of Cancer,* 91: 1580–90.

Armstrong, K., Putt, M., Halbert, C. H. et al. (2012) 'The influence of health care policies and health care system distrust on willingness to undergo genetic testing', *Medical Care,* 50, 5: 381–87.

Barnes, S. L. (2005) 'Black church culture and community action', *Social Forces,* 84: 967–94.

Bellcross, C. A, Lemke, A. A., Pape, L. S., Tess, A. L. and Meisner, L. T. (2009) 'Evaluation of a breast/ovarian cancer genetics referral screening tool in a mammography population', *Genetics in Medicine,* 11: 783–89.

Bliss, C. (2011) 'Racial taxonomy in genomics', *Social Science and Medicine,* 73, 7: 1019–27.

———. (2012) *Race Decoded: The Genomic Fight for Social Justice,* Stanford: Stanford University Press.

Bowen, M. S., Kolor, K., Dotson, W. D., Ned, R. M. and Khoury, M. J. (2012) 'Public health action in genomics is now needed beyond newborn screening', *Public Health Genomics,* 15: 327–34.

Bruinooge, S. S. (2003). 'American Society of Clinical Oncology policy statement update: genetic testing for cancer susceptibility', *Journal of Clinical Oncology,* 21, 12: 2397–2406.

Campbell, M. K. Hudson, M. A., Resnicow, K., Blakeney, N., Paxton A. and Baskin, M. (2007) 'Church-based health promotion interventions: evidence and lessons learned', *Annual Review of Public Health,* 28, 1: 213–34.

Carter-Edwards, L. Jallah, Y. B., Goldmon, M. V., Roberson J. T. Jr. and Hoyo, C. (2006) 'Key attributes of health ministries in African American churches: an exploratory survey', *North Carolina Medical Journal,* 67: 345–50.

Deleuze, G. and Guattari, F. (1987) *A Thousand Plateaus. Capitalism and Schizophrenia*, Minneapolis: University of Minnesota Press.

Epstein, S. (2007) *Inclusion: The Politics of Difference in Medical Research.* Chicago: University of Chicago Press.

———. (2010) 'Beyond inclusion, beyond difference: the biopolitics of health'. In I. Whitmarsh and D.S. Jones (eds) *What's the Use of Race: Modern Governance and the Biology of Difference.* Cambridge, MA: MIT Press.

Evans, D. G, Eccles, D.M., Rahman, N. et al. (2004) 'A new scoring system for the chances of identifying a BRCA1/2 mutation outperforms existing models including BRCAPRO', *Journal of Medical Genetics,* 41: 474–80.

Fullerton, S.M. (2011) 'The input-output problem: whose DNA do we study, and why does it matter?' In W. Burke and S. Goering (eds) *Achieving Justice in Genomic Translation: Re-Thinking the Pathway to Benefit.* Oxford: Oxford University Press.

Fullerton, S.M., Knerr, S. and Burke, W. (2012) 'Finding a place for genomics in health disparities research', *Public Health Genomics,* 15, 3–4: 156–63.

Gibbon, S. and Novas, C. (2008) *Biosocialities, Genetics and the Social Sciences: Making Biologies and Identities.* London: Routledge.

Hackworth, J. (2009) 'Neoliberalism, partiality, and the politics of faith-based welfare in the United States', *Studies in Political Economy,* 84: 155–80.

Halbert, C.H., Kessler, L., Collier, A. et al. (2012). 'Low rates of African American participation in genetic counseling and testing for BRCA1/2 mutations: racial disparities or just a difference? *Journal of Genetic Counseling,* 21, 5: 676–83.

Hall, M.J. and Olopade, O.I. (2006) 'Disparities in genetic testing: thinking outside the BRCA box', *Journal of Clinical Oncology: Official Journal of the American Society of Clinical Oncology,* 24, 14: 2197–2203.

Hall, M.J. Reid, J.E., Burbidge, L.A. et al. (2009) 'BRCA1 and BRCA2 mutations in women of different ethnicities undergoing testing for hereditary breast-ovarian cancer', *Cancer,* 115, 10: 2222–33.

Hasnain-Wynia, R., Baker, D.W., Nerenz, D. et al. (2007) 'Disparities in health care are driven by where minority patients seek care: examination of the hospital quality alliance measures', *Archives of Internal Medicine,* 167, 12: 1233–39.

Haynes, M.A. and Smedley, B.D. (eds) (1999) *The Unequal Burden of Cancer: An Assessment of NIH Research and Programs for Ethnic Minorities and the Medically Underserved.* Washington, D.C.: National Academy Press.

Huo, D. and Olopade, O.I. (2007) 'Genetic testing in diverse populations: are researchers doing enough to get out the correct message?' *JAMA: The Journal of the American Medical Association,* 298: 2910–11.

Joseph, G., Beattie, M.S., Lee, R. et al. (2010) 'Pre-counseling education for low literacy women at risk of hereditary breast and ovarian cancer (HBOC): patient experiences using the Cancer Risk Education Intervention Tool (CREdIT)', *Journal of Genetic Counseling,* 19, 5: 447–62.

Joseph, G., Kaplan, C., Luce, J. et al. (2012) 'Efficient identification and referral of low-income women at high risk for hereditary breast cancer: a practice-based approach', *Public Health Genomics,* 15: 172–80.

Kutner, M., Greenberg, E., Jin, Y. and Paulsen, C. (2006) 'The health literacy of America's adults: results from the 2003 National Assessment of Adult Literacy', Washington: National Center for Education Statistics. Accessed 16 July, 2013. http://nces.ed.gov/pubs2006/2006483_1.pdf

Lee, S.S. (2009) 'Pharmacogenomics and the challenge of health disparities', *Public Health Genomics,* 12, 3: 170–9.

Lincoln, C.E. and Mamiya, L.H. (1990) *The Black Church in the African American Experience*. Durham, NC: Duke University Press.

Lindor, N.M., Johnson, K.J., Harvey, H. et al. (2010) 'Predicting BRCA1 and BRCA2 gene mutation carriers: comparison of PENN II model to previous study', *Familial Cancer,* 9: 495–502.

Mozersky, J. and Joseph, G. (2010) 'Case studies in the co-production of populations and genetics: the making of 'at risk' populations in BRCA genetics', *BioSocieties,* 5, 4: 415–39.

Murphy, M. (2011) 'Distributed Reproduction'. In M. Casper and P. Currah (eds): *Corpus. An Interdisciplinary Reader on Bodies and Knowledge*. New York: Palgrave Macmillan.

NCCN Clinical Practice Guidelines in Oncology (NCCN Guidelines) (2013) *Genetic/Familial High Risk Assessment: Breast and Ovarian,* Version 2. Accessed 16 July, 2013. www.nccn.org

Nelson, A. (2011) *Body and Soul: The Black Panther Party and the Fight against Medical Discrimination.* Minneapolis: University of Minnesota Press.

Nielsen-Bohlman, L., Panzer, A.M. and Kindig, D.A. (eds) (2004) *Health Literacy: A Prescription to End Confusion.* Washington, DC: National Academies Press.

Olopade, O.I. (2004) 'Genetics in clinical cancer care: a promise unfulfilled among minority populations', *Cancer Epidemiology, Biomarkers and Prevention,* 13, 11:1683–6.

Omi, M. and Winant, H. (1986) *Racial Formation in the United States: From the 1960s to the 1980s.* New York: Routledge.

Parthasarathy, S. (2007) *Building Genetic Medicine: Breast Cancer, Technology and the Comparative Politics of Health Care.* Cambridge: MIT Press.

Pattillo, M.E. (1998). 'Sweet mothers and gangbangers: managing crime in a black middle-class neighborhood', *Social Forces,* 76, 3: 747–74.

Ponce, N.A., Afable-Munsuz, A. and Nordyke, R.J. (2007) 'Conceptualising the impact of genetic testing on cancer disparities in the USA', *International Journal of Healthcare Technology and Management,* 8, 5: 536–48.

Ponce, N.A., Tsui, J., Knight, S.J. et al. (2012) 'Disparities in cancer screening in individuals with a family history of breast or colorectal cancer', *Cancer,* 118, 6: 1656–63.

Regenstein, M. and Huang, J. (2005) 'Stresses to the safety net: The public hospital perspective', *Kaiser Commission on Medicaid and the Uninsured.* Washington, DC: Henry J. Kaiser Family Foundation.

Robson, M.E., Storm, C.D., Weitzel, J., Wollins, D.S. and Offit, K. (2010). 'American Society of Clinical Oncology policy statement update: genetic and genomic testing for cancer susceptibility', *Journal of Clinical Oncology,* 28, 5: 893–901.

Sankar, P., Cho, M.K., Condit, C.M. et al. (2004). 'Genetic research and health disparities', *JAMA: The Journal of the American Medical Association,* 291, 24: 2985–9.

Shields, A.E. and Crown, W.H. (2012) 'Looking to the future: incorporating genomic information into disparities research to reduce measurement error and selection bias', *Health Services Research,* 47, 3pt2: 1387–1410.

Shim, J.K. (2010) 'Cultural health capital', *Journal of Health and Social Behavior,* 51, 1: 1–15.

Taussig, K.S. (2007) 'Genetics and its publics: crafting genetic literacy and identify in the early twenty-first century'. In Burri, R.V. and Dumit, J. (eds) *Biomedicine as Culture: Instrumental Practices, Technoscientific Knowledge and New Modes of Life.* New York: Routledge.

U.S. Department of Health and Human Services (USDHHS) (2000) *Healthy People 2010*. 2nd ed., 2 vols., Washington, DC: U.S. Government Printing Office.

Washington, H. A. (2007) *Medical Apartheid: The Dark History of the Medical Experimentation on Black Americans from Colonial Times to the Present*. New York: Doubleday.

Weitzel, J. N., Clague, J., Martir-Negron, A. et al. (2013) 'Prevalence and type of BRCA mutations in Hispanics undergoing genetic cancer risk assessment in the southwestern United States: a report from the Clinical Cancer Genetics Community Research Network', *Journal of Clinical Oncology*, 31, 2: 210–16.

Middleword I

Historicizing biomedicine: toward a history of the present of BRCA

Martina Schlünder

In his seminal book *Discipline and Punish,* Michel Foucault (1975) explores the genealogies of the modern penal system. Focusing mainly on the eighteenth century, Foucault surprises readers with his intention to write the history of the present. Foucault surely was not interested in a Whig historiography in the sense that he understood the past as an inevitable pre-history of and progression to the present. He rather aimed to highlight the temporal complexities of historiography, which is always situated in and imbued with the present. Foucault understood the past as a space filled with historical fragments, which sometimes might help us to explain the present but even more to grasp its arbitrariness. Relying on Foucault's idea of the history of the present, I would like to explore what it means to historicize the 'time of BRCA'. In my contribution I look at the intersecting parts, at the topics, themes and figures which relate and connect the chapters and book sections in order to understand more about the broader picture of BRCA: how does BRCA fit into the history of biomedicine?

Biomedicine, more specifically the *term* 'biomedicine' has a confusing trajectory. In contrast to 'technoscience' it was coined by historical actors in the field of medicine and science, not by social scientists or historians. It emerged in the aftermath of World War I – for instance in Ludwik Hirszfeld's study of serological differences of blood groups – but gained momentum only after World War II, when the US-Atomic Energy Commission (AEC) established biomedical units or laboratories (Keating and Cambrosio 2003: 50–57). Biomedicine as a practice is entangled with the history of the Manhattan Project (the code name for the development of the first nuclear bomb) and the emergence of the Cold War and the nuclear age (Lenoir and Hays 2000). In this historical context, new structures of labor division and organization emerged: tightly managed research programs were established based on team work, defined goals and strict deadlines; close collaborations between several centres had to be managed over long distances; and infrastructures with inbuilt rules for communication, data management, standardization and regulation had to be created. Biomedicine then, is as much a product of new administrative techniques and political constellations as it is an effect of the molecularization and geneticization of medicine, or what historians of science often call the dominance of the lab and scientific knowledge over clinical practices and reasoning. It is rather the realignment of traditional relations between disciplines, professions, clinical practice, research, and its application. With the emergence of biomedicine, new spaces came into being, in disciplines, between disciplines, and in and between research institutions. Their affective economies of fear were dominated by the politics of first strike prevention, control, and the calculation of risks and survivor rates. Cancer, especially leukemia, played a major role as a research focus since the hematopoietic system is the first target of nuclear radiation. The analogies of the metaphors of Cold War and the war against cancer are telling and not at all coincidental.

Here is not the space to expand further details but it is important to introduce the history of biomedicine for two reasons:

1. In the course of the 1970s and 80s, the term 'biomedicine' migrated into the social sciences. On this trajectory it completely lost its historical context. Medical anthropologists usually refer to biomedicine as a synonym for western medicine per se without historicizing it. For a medical anthropologist like Arthur Kleinman, one could practice biomedicine already in the time of Descartes or the eighteenth century (Kleinman 1993), whereas historians of science and medicine continue to talk about biomedicine as something relatively new in the framework of western medicine. For historians of science, on the other hand, it seems difficult to think of medicine in other terms as western medicine. These different understandings often create confusions in the communication between the disciplines (Bruchhausen 2011).
2. In contrast to medical sociology and its analytical concept of biomedicalization (Clarke *et al.* 2010), history of science and medicine have not developed historical tools to explore the specificity of biomedicine (Löwy 2011). They either use the term very broadly for periodization – characterizing medical developments after World War II – or they narrow it too much for the description of laboratory innovations.

In order to understand more about the configuration of biomedical practices, their internal algorithms, and their particular history, I suggest looking at them as very specific spatiotemporal arrangements.[1] Historically, they are marked by their emergence as interstices, and it is important to notice here that they usually did not develop in neatly marked-off, well-defined disciplinary interstices but partly sprang up in the traditional academic disciplines themselves. They clustered around instruments or research topics, but at the same time practitioners still remained part of and interacted with the classical structure of academic research institutions, their internal distribution of power and their genealogical practices, and especially their hiring strategy regarding the kind of knowledge that has to be sustained (by teaching graduate students, etc.). The labor division and organization and the hierarchies and workflow in these interspaces,[2] however, were structured by other temporal economies and legacies. Here new spaces and temporal economies opened up to invest in different kinds of relations, intensifying and accelerating them.

Biomedical practices are not so much interested in the development of individual instruments or technologies but rather in techniques of connecting and separating, in splitting and splicing and the potential to change things, entities, and elements by including, gluing, fitting them in or clipping and cutting them out of their 'original' space, their 'habitat'. As we learn from this book, in-vitro fertilization (IVF), for instance, can easily change its place: by being put in the BRCA domain, IVF becomes anything but an infertility treatment (see Rubin, this volume). It is instead recommended to BRCA positive couples as a means to test the embryo's genetic status and prevent the birth of an affected child. Less than a thing in itself or an institution, biomedicine is a specific mode of doing things, of splitting and splicing, of ordering and arranging them.[3] More important than to state that we live in a relational and entangled world is to know and explore the 'politics of how and when': how and at what time things, instruments, and people are connected, disconnected, and realigned, and how this rearrangement changes the links in the chain. How, for instance, do we understand the practical connections and reconnections between patients, hospitals and labs particularly as they are shaped by a shifting emphasis on genes and their materialities? When is it no longer understood as a single spot where mutation takes place but rather a highly dynamic process of pathways and signals? It does not only affect the clinical practice but all links of the chain are moved around. What happens as a result to genetic counseling in India, in Brazil, elsewhere? I do not intend to emphasize here that all innovations always emerge from the laboratory. I rather suggest that we focus our analyses on the making of relations and connections and the kinds of things, entities, and subjectivities that are produced by linking them. In a complex structure it makes little sense to look only after causal explanations for change. We must be aware that modifications in the chain can induce multiple and often contradictory effects at the same time. How does a technology like the Internet reconfigure the place and the reality of patients? Boundaries are blurred and patients remain patients, but simultaneously they are consumers and active research participants. What does that offer to them: more freedom or more exploitation, or maybe both? Understanding biomedical practices as a socio-technical arrangement (l'agencement) inspires us to think about relations and connections in different ways and helps to question the traditional research practice of separating nature and culture, the economy, the state, society, and academia in neatly clear cut, rigid blocks that does not allow for analyzing their dynamic distribution and the ways connections are built and made among them. It facilitates conceiving of these blocks as dispersed phenomena throughout biomedical practices.[4] That does not mean that it is impossible to analyze or historicize them. The whole layout of biomedicine changed considerably between the nuclear age and the post-Cold War era of neoliberalism and globalization.

The book offers a set of different approaches to the complex arrangement of biomedicine by exploring configurations of breast cancer genetics. The contributions follow patients, possible future patients, clinical practitioners, researchers, scientists, pharmaceutical companies, and DTC (direct-to-consumer) personal genetic testing companies through multiple BRCA networks highlighting gender perspectives, genealogical practices and their entanglements with biomedicine, risk calculation, identity politics, and the colonial and fascistic pasts of non-western and western countries in a transnational and comparative framework. Even if each chapter gives preference to specific entries and actors in the field, they have to be understood as a multiple access into one complex formation. In what follows, I assemble and draw the contributions of all sections together in order to explore their common topics, subplots, and tropes.

Historicizing health and disease

The most important epistemic change from medicine to biomedicine is the reconfiguration of the relation between the normal and the pathological with an increasing emphasis on health instead of disease (Clarke *et al.* 2010; Keating and Cambrosio 2003). Prioritizing health produces its own paradoxes. The risk, the possibility of becoming sick spreads and produces similar effects *as if* something (a pathological event) has already happened. The reactions to a positive test for a BRCA mutation range from understanding BRCA already as a 'near cancer experience' (Pelters, this volume) to 'look[ing] at somebody with BRCA as healthy' (Rubin, this volume). There is, however, a growing will to intervene in bodies without symptoms, bodies that are still healthy and 'normal' but under a specific statistical threat of becoming sick. The most feared effects and side effects of radical cancer treatments are forestalled and brought forward in preventive mastectomies or oophorectomies. In the culture of 'as if', the boundaries between health and disease are increasingly blurred. Instead of expanding the territories of health, a pathological maelstrom seems to flood and shrink it, reducing our understanding of health to the absence of genetic risks (see Rubin, this volume).

In his groundbreaking book *Genesis and Development of a Scientific Fact* (1935/1979), Ludwik Fleck ponders over the idea that diseases might not exist – only sick people each of them ill in their own ways. Diseases, he suggests, could be seen as historical abstractions, very important ones and essential for medicine to intervene on. Diseases thus can be understood as historical attempts to subsume, to pool, and to order bodily phenomena and not getting shipwrecked in the sea of individual biological variation and difference. These abstractions can only be understood as historically and socially grounded, thus open to permanent transformation as much as living beings. If we understand biomedicine as a 'l'agencement', a historically situated socio-technical arrangement and a dispersed phenomenon, then all parties involved are affected by this movement of permanent changes. Diseases are no exceptions and change as much as our bodies and environments; meanwhile for doctors and scientists, breast cancer has lost its uniqueness and is more and more perceived as a 'heterogeneous group of different diseases' (Bourret *et al.*, this volume). Fleck's thought experiment to differentiate between sickness and sick people also helps to understand how difficult it is to speak about biological difference. Diseases as materialized abstractions have a similar origin and meet a similar need as other concepts like race, ethnicity, population, and sex and gender, which try to order unclear and messy biocultural aggregations. They 'cohabitate' the uneven grounds where culture and nature mingle without completely mapping on to each other, and all of them are imbued with their own historical trajectories which were and never will be innocent ones (see Joseph and zur Nieden, this volume). It is not an easy task to historicize them in a way that enables us to understand our messy present better, and not every handling of the past is a historicization as the story of the emergence of the 'Ashkenazi founder mutations' vividly illustrates (see Mozersky and Gibbon, this volume; zur Nieden, this volume). Every contribution of this volume struggles with the task to historicize the inherited abstractions and their materialization in our present and conceptualize new ones which might be able to keep at bay the social hierarchies, identity politics, and strategies of exclusion which seem to come with them.

Temporal topologies in biomedicine

In his conversations with Bruno Latour, philosopher Michel Serres conceives time as a topological structure, and as a space, and he explains it with his crumpled handkerchief (Latour and Serres 1992). Time is folded, full of gaps, discontinuities, unexpected turns and connections and not something that flows continually. Following Serres, we can understand time as heterogeneous and complex, something we all have to manage, to translate, to work with in order to transform it into a smooth, linear, homogeneous or chronological 'river'. Whereas the impact of the future in biomedicine has already attracted some scholarly attention (Adams *et al.* 2009), this volume builds upon Serres's idea of time as a spatiotemporal process. This edited volume is not so much interested in researching singular temporal kinds like the anticipation of the future in the present, or the past re-enacted by genealogical practices in modern genetics. It rather explores the complex temporal topologies and landscapes of BRCA. Serres's idea resonates well with the concept of *l'agencement* and helps to investigate not only the times of BRCA, but also to catch a glimpse how much our own research is embedded in it. Simultaneously, it allows us to recognize how time is used as a major resource and material in biomedicine, something that accelerates life in incubators and slows it down in freezers, that loops and transcends even the limits of an individual's life by 'storing the present for the future through biobanking' (see Lee, this volume). Nonetheless, while, movements in time might be considered as an acceleration: a 'race' or indeed a slowing down, it is also important to consider how biomedicine works to transgress common sense temporalities, by allowing, for instance, living material (tissues, information) to survive an individual's death or through the process of creating 'previviors' (see Pelters, this volume), the anticipated survivor of a cancer who never actually comes into being, or, indeed, by producing drugs, which wander around searching for a fitting disease they can cure (see Bourret *et al.*, this volume). More twisted temporalities emerge in the disconcertment (see Verran 2001) of decision making, for instance about the question of whether health is the main goal of a life or only one among other human goods. When parents with a positive test for BRCA mutations have to choose if they want to test their unborn baby (by PGD) or not they often loop in time and ask themselves the same question from the position of their parents: 'If my mother had this opportunity, maybe I wouldn't be here?' or they explore the temporal landscapes of subjunctives: 'Would I have chosen never to be born? Would I say my life hasn't been worth living because of it?' (see Rubin, this volume). Even more layers of involuted time are to be found in the postcolonial presence of India. Here, breast cancer is understood as the embodied pathology of modernity and simultaneously as an expression of a malignant temporal epoch of Hindu cosmology (see MacDonald, this volume). Cancer in India appears as a disease symbolizing the transition of the country: understanding it as a disease of the modern life style, it is nevertheless not discussed in the terminology of genetics but in the still hegemonic discourse of infectious diseases, for example when people talk about the disease as 'spreading' or that one is at risk of 'catching' it.

The transnational and comparative approach allows fascinating insights in the 'affective economies' in the times of BRCA. Feminist theorist Sara Ahmed (2004) suggests understanding emotions as constituted by these economies. Emotions do not reside in the individual's psyche but rather are produced and valued by the circulation between individuals in affective economies. Even though the risk of attracting breast cancer is not discussed in a genetic discourse in India, Alison MacDonald's chapter illustrates emphatically how the dominant emotions of fear and anxiety emerge and circulate 'in wider networks of kin relations'. Here we learn about another version of the 'bioeconomy', which seems to build the other side of the coin: instead of hypes and hopes and a climate of speculation about new options to economize 'products' from living materials or data extracted from it, we look here at an 'ethos of concealment' where the suspicion of cancer in a family threatens potential marital prospects and thus effects the economic security of women and their families.

From Sandra Lee's chapter we learn that the most important political question in the field of biomedicine might be situated in the problem of how we conceptualize the relation between the individual and the collective, or how we intervene in the neoliberal practices of individualization. Her suggestion to circumvent the politics of personalized medicine with the establishment of something so old and historic like 'the commons' also points to the importance of historicizing present biomedical practices. Historicization is by no means a task reserved for historians. Here again it helps to take a closer look at the different actors in the chapters of this volume, for instance at the capability of the women in the 'Family History Project' (see Joseph, this volume) to historicize their pasts, i.e., their experiences by abducting the offer of an 'at-risk subjectivity' into the affirmation of their collective life-long experience of being racially and socially discriminated against.

There may be a lot of different ways to historicize, which we still have to discover as a way to describe, analyze, reflect, and alter our mobile (and maybe multiple) positions in the dynamic sociopolitical arrangement – the 'l'agencement' – of biomedical practices. Understanding biomedicine as distributed or as one among other dispersed sociopolitical phenomena in postindustrial, neoliberalized societies means that we cannot claim a neutral and innocent position outside this arrangement in order to do our jobs as social scientists or historians. We still have to unravel how to interact with these dispersed, mobile, and complex arrangements. One option might be – like biomedicine – to break away from firm, fixed, and disciplined positions to develop a more itinerant, ambulant historiography or anthropology so that we can follow the trajectories of a gene, its concepts and materializations, and its (possible) diseases across the intersections of what were once called society, politics, economy, and nature.

Notes

1. The term "arrangement" has a mundane connation but also refers to the concept of "l'agencement" coined by theorists Gilles Deleuze and Félix Guattari to explore and describe socio-technical changes in postindustrial societies as not static and structural but rather as highly dynamic and procedural (Deleuze and Guattari 1987).
2. Keating and Cambrosio called them "biomedical platforms" according to the term their actors used in order to describe their activities (2003). I prefer here to stick to the more abstract concept of socio-technical arrangement or l'agencement in order to explore the options how to expand it for further research.
3. One of the best explorations of contemporary biomedicine was the exhibition "Split and Splice" at the "Medical Museion," in Copenhagen 2009; see "Split + Splice. A User's Guide," 2009.
4. An excellent example for analyzing biological procedures as dispersed and distributed phenomena is Murphy 2011.

References

Adams, V., Murphy, M. and Clarke, A. E. (2009). 'Anticipation: technoscience, life, affect, temporality', *Subjectivity,* 28, 1: 246–65.

Ahmed, S. (2004) 'Affective economies', *Social Text,* 22, 2: 118–39.

Bruchhausen, W. (2011) 'Biomedizin in sozial- und kulturwissenschaftlichen Beiträgen. Eine Begriffskarriere zwischen Analyse und Polemik', *NTM. Zeitschrift für Geschichte der Wissenschaften, Technik und Medizin* 18: 497–522.

Clark, A., Mamo, L., Fosket, J. R. and Fishman, J. R. (2010) *Biomedicalization: Technoscience, Health, and Illness in the U.S.* Durham, NC: Duke University Press.

Deleuze, G. and Guattari, F. (1987) *A Thousand Plateaus. Capitalism and Schizophrenia.* Minneapolis, MN: University of Minnesota Press.

Fleck, L. (1935; trans. 1979) *Genesis and Development of a Scientific Fact.* Chicago: University of Chicago Press.

Foucault, M. (1975) *Discipline and Punish: The Birth of the Prison.* New York: Random House.

Keating, P. and Cambrosio, A. (2003) *Biomedical Platforms.* Cambridge, MA: The MIT Press.

Kleinman, A. (1993) 'What Is Specific to Western Medicine?' In W. Bynam and R. Porter (eds.), Companion Encyclopedia in the History of Medicine, Vol. 1, pp. 15–23. London: Routledge.

Latour, B. and Serres, M. (1992) *Éclaircissements: cinq entretiens avec Bruno Latour,* Paris: Bourin.

Lenoir, T. and Hays, M. (2000) 'The Manhattan Project for Biomedicine'. In P. Sloan (ed.) *Controlling Our Destinies* pp. 29–62. Indiana: University of Notre Dame Press.

Löwy, I. (2011) 'Historiography of biomedicine: 'bio,' 'medicine,' and in between', *Isis* 102, 1: 116–22.

Murphy, M. (2011) 'Distributed Reproduction'. In M. Casper and P. Currah (eds) *Corpus. An Interdisciplinary Reader on Bodies and Knowledge.* New York: Palgrave Macmillan.

Split + Splice. Fragments from the Age of Biomedicine, User's Guide for the Exhibition at Medical Museion Kopenhagen 12.6.-13.12.2009.

Verran, H. (2001) *Science and an African Logic*. Chicago: University of Chicago Press.

Section II

Risk, personhood and subjectivity

4 Situating breast cancer risk in urban India

Gender, temporality and social change

Alison Macdonald

Introduction

This chapter explores cultural articulations of breast cancer risk in relation to the ethnographic context of India – specifically, the activities of breast cancer patient activist organizations. In the chapter, I examine constructions of risk at the intersection between perceptions of social change and modernization and pre-existing notions of gender, which are being mobilized in novel ways within an emergent field of preventative medicine in urban India. Currently, there is minimal emphasis on the potential risk posed by the hereditary component of breast cancer within these activist groups. Therefore, the ensuing analysis considers this 'absence', or subordination, of BRCA-related knowledge in light of the activities and sense-making practices of patients and volunteers where conceiving and confronting 'risk' – as part of advocating breast cancer preventative health care practices – frames (and is framed by) appeals to temporalities of social change and modernity as they relate specifically to gendered livelihoods, health and the family. In this chapter, I situate these ethnographic particularities in relation to an increasingly globalizing arena of transnational genetic technologies in order to further re-frame and problematize BRCA-related knowledges and practices (see Gibbon *et al.* 2010).

Breast cancer in India

The incidence of breast cancer is rising in Indian women. In 2008 it was estimated that there were 115,251 newly diagnosed cases of breast cancer, and this is estimated to rise to 200,000 in 2030 (Ferlay *et al.* 2010). Recent data from the National Cancer Registry Programme[1] shows that breast cancer has emerged as the leading site of cancer among women (NCRP 2009; see also Argawal and Ramakan 2008). However, despite the increasing burden of breast cancer, public health initiatives remain limited. There is currently no nationwide screening system, and this, together with a lack of cancer awareness and a heightened fear of the disease, results in the majority of patients presenting at an advanced, and therefore often incurable, stage of the disease (see NCCP 2002). Although every state has a regional cancer centre, the delivery and provision of these state oncology services are widely disparate. The availability and affordability of treatment can vary dramatically both between and within states, with the poorer states emerging as grossly underserved. In rural areas especially, there is often little access to any cancer diagnostic and curative facilities, and patients must travel long distances to city centres to access treatment. Urban areas like Mumbai have a wide range of medical establishments, and although there is a fair amount of government tertiary health care centres, many of these are still ill-equipped for oncological care because they lack the polyvalent and specialist oncological services required for diagnosing and treating cancer. This is further exacerbated by a lack of qualified and specialized trained staff. Furthermore, cancer treatment is particularly costly, with many second-line drugs and treatments, such as radiotherapy, reaching up to three times the annual income of a rural family. In this context, therefore, the experience of cancer is shaped by socio-economic positioning and mediated through structural conditions that heavily dictate the ways in which cancer is experienced by patients and their families.

Emerging urban breast cancer activism

Given the paucity of state facilities, a large proportion of public health advocacy surrounding breast cancer is carried out by urban non-governmental organizations (NGOs) and charities. While these organizations are few and far between nationally, they are extremely proactive and operate first and foremost in relation to the specific socio-economic context in which patients are trying to access and manage the multiple practicalities of receiving oncological treatment. This includes engaging in various activities – from opportunistic screening and detection camps, to raising awareness and fundraising for free medication. I conducted ethnographic research between March 2009 and August 2010 with three organizations operating in Mumbai in the northwest state of Maharashtra.[2] There, I worked with a prominent, large-scale NGO that operates as multifaceted aid-dispensing agency providing cancer awareness, cancer screening and diagnostics. It also engages in large-scale fundraising projects and contributes to public health policy, intervention and advocacy. At the same time, I also conducted fieldwork with two smaller volunteer-based groups that work exclusively for breast cancer patients and have been organized by previous breast cancer sufferers. These groups have emerged in the last ten to fifteen years and operate on a much smaller scale than other large cancer NGOs. Their outreach is local and their funding capabilities extremely limited. These organizations are wholly dependent on word of mouth – either through their members and volunteers, who tell their friends and family, or via the patients themselves. They primarily seek to provide post-operative emotional support (what is described as social 'rehabilitation') and provide a range of biomedical and financial information to patients and their families. Some also offer financial aid by distributing free medication, such as Tamoxifen, to needy patients within the government institutions. These groups originated from the women's own experiences of suffering with breast cancer as they mobilized around rudimentary provisions of care and a dire lack of patient-centred information. Given the underserved cancer wards and hospitals where doctors are overwhelmed with patients, a crucial part of the volunteers' activities is acting as brokers for all cancer-related information between patients, their families and the doctors.

While these groups could be described as contributing to an emergent field of cancer activism in Mumbai, they are not coming together to form a larger social lobby or indeed a wider breast cancer movement of the kind seen to proliferate in Euro-America, particularly in the UK and US. Here, activism has facilitated and attracted a particular kind of 'voice and visibility' within both public and biomedical/scientific domains (Kaufert 1998; Klawiter 2000a) and it has also now diversified and created different arenas of political lobbying, including environmental or 'green' activism (Klawiter 2000b; Ley 2009) or advocacy driven by scientific research and 'hope and hype' around BRCA-related research (Gibbon 2007). In Mumbai however, it is only in 'pockets' of the city – in hospitals, clinics, NGO offices and volunteers' homes – that one sees or hears about breast cancer. Cancer organizations in Mumbai are not advocating a cure for cancer, activists are not influencing or funding scientific research, and the public are not pinning pink ribbon badges in a celebration of solidarity to fight against the disease. Rather, charitable and public health initiatives around breast cancer are currently squarely focused on rolling out, albeit in diverse and disjointed ways, awareness messages concerning disease symptoms and practices of early detection and prevention. Although breast cancer activism is frequently glossed as a 'globalizing' sphere, ethnographic specificities continue to make plain that activist practice speaks to divergent priorities and specific aims (see also Klawiter 2000a).

This takes particular saliency when exploring the role of BRCA technologies and related knowledges and practices in India. This arena has developed significantly within the Euro-American context and continues to evolve, as other nongenetic and epigenetic factors are increasingly seen to play a role. Thus, ongoing limitations and challenges to BRCA testing continue to unfold. In a wider viewpoint of the 'global', this is further intensified, as comparative perspectives reveal cultural and institutional specificities around such developments that simultaneously illustrate the 'unevenness' of complex global intersections (see Gibbon *et al.* 2010). This is nowhere more apparent than in the context of India. The Indian government has an increased interest more generally in the potential and promise of scientific research and genomic science, as the state and research community seek to reposition India's status as a biotechnological 'global' player (Bharadwaj and Glasner 2009; see also Gottweis 2009; Sunder Rajan 2006). The Indian Council of Medical Research (ICMR) has funded the Advanced Centre for Treatment, Research and Education in Cancer (ACTREC), which includes a Cancer Research Institute in Mumbai.[3] At the time of research, BRCA testing was available here and at a few other select centres in India, including the large private biotech company Reliance Life Sciences in Navi Mumbai.[4] However, the degree of genetic involvement in cancer in India is only just beginning to emerge (see, for example, Sarin 2006). Likewise, the 'hype' around cancer genetics has yet to fully trickle down to the delivery and provision of cancer care on the ground. Here, BRCA-related knowledges and practices take a backstage role in the quotidian grassroots activities of the voluntary cancer organizations where social and economic complexities surrounding accessing care and the fear of the disease dictate and constrain the way the volunteers respond to patients needs. It is in this specific context of the grassroots activities of the activist patient groups, and the interactions between volunteers and patients, that questions concerning disease risk, causality and temporalities of social change will be discussed and explored.

Situating BRCA, risk and disease 'transferability'

When I brought up the issue of BRCA testing with NGO professionals and charity volunteers – for example, where and how one could be tested for a heritable predisposition – many were unsure of the details or did not know about BRCA-specific technologies at all. Those who did were quick to tell me that this was not a priority and bracketed it off from their own grassroots activities of providing the basic provisions of care. The test alone can cost anything between 54,000–70,000 rupees (roughly £600-£800), which immediately restricts this option to the wealthy echelons of society. This is one of the most significant issues currently shaping the low uptake of cancer genetic intervention. This was highlighted to me by one of the few genetic counsellors in India during an interview in her fairly upmarket private clinic in the south of Mumbai. She reiterated financial cost as one of the major factors influencing a family's decision to actually have the test. She explained that, since her return to India in 2008 from the US (where she received her training), she has had ten women referred to her with a suspected genetic disposition to breast cancer, and that after an initial consultation, none of these women chose to have the test. This, she stated, was most likely because of the sheer cost involved in testing. Also, she explained that many people are currently in a position where they can be adequately informed through family history rather than having to bear the cost of having this confirmed by a genetic test.

At the same time, however, the articulation of genetic heritability between patients and volunteers, and among the volunteers themselves, is frequently overshadowed by a more general concern for the 'transmission' of breast cancer. While I encountered multiple, shifting and varied conceptualizations of cancer aetiology and causality, the 'transferable' risk of breast cancer – however variously conceived – means cancer is often considered to be 'spreading' (*phaĩl raha haĩ*), 'catching' or contagious, primarily possessing the ability to pass through and move between persons. This becomes particularly salient in the context of the family. For example, many women and their families believe that it can spread from a patient to her child through breast milk, or else through the contact of maternal blood to her foetus. It can also be transferred through sexual intercourse and the sharing of food and utensils. In the voluntary organizations and the state cancer hospital, patients frequently posed these kinds of questions to volunteers, voicing an underlying anxiety concerning the principle of motility and transmission, particularly between members of the family. This becomes particularly salient for daughters of mothers with breast cancer, as the mothers themselves would often articulate a fear that, if they have had cancer, their daughters will now also be susceptible, without necessarily specifically pinpointing a heritable component. The 'mechanics' of biological transferability were rarely discussed in the interactions between patients and the volunteers. Rather, the discussion of the transferability of breast cancer is often glossed over by the volunteers, who try to minimize the fear that cancer is potentially 'in the family', which is expressed by many patients and their families when they visit. The significance of this fear manifests in a concern that the marital prospects of a daughter might be somehow spoiled. Given that most marriages are still arranged in India, and also according to the still existing restriction of a preference for a caste group and ethnic community, the onus is very much on finding a 'good match' for a daughter according to certain criteria. The revelation of breast cancer in the family therefore potentially threatens this process by blighting the suitability of a family within their community in ways that have led patients, NGO volunteers and health professionals to describe breast cancer as 'stigmatizing' or 'tabooed'. Thus, the notion of cancer as 'spreading' is not something easily discussed by patients and their families, and in turn it contributes to an ethos of concealment within the family, kin networks and the wider community (see Macdonald 2013).

The genetic counsellor also highlighted this issue when I asked her about the anxiety that surrounds cancer as a transferable disease. She agreed, explaining: 'First of all is that genetic testing has not really been culturally taken up as something that people are open to. A genetic test means something is wrong with my genes, which means there is something wrong with my family.' She then emphasized the gravity of having this validated with a scientific 'stamp', as she suspected people would not want others to know. This was echoed at a cancer genetics seminar I attended at one of the private hospitals in the centre of the city. It was hosted by the coordinator of a genetics clinic at ACTREC. Again, the geneticist pointed to the potential complications of having cancer 'in the family' with particular reference to marriage practices. She gave the example of one family who refused to go ahead with a marriage because they were concerned that there was 'too much' cancer in the proposed girl's family, and that this meant the girl would also be susceptible. In response, the girl's family asked the genetic clinic coordinator to speak with the boy's family in order to explain and dispel their fears and ease any concerns.

In this way, disease 'risk' – be this articulated as genetic or not – emerges as an interpersonal anxiety arousing 'biomoral' concern for a bodily transgression (see also Cohen 2001) that is located interpersonally as 'off' the body within a wider network of kin relations (see Das and Addlakha 2001). In the patient organizations, volunteers are often at pains to dispel the immense fear articulated by patients when they come to visit in relation to these concerns. They often profile patients according to how much they appear to know about the 'seriousness' of their disease status, including their ability to deal with and take on board medical information, to such an extent that, even if patients ask why cancer happens and if it is inherited or catching to their daughters, this is brushed over and quashed immediately in order to minimize any undue anxiety and fear.

Gendering of risk and temporalities of social change

Coterminous with concerns regarding disease transferability and disease risk, conceptualizations of breast cancer risk are also constructed and confronted via the intertwining of gendered values/practices and ideologies related to the emergent temporality of life *ājkal* (nowadays). Given the lack of aetiological knowledge, the causality of cancer is open to variable socio-cultural interpretation, and anthropological studies have highlighted a particular association between the disease and certain kinds of modernist conditions and practices (see McMullin and Weiner 2008). For example, this may be not only through changes in lifestyle, such as those associated with environmental pollutants (Karakasidou 2008) or diet (Weiner 2008), but also changes associated with wider neoliberal policies, practices and ideologies (Chavez 2008). Cancer has even been described as a pathology of the 'postmodern body' that is surrounded by and containing rapid, flexible change and is reflective of and underpinned by globalization and late capitalist, changing socio-economic structures (Weiss 1997: 469).

I frequently encountered notions of breast cancer in Mumbai linked to social change and flux. Among health professionals in Mumbai, breast cancer is also connected to changing patterns of life, particularly in the urban areas where ideas surrounding detrimental 'lifestyle' practices – such as physical inactivity, smoking tobacco, chewing *paan* (a form of tobacco), eating 'junk' foods, cooking with an abundance of *ghee* (clarified butter), drinking alcohol and eating meat – are often at the fore of public health prevention campaigns. For breast cancer specifically, these lifestyle choices are also gendered and relate particularly to urban women's reproductive life cycles.[5] Within the activist organization, this is articulated as a change in gender roles and lifestyles, whereby the 'emancipation' of women, through education and the pursuit of careers, delays the age of marriage, the age of first childbirth and the length of breastfeeding (all of which are considered to be protective against breast cancer).

This is a particularly complex arena, as lifestyle changes associated with perceptions of modernization feed into the novel realm of emergent preventative medicine within the activist groups in ways that are seen as reinforcing more 'traditional', or pre-existing, values concerning questions of gendered health and well-being. Here, an ambiguous discourse is emerging around the challenges, contradictions and possibilities of the 'modern' Indian woman's current lifestyle. For example, in an awareness lecture delivered by an NGO volunteer, I sat and listened while she explained to a group of coy middle-class female employees of a corporate bank that there is an urban/rural divide in cancer incidence in India, emphasizing that there is more breast cancer in the city. But, she exclaimed, 'How different can we be from our sisters in the villages?' The volunteer went on to describe the 'modern Indian woman' who lives in the city and whose lifestyle is 'Westernized' because of her diet, lack of exercise, education and career orientations. She contextualized this scientifically, explaining that it is about the reproductive hormones, because longer periods of fertility mean more exposure to oestrogen, which in turn can increase the risk of breast cancer.

This emphasis on changing temporality has consequently fed into discourses and practices of preventative medicine. Many of the volunteers who previously had breast cancer themselves, for example, articulated this concern for their daughters' future. I heard them explaining to women suffering with breast cancer that they must marry their daughters off early, because not having children quickly can pose a potential risk for cancer. I once even overheard a volunteer on the phone to a young woman whose mother had just been diagnosed with cancer, telling her to have a baby to 'protect yourself'. When I brought this issue up with Anupama, a previous breast cancer sufferer and long-standing volunteer with one of the pioneering breast cancer charities in Mumbai, she explained it to me as follows:

> For our daughters . . . we get them married at the right age like my daughter is going to be turning 24 now and I have started looking out for her because if I get her married in the next year she will be 25 and by the time she has her family and have kids she should be done with all her pregnancies by 28, 29 years of age, breast fed and all and keep at her ideal body weight.

In her interaction with patients, Anupama gave them the same advice. One morning while she was massaging a woman with advanced lymphoedema in her arm after her mastectomy surgery, Anupama was asked what causes breast cancer. She explained that there is no one single cause, but there are 'risk factors' that could increase one's chances of getting breast cancer and positioned this in relation to the life course of young women. In emphasis of this, she said the best strategy is to get 'our daughters' married at 24–25, finish having a family by 28, breast feed and stay slim. Thus, in the voluntary patient organizations, not only are contemporary temporalities of social change conceived as influencing the risk of breast cancer, but gender is also implicated, for the ambiguity of young women now marrying 'late' re-inscribes older patterns of kinship practice and gendered values in novel ways in the emergent discourse of breast cancer prevention.

What is also significant is the way in which the biomedically defined risk factors also glide into another parallel discourse concerning culturally elaborated notions of society *ājkal* (nowadays). In a private medical clinic, while I was accompanying a volunteer on her rounds of the chemotherapy patients, I had a conversation with a family while their mother was undergoing chemotherapy. We were sitting together, and the topic of conversation turned to the possible causes of breast cancer, prompted by the husband's queries, as he pointed specifically to changes happening in urban cities, especially where children are moving away and the family is more dispersed. This in turn presents a problem for mothers, who have no one to care for. He explained that this causes them to take 'tension' and become susceptible to suffering and disease. Together, he and his son marvelled at the difference between life in the city and life in the village, where they claimed the family is more cohesive and robust. In turn, this prompted questions about cancer incidence in the villages. The volunteer explained that there was less breast cancer in the villages than in the city and they nodded, as if this was what they had expected to hear. 'There are two Indias,' the husband said, and then added, 'but of course it should be one!' The son then pointed out that urbanization in the last twenty years has had good effects in India, especially regarding computers and IT (information technology), but then stated that this has also had side effects, and he pointed to his mother lying on the metal bed with the IV drip attached to her arm.

The concern regarding modernization is positioned here not in relation to 'life-style' factors, but rather in relation to the debilitating consequences of modernity as impacting the heart of the Indian family whose disintegration is in turn making women worried and sick (see also Cohen 1998). Many women experiencing breast cancer whom I spoke to and formally interviewed are aware of the biomedically defined risk factors for breast cancer, yet they often expressed frustration, ambiguity or indifference in their evaluation of these potential 'risks' in relation to their own diagnosis and personal lives. Frequently however, I encountered the notion that the causality of breast cancer is linked to problems of stress or 'tension', specifically the mental tension that can occur in relation to many different distressing situations. I often encountered this explanation from women who described prolonged difficulties, such as attempts to manage economic hardship, which caused them to have *chintā* (worry, anxiety) about the welfare of their families, the health of their children, or as a result of domestic discord within the context of the joint family,[6] which in turn they perceived as making them susceptible to breast cancer. Sometimes these changes were also linked to the current epoch of *kaliyug,* the last of the four cycles of time in Hindu cosmology.[7] The invocation of *kaliyug* has been noted to encode and explain many of the dilemmas of everyday life in India as they pertain to the (often) negative aspects of modernity, including contexts of illness and health (see Cohen 1998; Copeman 2009; see also Pinney 1999). In a similar way, *kaliyug* was described to me as a *kharāb* (bad) time, emphasized as a period of inherent imbalance that increases the potential for suffering because people are becoming more restless and agitated due to the increase in desires or the feeling of *asaktī* (attachment, involvement) with the increasingly material and selfish world in which children turn away from the family and lose respect for their elders and each other. Therefore, living in such a world increases the potential for one to acquire 'tension', which in turn impacts the body, leading to *bimari* (illness, disease).

In this light, it is particularly interesting to note the way in which the risk and causality of an emergent disease such as breast cancer is conceptualized and confronted through indigenous cosmologies of temporality, in which 'modernity' is seen to play a prominent role in people's evaluations of the causality of their disease. At the same time, this becomes interwoven with contemporary gendered values and practices. This resonates with recent studies that have described the 'feminization', or gendering, of breast cancer genetic risk in which tensions and paradoxes concerning female nurturance, motherhood and proactive individuality shape health awareness and disease risk management (see Gibbon 2006, 2007; Hallowell 1999; Kampriani 2009). Together with an emphasis on temporality, this goes a long way in initially situating breast cancer 'risk' within the context of an emerging field of preventative health care in urban India.

Conclusion

While the voluntary associations advocating breast cancer care and awareness do not currently revolve around the scientific research community and predicative testing, they are responding to a more general risk of breast cancer in particular ways. In this chapter, I have focused on how such risk is confronted and constructed at the intersection between gendered expectations and values, the family and emergent perceptions of temporality and social change in urban India. On the one hand, 'risk' has been explored in relation to the 'feminization', or gendering, of breast cancer genetic risk, which is coterminous with an overarching concern regarding social change and malignant temporality in which preoccupations with 'modern' lifestyles are seen as impacting the health of the nation. On the other hand, the ethnographic particularity of India presents another angle from which to begin to confront BRCA-related knowledges and practices in relation to a comparative globalizing arena. While the clearly increasing interest in genetic and genomic science occupies national agendas in ways that speak to international trends, at the same time such concerns are subordinated in the everyday practices surrounding the advocacy of breast cancer detection and care where economic restrictions, diverse perceptions of the causality of disease and the incessant fear that surrounds the disease come to the fore. In this sense, this chapter offers the 'absence' of BRCA-related practices – as it intersects with local perceptions of breast cancer risk more generally – as a pertinent contribution through which to explore and situate the scope and reach of the transnational movement of BRCA technologies as they emerge locally, while at the same time informing the wider comparative project by further illuminating the nuances, disjunctures and instabilities that lie therein.

Notes

1. Comprehensive data available on cancer trends in India are scarce, but the most credible information concerning a large proportion of the population is available from the hospital- and population-based registries organized through the National Cancer Registry Programme (NCRP) of the Indian Council of Medical Research (ICMR).
2. Funding for this research was provided by the Economic and Social Research Council, UK (ESRC). I am grateful to the editors for their thoughtful comments on drafts of this chapter and to members of the BRCA network for many invaluable discussions.
3. CTREC serves as the apex national referral centre for comprehensive clinical and laboratory genetic services and genetics research for all major cancer predisposition syndromes, including BRCA1 and BRCA2, and has a dedicated daily Genetics Clinic and a Cancer Genetics Lab. It forms part of the Tata Memorial Centre (TMC), which includes Tata Memorial Hospital in Mumbai. The TMC is an autonomous grant-in-aid institution of the Department of Atomic Energy, Government of India.
4. Reliance has been testing for BRCA1/2 mutations in Mumbai using methodology similar to Myriad for the past eight years. The price of the test is around 54,000 INR (£595).

5. While these risk factors were often alluded to by health professionals and volunteers, they by no means represent a clear-cut picture of the nature of cancer aetiology in India. The patterns and trends of the Indian cancer profile (which is itself multi-dimensional and specifically differentiated, given the size and diversity of the country) are only beginning to emerge.
6. Commonly, kinship and residence patterns in India dictate that a bride lives with her husband and in-laws in patrilocal residence. This means that one encounters large families, consisting of a son, his brothers and their wives and children, living together with their own parents in what is described as a 'joint family' setting.
7. *Kaliyug* is the age of vice – a morally turbulent time characterized by spiritual degeneration, dissention, turmoil, doubt and delusion.

References

Argawal, G. and Ramakan, P. (2008) 'Breast cancer care in India: the current scenario and the challenges for the future', *Breast Care,* 3, 1: 21–27.

Bharadwaj, A. and Glasner, P. (2009) *Local Cells, Global Science: The Rise of Embryonic Stem Cell Research in India.* London: Routledge.

Chavez, L. (2008) 'Wasting away in Neoliberal-ville: Mexican immigrant women's views of cervical cancer, social inequality, and gender relations'. In McMullin, J. and Weiner, D. (eds) *Confronting Cancer: Metaphors, Advocacy, and Anthropology.* Santa Fe: School for Advanced Research Press.

Cohen, L. (1998) *No Aging in India: Alzheimer's, the Bad Family and Other Modern Things,* Berkeley: University of California Press.

———. (2001) 'The other kidney: biopolitics beyond recognition', *Body and Society,* 7, 2–3: 9–29.

Copeman, J. (2009) *Veins of Devotion: Blood Donation and Religious Experience in North India.* New Brunswick: Rutgers University Press.

Das, V. and Addlakha, R. (2001) 'Disability and domestic citizenship: voice, gender and the making of the subject'. *Public Culture,* 13, 5: 511–531.

Ferlay, J., Shin, H. R., Bray, F., Forman, D., Mathers, C. and Parkin, D. M. (2010) 'Estimates of worldwide burden of cancer in 2008: GLOBOCAN 2008', *International Journal of Cancer,* 127, 12: 2893–917.

Gibbon, S. (2006) 'Nurturing women and the BRCA genes: gender activism and the paradox of health awareness', *Anthropology and Medicine,* 13, 2: 157–71.

———. (2007) *Breast Cancer Genes and the Gendering of Knowledge: Science and Citizenship in the Cultural Context of the 'New' Genetics.* Hampshire: Palgrave MacMillan.

Gibbon, S., Joseph, G., Kalender, U. et al. (2010) 'Perspectives on globalising genomics: the case of "BRCA" breast cancer research and medical practice, *BioSocieties,* 4, 5: 407–14.

Gottweis, H. (2009) 'Biopolitics in Asia', *New Genetics and Society,* 28: 201–4.

Hallowell, N. (1999) 'Doing the right thing: genetic risk and responsibility'. In Conrad, P. and Gabe, J. (eds) *Sociological Perspectives on the New Genetics.* Oxford: Blackwell Publishers.

Karakasidou, A. (2008) 'The elusive subversion of order: cancer in modern Crete, Greece', In McMullin, J. and Weiner, D. (eds) *Confronting Cancer: Metaphors, Advocacy, and Anthropology.* Santa Fe: School for Advanced Research Press.

Kampriani, E. (2009) 'Between religious philanthropy and individualised medicine: situating inherited breast cancer risk in Greece', *Anthropology and Medicine,* 16, 2: 165–78.

Kaufert, P. (1998) 'Women, resistance and the breast cancer movement'. In Lock, M. and Kaufert, P. (eds) *Pragmatic Women and Body Politics.* Cambridge: Cambridge University Press.

Klawiter, M. (2000a) 'Racing for the cure, walking women and toxic touring: mapping cultures of action within the Bay Area terrain of breast cancer'. In Potts, L. K. (ed.) *Ideologies of Breast Cancer: Feminist Perspectives.* London: MacMillan Press.

———. (2000b) 'From private stigma to global assembly: transforming the terrain of breast cancer'. In Burawoy, M. and Gowan, T. (eds) *Global Ethnography: Forces, Connections and Imaginations in a Postmodern World.* California: University of California Press.

Ley, B. (2009) *From Pink to Green: Disease Prevention and the Environmental Breast Cancer Movement.* New Brunswick, NJ: Rutgers University Press.

Macdonald, A. (2013) *Breast Cancer Survivorship in Urban India: Self and Care in Voluntary Groups.* PhD thesis, University College, University of London.

McMullin, J. and Weiner, D. (eds) (2008) *Confronting Cancer: Metaphors, Advocacy, and Anthropology.* Santa Fe: School for Advanced Research Press.

National Cancer Control Programme (NCCP) (2002) *50 Years of Cancer Control in India,* edited by S. P. Agarwal, Y. N. Rao and S. Gupta, Ministry of Health and Family Welfare, Government of India, New Delhi.

National Cancer Registry Program (ICMR) (2009) *Time Trends in Cancer Incidence Rates: 1982–2005.* Bangalore, India.

Pinney, C. (1999) 'On living in the Kal(i)yug: notes from Nagda, Madhya Pradesh', *Contributions to Indian Sociology,* 33, 1–2: 77–106.

Sarin R. (2006) 'A decade of discovery of BRCA1 and BRCA2: are we turning the tide against hereditary breast cancers?' *Journal of Cancer Research Therapy,* 2: 157–8.

Sunder Rajan, K. (2006) *Biocapital: The Constitution of Post-genomic Life.* Durham, NC: Duke University Press.

Weiner, Diane. (2008) 'Changing views of cancer: three decades of Southern California native perspectives'. In McMullin, J. and Weiner, D. (eds) *Confronting Cancer: Metaphors, Advocacy, and Anthropology.* Santa Fe: School for Advanced Research Press.

Weiss, Meira. (1997) 'Signifying the pandemics: metaphors of aids, cancer, and heart disease', *Medical Anthropology Quarterly,* 11, 4: 456–76.

5 Gender trouble?

Queering the medical normativity of BRCA femininities

Britta Pelters[1]

Introduction

BRCA discourses are necessarily gendered at a number of levels. Take, for instance, the words 'breast cancer genes'. Reading this phrase conjures up a number of images and ideas: images of suffering in the word 'cancer', of familial potential in 'genes' and of women in 'breasts'. Indeed, breasts are perhaps *the* iconic image of femininity, as is demonstrated by a simple image search on Google for 'breast', which generates countless images of women and their breasts, but virtually none of men. Arguably, breast cancer genetics has become directly, or indirectly, associated with femininity, thanks to the abundance of pink ribbon campaigns that construct 'breast cancer' as the archetypal women's disease. Likewise, genetics and genes are associated with mothers and women as their reproductive centre and source (Steinberg 1996).

To date, social scientists and ethicists, especially, have addressed gendered effects in the field of BRCA. On the one hand, they have studied the effects of gender on agency and responsibility following the disclosure of genetic information (d'Agincourt-Canning 2001, 2006; Hallowell *et al.* 2003), pointing at women as 'genetic housekeepers' and 'primary receivers of the discourse of genetic responsibility' (Kollek and Lemke 2008: 253).[2] On the other hand, Hallowell (1998, 1999), for example, describes how women make decisions regarding risk-reducing surgery by weighing the costs as well as benefits. The results of risk-reducing surgery can then be depicted as creating and managing a look considered feminine and as experiencing a special material embodiment. Hallowell thus points to the intricate ways in which organs are linked to constructions of femininity, whereas the former outcomes present individual negotiations of the traditional female role as a caregiver, especially in health. Women are thus positioned at the centre of attention, which confirms the observation of a gender bias in both BRCA research and practice (Happe 2006). Yet the question remains whether these femininities challenge the normative scope of what is constructed as feminine in medicine and thus whether they expand the meaning of womanhood.

In this chapter, I will contrast notions of BRCA femininities as produced by the medical gaze (Foucault 1973) with those that are presented in personal narratives of BRCA-positive women. Based on biomedical articles accessible on Pubmed which concern the impact of different prophylactic surgical procedures on femininity, I will demonstrate that, within this context, femininity must necessarily be seen in terms of a vulnerability to loss due to a biomedical narrative which is based on normative assumptions about gender functionality. This medical interpretation will be contrasted with personal narratives of BRCA femininities, narratives that address this normative 'blind spot' by integrating the BRCA narrative into a personal narrative of femininity in a way that follows a notion of gain. The gender functionality of the medical system is thus complimented by personal gender regulation as a second valid norm for constructing sex/gender[3] in the BRCA field.

Within the scope of this norm, women may become, to a certain extent, liberated from the confinements of the feminine body, confinements that even seem to have an impact on the scope of adopted social roles. Broadening the potential of 'lived femininity' by using technological possibilities, such as the BRCA arsenal, evokes associations with the myth of the cyborg (Haraway 2006), an irreverent being who 'is about transgressed boundaries, potent fusions, and dangerous possibilities' (121). The cyborg could open the door to a 'post-gender world' (118) by delightfully constructing new ways of producing, reproducing and imagining – ways that challenge the 'natural order of the sexes by challenging the idea of nature as an entity separate from both culture and technology. The fusing potential of the cyborg could lead to the creation of hybrid femininities, including already existing and new ideas which could have an impact on the way women are expected to be and behave in their social milieu (such as their family), making other constructions of femininity available to non-BRCA-positive women as well.

I thus argue that the gender-regulating BRCA-positive woman holds a queering potential which could broaden the chances for the presentation and embodiment of femininity, not only for herself but also in general. This personal gain may therefore, in the end, turn out to be a normative and collective one.

The biological is social: theoretical cornerstones and empirical data that matter

This chapter is based on a post-structuralist understanding of sex/gender (Butler 1990, 1993). Sex has initially been defined, and is still often referred to, as the biological 'sex of the body' related to bodily features – such as body shapes and sexual organs – which are seen as 'natural' physical attributes of either male or female individuals. In contrast, gender is understood as the social gender role that defines expressions of femininity and masculinity (Wilchins 2004). As such, it has long been regarded as a product of an interactive learning process; a product deemed 'man' and 'woman'. Gender is a constant social construction whose result is determined by the actual socio-cultural context in which it is performed. This 'doing gender' (Lorber 1999) leads to a gender status hierarchy that stabilizes social structures. Judith Butler has argued that not only gender, but also sex can be regarded as a social construction, as a product of repetitive performative acts in the context of a certain discourse. In other words, it is not sex that determines gender but the opposite, meaning gender determines sex – or more correctly, our social and cultural notions and assumptions about what makes a man or a woman determine sex. Moreover, both sex and gender exist within the imaginative frame of a necessary and thus normative heterosexuality as the righteous direction of desire, a constellation that is known as the heterosexual matrix.

Consequently, we have an essentialist dichotomy that dictates that there are objectively two, and only two, essentially different biological sexes: male and female. A series of binaries determines what characteristics are to be expected of the positions of 'a real, feminine woman' and 'a real, masculine man'. Whereas femininity is associated with attractiveness, nurturing and caring, softness, passivity, submission and emotionality, masculinity is characterized by power, providing and protecting, toughness, activity, dominance and rationality – all of which are more highly valued than feminine features in Western societies. Thus, most Western societies rank masculine men 'naturally' higher than their feminine women counterparts (Wilchins 2004). These binaries are consolidated in seemingly objective descriptions, such as the portrayal of the reproductive process in medical textbooks. These depict exactly these representations of femininity and masculinity in the roles and features of the egg and the sperm (Martin 1991) – for example, the apparent feminine passivity of the egg is contrasted with the masculine activity of the sperm, traits that can be retrieved in women's descriptions of reproductive experiences (Martin 1989) and which thus (re-)produce gender characteristics.

As female breasts have come to be seen as extremely important for the common representation of femininity and thus BRCA femininities, their symbolic significance and functionality needs to be addressed. Breasts have both a relational contact function that is connected to their acting as representations of the female potential for nurturing (within the mother–child relationship) as well as a sexual power (in a necessarily heterosexual relation with a male partner) (Olbricht 2002). Despite their powerful, even aggressive potential, breast-mediated lust, sexual arousal and attractiveness have been perverted in public, just as breasts are sexually objectified by the porn industry, advertisements and 'everyday' media (Kilbourne 1994; Wolf 2002) and have become objects for the dominant male gaze (Young 1990). The sexualization of women's bodies results in women needing to discipline their bodies by seeking to control their proper feminine image to ensure it has an 'appealing exterior' with presumably seductive qualities, a task which is experienced as both natural and important to a woman's feminine identity (Bartky 1990). The need to control the body – and the corresponding fear of a loss of control – keeps women busy with diets and fitness and thus limits their chances of gaining power in society (Kilbourne 1994), even if a 'seductive' body can be used as a powerful tool in private. A woman may deliberately choose an object status to get her own way but only at the price of a) dependence on (male) others and b) appearing passive, thus confirming the image of the reliant woman.

In contrast to breasts, ovaries are regarded as representing reproductive capacity. Due to their position inside the body, they can be considered far less obviously connected to feminine identity and therefore more amenable to objectification, even by women themselves (Hallowell 1998). However, research has demonstrated that ovaries are indeed associated with the construction of feminine identity in very complex ways (Hallowell and Lawton 2002).

Table 5.1 Pubmed hits according to search terms (October 2012)

	Gender identity	*Gender*	*Femininity*	*Body image*	*Psychosocial*
BRCA	0	8	2	9	36
Breast cancer genes	0	0	0	0	3
HBOC	0	4	0	1	12
Hereditary breast cancer	0	0	0	4	18
Hereditary ovarian cancer	0	0	0	0	2

Based on the understanding that femininities are conventions constructed in discourses, language – and its latent normative content – is of the utmost importance for the following analysis. A general hermeneutical stance that aims at investigating the structural traits of situations is thus combined with a perspective informed by intersectional norm-critical education (Bromseth and Darj 2010), which I apply to analyse normative assumptions concerning femininity. Developed out of queer education, norm-critical education aims at determining commonly valid norms as well as their underlying narratives and their orders of power. Norms are described as 'implicit and generally valid rules for how we are supposed to act towards each other and think concerning different questions' (Brade *et al.* 2008: 18). Norm-critical education thus broadens the focus beyond sex/gender and sexual norms in order to take a broad range of normative, intersecting socio-cultural categories (class, disability, age, etc.) into consideration.

The empirical material I will focus on in this chapter consists of two types of text data: medical articles listed on the Pubmed database and interview data. I chose Pubmed because of its wide currency in the field of biomedicine and public health. The articles listed in Pubmed are representative of the knowledge on which the biomedical field relies. The articles included in this analysis were found by doing searches with the following terms: 'BRCA', 'breast cancer gene', 'hereditary breast and ovarian cancer' and 'familial breast and ovarian cancer' in combination with 'femininity', 'gender', 'gender identity', 'body image' and 'psychosocial consequences'.[4] The total number of hits is displayed in Table 5.1.

The search was directed at articles that discuss the effects of BRCA or HBOC on gender and not, for example, gender as an influential factor for making decisions. Using this selective strategy resulted in only nine articles. It can be concluded that gender issues are highly underrepresented in the available medical literature.

The normative scope of the Pubmed articles and the norm of gender functionality

Of the reviewed biomedical articles that discuss femininity in the context of BRCA, most – Campfield Bonadies *et al.* 2011; den Heijer *et al.* 2004; Friedman and Cramer 2005; Kwong and Chu 2012; Lostumbo *et al.* 2010; Nelson *et al.* 2005; Unukovych *et al.* 2012; Vadaparampil *et al.* 2006, 2007 – do not question assumptions about sex/gender within the heterosexual matrix. This is due to their theoretical underpinnings and failure to include transgender or transsexual people's experiences, for example; they therefore stabilize these assumptions. While the sex- and gender-related issues in these texts are centred on prophylactic surgery and the importance of material changes to the body, they ignore other possible 'genderizable' features – such as agency (in health promotion) or responsibility (during counselling) – as being relevant to femininity, although this would have been possible at other processual points.[5] This material focus seems to be acknowledged by the scope of the contexts and effects in which the terms 'sex' and/or 'gender' are mentioned. These consist, for example, of body image, sexual functioning, satisfaction with surgical results, feelings of physical or sexual attractiveness, impact on libido and menopausal symptoms (Campfield Bonadies *et al.* 2011; Friedman and Cramer 2005; Lostumbo *et al.* 2010; Unukovych *et al.* 2012; Vadaparamil *et al.* 2006, 2007). All of these affect feminine sexual and reproductive potential and resonate with the two stereotypical images of 'the mother' and 'the seductress'. They are ultimately understood as physical, as the following quote demonstrates:

> Frost 2005 found a number of adverse physical effects among women who had CPM [contralateral prophylactic mastectomy]: 33% reported their body image was negatively affected; 26% felt less feminine; 23% had an adverse effect on their sexual relations; and 12% reported adverse effects on their emotional stability.
>
> (Lostumbo *et al.* 2010: 14)

This typical quote hints at the common use of quantitative psychometric measurements in these studies (all references but Kwong and Chu 2012 and Matloff *et al.* 2009) as data that are regarded as addressing an 'emotional or social function' (Lostumbo *et al.* 2010: 13). If we look at the quote, the changes of functionality mentioned only seem to exist as an adverse loss or diminishment, whereas the remaining percentages are not described in detail. This implies that there are no changes in theses cases. Here, functionality is obviously not affected, which seems to represent the best a woman can hope for in the case of opting for risk-reducing surgery. This observation resonates with the intrinsic logic of the investigative scenario presented and is acknowledged in other accounts as well (den Heijer *et al.* 2004; Lostumbo *et al.* 2004; Nelson *et al.* 2005; Vadaparampil *et al.* 2006, 2007). One example is another study (Frost *et al.* 2000, which was mentioned in Lostumbo *et al.* 2010 but did not appear in the Pubmed search) which explicitly reports beneficial effects. And yet, its argumentative structure stresses negative surgery outcomes as actually more important (in contrast to positive outcomes) by mentioning them at the very end in a sentence that starts with 'however', which puts special emphasis on them:

> The majority of women reported no change/favorable effects in levels of emotional stability (68%/23%), level of stress (58%/28%), self-esteem

> (69%/13%), sexual relationships (73%/4%), and feelings of femininity (67%/8%). Forty-eight percent reported no change in their level of satisfaction with body appearance; 16% reported favorable effects. However, 9%, 14%, 18%, 23%, 25%, and 36% reported negative effects in these 6 variables, respectively.
>
> (319)

The article by Matloff *et al.* (2009), appears to be different from the rest in that it depicts the impact of BRCA information on a woman's lifecycle. From puberty on, however, girls are presented as being 'vulnerable to an array of anxiety, fear, anger, depression, and ambivalence in the context of breast development and sexual maturation' (15). Although the article covers counselling and does not focus solely on risk-reducing surgery, this tendency to emphasize the ominous effects of BRCA information – such as a threatening loss – on sexual self-image, intimate partnerships and sexual functioning continues in the main text, even if the given case examples do present a more balanced picture. This is reflected in the authors' concluding advice:

> Information regarding how to manage menopausal side-effects, as well as pre- and postsurgical sexual rehabilitation counseling, should be available to patients and partners. Although prophylactic BSO [bilateral salpingo-oophorectomy] and BM [bilateral mastectomy] are highly-effective tools in reducing cancer risk in female BRCA carriers, the effects of these choices on sexual self-image and sexual functioning should not be underestimated.
>
> (18)

Thus, even in this more differentiated article, an internal logic of loss and a femininity that focuses on the female body in the context of reproduction and sexuality is apparent.

Framing the data this way indicates an intelligible normative background of femininity that is inextricably intertwined and intersected with societal stereotypes. The biomedical norm of gender functionality in these articles reflects and reiterates a general societal norm. Femininity is hereby seen as depending on having the 'right' organic equipment to promote both a functional feminine appearance (breasts) and a reproductive functionality (ovaries), according to the notion of the existence of two biological sexes. Both outer and inner organs are supposed to complement each other in a synergetic way. They are understood as the inevitable conditions determining sex/gender and as confirming the dichotomous norm as a 'natural sex/gender order'. Because they relate to sexuality and reproduction, they also resonate with, and reproduce, the feminine gender stereotypes of the nurturing and caring 'mother' and the sexually objectified 'seductress' in a heteronormative relational context. This is where the biomedical and societal discourses become intertwined and enhance one another.

Accordingly, the removal of at-risk organs is interpreted as a threat to femininity; it is an adverse event – a potential loss, rather than a potential gain in the quantitative culture of biomedicine. This loss is phrased in terms like 're-moval', 're-construction' and 're-placement'. The use of these terms individually and in combination suggests that something essential (breast tissue, hormones) is taken away that needs an artificial substitute (silicon, chemicals) while pointing out that the 'natural state', while preferable, has to be sacrificed for the greater good of health. The reconstructed woman is consequentially compromised, as she is healthy but no longer wholly feminine. Genetic irregularities, such as carrying a BRCA variation, consequentially need to be portrayed as negative events within the biomedical literature, rendering any benefits of being BRCA-positive hardly imaginable. Thus, in light of the norm of gender functionality, the aim of medical intervention seems to be to maintain or even maximize femininity by (re-)constructing it – in other words, by producing the 'necessary' female organic equipment through a succession of prophylactic and reconstructive surgeries (or hormone replacement 'therapies'). In terms of reconstructed femininity, how the diseased cancer survivor and the BRCA-positive cancer 'previvor' are presented correspond to each other (Sulik 2011), highlighting the image of BRCA as a near-cancer experience. The figure of the 'she-ro', the female hero who bravely fights breast cancer, with her 'femininity, sexuality and desirability (. . .) intact' (Klawiter 2004: 848) despite surgical interventions – fighting not only for survival, but for a better life as a consequence of a cancer-derived transformation (Sulik 2011) – seems to represent both a neoliberal version of stereotypical femininity and a feminized version of the health-conscious citizen whose pursuit of happiness has turned into the pursuit of health in order to live a good life (Crawford 2006).

Gaby's feared 'loss' versus Lisa's and Anke's 'gain': three cases of BRCA femininity

The cases presented here are based on interview data consisting of narratives collected during episodic single interviews (SI) and family interviews (FI). These were conducted in Germany in 2007 as part of a PhD project (Pelters 2012). In this project, I examined the phenomenon of 'doing health', meaning constructing situated health standpoints based on new information relevant to health, like BRCA test results, by using an evaluative filter determined by relational and transgenerational resources, biographical situation and interpretational and operational knowledges. The interviewees were white, heterosexual, West German BRCA-positive women who had received their BRCA test results at least two years before the interview.[6] They also had at least one relative affected by cancer who had survived the disease for more than 15 years or was still alive at the time of the interview. Moreover, the women participated in prevention or early detection measures offered by their HBOC clinic, through which the women were contacted. The cases have been hermeneutically analysed and reconstructed. In the following, I will first discuss one woman as an example of the confirmed norm of gender functionality before presenting two women who use their BRCA status to construct an alternative femininity that suits them.[7]

Gaby Böttcher (single, one child)

On the maternal side of Gaby Böttcher's family, HBOC has fatally affected many members, with Gaby's mother being the last casualty. Her mother's life with cancer was characterized by a failed marriage, social withdrawal and solitude. Drawing on a relational understanding of health, Gaby deems these aspects as responsible for the cancer's progress.

BRCA-positive, Gaby (test age 37) struggles to be her mother's opposite, to remain healthy and live a good life. In order to achieve this, she has developed a relational, outgoing lifestyle for which parties and male attention are of extreme importance. She benefits from an inherently female presence, to which she says: 'I appear female enough, apparently.' She sees this as her chance for a heterosexual partnership that will allow her to experience both a successful femininity and social integration, with health-promoting effects. Both of these things counteract her mother's failures as a woman and as a cancer patient, which points at an interdependency between health and femininity in this case.

After taking the BRCA test, it was vehemently suggested that she have an oophorectomy, and she has strongly considered consenting to a surgery. The surgery would deprive her of her relational possibilities because it would threaten her feminine potential, as Gaby locates this in her ovaries: 'you are not allowed to look at it [oophorectomy] like "What is a woman?" (. . .) I simply have to look at it from a health angle, you aren't allowed to put it as something like ovaries [=] symbols of fertility' (SI). To undergo surgery would mean a (health-)threatening loss of her feminine and social potential, which seems to follow normative assumptions that are in line with the norm of gender functionality. This is because Gaby depends on having a complete organic 'set-up' for her to be able to regard herself as a real woman and to attract men and start a serious relationship.

Anke Brause (test age 43) and Lisa Schall (test age 20) are BRCA-positive members of a family that has several members who were affected by HBOC. Of these, only Anke's mother and Lisa's grandmother Johanna survived the cancer. During the cancer period, the family developed a pragmatic, preventively functional way of dealing with their bodies that aims at performance and presentability.

Anke Brause (married, no children except goddaughter Lisa)

Because of the BRCA-positive test results, Anke has had an oophorectomy and has since been using the offer of intensified breast screening together with the rest of the female BRCA-positive family members. To her, the oophorectomy is merely a sequel in her ongoing liberation from too much femininity, which peaked three years prior to the BRCA-test when she underwent breast reduction from cup size J to C. She chose this therapeutic breast surgery to overcome the back pains and the slipped disk she regularly suffered. She also wanted to remove the sexually objectifying attention she was unable to avoid completely. Thus, when Anke describes her original breasts as 'two kilograms left and right' (FI), she depicts a load that is not only physical but also psychological. Her tendency to wear large, flamboyant hats, which presumably diverted objectifying gazes, and the following quote from the family interview[8] point at her longing for a body that can be experienced as appropriate:

Anke: I had a breast reduction in 2001, if I had had the diagnosis [BRCA+] before that, you could have counted me in [for PM] directly (. . .)

Lydia: But with a reconstruction, right?

Anke: No! (. . .) You have such a thing for twenty-to-twenty-five years, then you'll also be happy when it's gone (raised voice) because then I could run around without a bra and wouldn't need a bra and then I could even wear those light dresses

Lisa: And how does that look like, with no boobs?

Anke: How would I know?

Lisa: Then you have a belly and no boobs, or what?

Anke: So what?

Lisa: That's horrible (. . .)

(FI)

This quote also shows that Anke's preference for a bodily liberation is not necessarily over yet, something she confirms in the SI when she says she is considering a future prophylactic mastectomy. Being entirely 'breastless' does not seem to be problematic to Anke, even if it does to other family members.

Anke's breast reduction resulted in the end of her back problems, and she began to feel sexually attractive. She celebrated and staged this by going on a much longed-for shopping trip to buy expensive lingerie that contrasted with her former limitation of only being able to purchase corset-like undergarments from the medical supply store. This framing points at her breast reduction as a crucial step toward becoming a self-sufficient, proactive woman in charge of her own body and life.

Anke subsequently understands the oophorectomy as having provided her with another opportunity to continue this trend toward freeing herself from 'too much' (SI) femininity, namely by liberating her from very painful menstruation, which Anke attributed to 'way too many female hormones' (SI):

> (. . .) this may sound harsh but this gene, the mutated one, was not that bad because I finally had a reason to get rid of my menstruation, you have to know that I had four days of migraines every month and I needed to get up three times a night to change a tampon.
>
> (SI)

Thanks to this process of constructing a self-determined femininity, Anke now has a body to which she can finally connect and relate. She states, 'I simply love it [her body], it exists so that I can have a good life' (SI). She has therefore gained agency through her BRCA status, which even allows her to confront screening with a new-found trust in her own bodily knowledge. Anke can thus be regarded as working with the knowledge of her BRCA status in a way that enables her to regulate her gender and provides her with a 'bearable' amount of femininity. In her case, 'less' seems to be perceived as 'better' and therefore 'more'.

Lisa-Aziza Schall (engaged, no children)

Before taking the BRCA test, Lisa apparently had a rather insecure, ambivalent femininity which seemed to be derived from the sexualized position of the 'seductress' ascribed to her by other family members. Her aunt Anke described how Lisa could twist her uncle around her finger as a child to get the toy she wanted, and Lisa's mother, Lydia, said her daughter had had the 'right touch with men' (SI) since the age of four, when Lisa made contact with a man during their holidays whom Lydia later married. Thus, according to the family narration, from an early age Lisa was used to using her looks, her emotionality or her ability to appear helpless in her encounters with men. This strategy located her in a seemingly passive, needy and rather subordinate position within the binary gender hierarchy. Although it provided her with a competitive advantage over other girls and an indirect and powerful tool when dealing with boys and men in her heteronormative world, it also prohibited her from meeting men on equal terms. However, Lisa presents herself as wanting to establish relationships with boys and men in ways which are not characterized by a hierarchy, but by an equality between the two parties because they are unaware of belonging to 'the opposite sex' and of all the gendered expectations which come along with that – a hope which has obviously not been fulfilled:

> I always had more male friends because I think a lot of girls have been jealous of me as I was a fair *blonde* very *beautiful* (. . .) I simply had more buddies (. . .) there was only that one stupid effect that they sooner or later got a crush on me.
>
> (SI)

Because of her positive BRCA test, Lisa opted for screening. In her narrative, she even links her decision to take lessons in karate to her being BRCA-positive. This apparently resembles her reaction to her grandmother's last bout with cancer, after which she tried tae kwon do, and reveals both a pragmatic pattern of dealing with cancer and fits with her general operational strategy: gaining control through (competitive) fighting. Another example of this strategy is her way of framing her anorexic teenage struggle for body control in terms of a competition with her cousin. Lisa can thus be regarded as (at least additionally) using martial arts as a way of disciplining herself and as a way of staging the fight against her 'enemy' (FI), cancer, already in advance:

> I do martial arts, and that helps me, too, because I have the feeling I can fight it [cancer risk] . . . even if I don't feel like it [martial arts training] I tell myself, 'No, you have to go, because it is for your body and against the cancer.'
>
> (FI)

Because karate represents and highlights many features which are seen as masculine – power, toughness, activity, competitive dominance – it also provides a means through which Lisa seems to be able to return to her preferred buddy-state with men, a relation which is characterized by gender equality, not hierarchy. However, this time these relationships are not achieved through both sides ignoring gendered differences, something which proved to be an unstable arrangement in the past due to the 'constant falling in love' which put an end to being buddies, which Lisa complained about. Her being an equal buddy is instead the result of her active achievement of an acknowledged position and thus, in a way, the activation of her own masculine potential in the masculine-connoted sphere of the local karate club in her rural area, which – according to its website – seems to have started to attract more female members since Lisa joined. This constellation makes her gender performance much more self-sufficient and successful in terms of its effect on self-identity.

> (. . .) in karate, most of them are blokes, and with them, I am more buddy-like, in the beginning, they surely regarded me as a woman or a girl (. . .) but in the meantime, they regard me as a buddy, too, I suppose.
>
> (SI)

This masculine performance seems to be balanced by staging femininity through both a very feminine-looking appearance and a secure heterosexual relation that allows her to still prove that she is 'a real, feminine woman' and not risk her societal position inside the heterosexual matrix. As a result, Lisa has developed a more masculine-connoted femininity that can be regarded as empowered compared to the sexually objectified stereotype she both used and depended on in the past. She has converted her BRCA test results into an activity that is presented as expanding her performance range of gender expression and thus her gendered privileges. She thereby seems to have diversified what power and modes of expression 'femininity' can cover and has used the test results in a gender-regulative way, as does her aunt.

Conclusion

Whereas the example of Gaby's loss confirms the validity in society of a naturalized understanding of femininity based on the norm of gender functionality, Lisa's and Anke's gain questions and diversifies, in other words queers, this normative view of femininity. Lisa and Anke use BRCA-related knowledge and practices as well as their technologically established degrees of freedom in order to overcome the boundaries of a given 'female nature' and to regulate their sex/gender potential according to their own needs. This leads to an alternative femininity that suits them. Thus, technoscience in the form of BRCA testing and management has presented them with a means with which to liberate themselves from the boundaries of sex/gender which society and their social milieus had in store for them.

If we return to the concept of the cyborg (Haraway 2006) – a hybrid figure that fuses nature and technology, fiction and social reality – a hypothesis for understanding the liberating potential of technoscientific genetic data becomes tangible. The successful description of gendered bodies using a coding technology decodes the 'naturalness' of the body as something produced or even artificial, as a piece of information processing. In this moment of distancing or even alienation, hidden ideas of self-formation formerly classified as 'non-female' can be liberated from this label and perceived as legitimate due to the levelling of gender differences by the technoscientific code. New femininity formations emerge which transgress the old male/female dichotomy in the women's social milieus. Through the enactment of these formations, they rewrite the gendered space of possibility into a more fused version, at least to a certain extent. This may be understood as a very practical, performative implementation of Haraway's statement: 'Writing is preeminently the technology of cyborgs' (142).

One look at the actual queering effects shows their dependence on context. Whereas Anke questions normative assumptions about how a woman should look in her family, Lisa expands the limits of when she needs to be regarded (and to regard herself) as a woman in her karate environment. However, both women do not understand themselves as some sort of 'gender warriors' but are rather 'ordinary' cis-women – cis-people being 'individuals who have a match between the gender they were [legally] assigned at birth, their bodies, and their personal [gender] identity' (Schilt and Westbrook 2009: 461). They are thus cis-women who perform their sex/gender-regulating activities embedded in quite common lives. I understand this as a factor that enhances the validity and pervasiveness of the gender-regulating norm as an alternative to the norm of gender functioning. The new gender narratives dismiss the norm of gender functionality even if, or precisely because, Lisa and Anke are miles away from postgenderism. The potential for transgression that comes with being something different from or beyond 'the usual' appears to be powerful because it represents something not too different. Familiarity seems to promote change if it is amended by an attractive new narrative – the narrative of health with its promise of a good life. This is a subversive challenge to normativity within this hybrid state (Tuider 2004). As such, it is directed both at the biomedical interpretive authority, which is unaware of or unwilling to see and promote this alternative way of dealing with BRCA, and at the image of femininity within the women's social milieus. Thus, through this subversion of 'lived femininity', a personal gain becomes a collective one.

Notes

1. I would like to thank Nina Hallowell, Kristen Abatsis McHenry and the editors for their valuable comments.

2. All translations here are mine.
3. I choose this way of writing to express that sex and gender are understood as the same with regard to them both being constructs (see theoretical background).
4. Articles on risk-reducing surgery were deliberately excluded from the search to prevent a self-fulfilling prophecy. Their exclusion might, however, have led to the loss of more differentiated articles.
5. In the counselling and testing phase, the caring, relationally responsible type of femininity could, hypothetically, be stressed due to the exchange of familial information. Health-promoting activities (dieting, stress reduction, etc.), however, could emphasize the features of an 'altruistic', in other words relationally responsible and caring, type of femininity, while also playing to women's ambivalent, even 'egoistic' efforts of bodily control (Kilbourne 1994). Efforts to control the body especially question the idea of a 'real woman' as passive and soft due to the emphasis on agency and (will) power.
6. *A posteriori* interview data present a re-narration at a time when the actual experience has been transformed by its integration into a consistent narrative of the self, which could pose as a limitation. However, the data are regarded as significant because they represent the reality on which the person acts and determine further experiences.
7. Due to the limited scope of this publication, these cases have been extremely shortened. The reader can refer to Pelters (2012) for a complete in-depth analysis.
8. Participants were Anke, her goddaughter Lisa, her sister Lydia and her mother Johanna.

References

Bartky, S. L. (1990) *Femininity and Domination: Studies in the Phenomenology of Oppression*. New York: Routledge.

Brade, L., Engström, C., Sörensdotter, R. and Wiktorsson, P. (2008) *I normens öga. metoder för en normbrytande undervisning*. Stockholm: Stiftelsen Friends.

Bromseth, J. and Darj, F. (2010) *Normkritisk pedagogik. Makt, lärande och strategier för förändring*. Uppsala: Centrum för genusvetenskap, Uppsala universitet.

Butler, J. (1990) *Gender Trouble: Feminism and the Subversion of Identity*. New York: Routledge.

———. (1993) *Bodies that Matter: On the Discursive Limits of 'Sex'*. New York: Routledge.

Campfield Bonadies, D., Moyer, A. and Matloff, E. T. (2011) 'What I wish I'd known before surgery: BRCA carriers' perspectives after bilateral salipingo-oophorectomy', *Family Cancer*, 10, 1:79–85.

Crawford, R. (2006) 'Health as a meaningful social practice', *Health*, 10, 4: 401–20.

d'Agincourt-Canning, L. (2001) 'Experiences of genetic risk: disclosure and the gendering of responsibility', *Bioethics*, 15, 3: 231–47.

———. (2006): 'Genetic testing for hereditary cancers: the impact of gender on interest, uptake and ethical considerations', *Critical Review of Oncology and Haematology*, 58, 2: 114–23.

den Heijer, M., Seynaeve, C., Timman, R. et al. (2012) 'Body image and psychological distress after prophylactic mastectomy and breast reconstruction in genetically predisposed women: a prospective long-term follow-up study', *European Journal of Cancer*, 48, 9: 1263–8.

Foucault, M. (1973) *The Birth of the Clinic: An Archaeology of Medical Perception*. London: Tavistock.

Friedman, L.C. and Kramer, R.M. (2005) Reproductive issues for women with BRCA mutations', *Journal of the National Cancer Institute Monographs*, 34: 83–6.

Frost, M.H., Schaid, D.J., Sellers, T.A. et al. (2000): 'Long-term satisfaction and psychological and social function following bilateral prophylactic mastectomy', *JAMA*, 284, 3: 319–324.

Hallowell N. (1998) 'You don't want to lose your ovaries because you think "I might become a man". Women's perceptions of prophylactic surgery as a cancer risk management option', *Psycho-Oncology*, 7, 3: 263–75.

———. (1999) 'Reconstructing the body or reconstructing the woman? Perceptions of prophylactic mastectomy for hereditary breast cancer risk'. In Potts, L. (ed.), *Ideologies of Breast Cancer*. Basingstoke: Palgrave Macmillan.

Hallowell, N. and Lawton, J. (2002) 'Negotiating present and future selves: managing the risk of hereditary ovarian cancer by prophylactic surgery', *Health*, 6, 4: 423–43.

Hallowell, N., Foster, C., Eeles, R., Ardern-Jones, A., Murday, V., Watson, M. (2003) 'Balancing autonomy and responsibility: the ethics of generating and disclosing genetic information', *Journal of Medical Ethics*, 29, 2: 74–83.

Happe, K.E. (2006): 'Heredity, gender and the discourse of ovarian cancer', *New Genetics and Society*, 25, 2: 171–96.

Haraway; D. (2006) 'A cyborg manifesto: science, technology, and socialist-feminism in the late 20th century'. In Weiss, J., Nolan, J., Hunsinger, J. and Trifonas, P. (eds) *International Handbook of Virtual Learning Environments*. Dodrecht: Springer.

Kilbourne, J. (1994) 'Still killing us softly. advertising and the obsession with thinness'. In Fallon, P., Katzman, M.A. and Wooley, S.C. (eds) *Feminist Perspectives on Eating Disorders*. New York: Guilford Press.

Klawiter, M. (2004) 'Breast cancer in two regimes: the impact of social movements on illness experience', *Sociology of Health and Illness*, 26, 6: 845–74

Kollek, R. and Lemke, T. (2008) *Der medizinische Blick in die Zukunft: Gesellschaftliche Implikationen prädiktiver Gentests*. Frankfurt/Main: Campus.

Kwong A. and Chu, A.T. (2012) 'What made her give up her breasts: a qualitative study on decisional considerations for contralateral prophylactic mastectomy among breast cancer survivors undergoing BRCA1/2 genetic testing', *Asian Pacific Journal of Cancer Prevention*, 13, 5: 2241–7.

Lorber, J. (1999) '"Night to this day": The social construction of gender'. In Ferguson, S.J. (ed.) *Mapping the Social Landscape: Readings in Sociology*. Mountain View: Mayfield Publishing.

Lostumbo, L., Carbine, N. and Wallace, J. (2010) 'Prophylactic mastectomy for the prevention of breast cancer', *Cochrane Database of Systematic Reviews*, 11: Art. No.: CD002748. doi:10.1002/14651858.CD002748.pub3.

Martin, E. (1989) *The Woman in the Body*. Milton Keynes: Open University Press.

———. (1991) 'The egg and the sperm: how science has constructed romance based on stereotypical male-female roles', *Signs*, 16, 3: 485–501.

Matloff, E.T., Barnett, R.E. and Bober, S.L. (2009) 'Unravelling the next chapter: sexual development, body image, and sexual functioning in female BRCA carriers', *Cancer Journal* 15, 1: 15–18.

Nelson, H.D., Huffman, L.H., Fum R., Harris, E.L., Walker, M., Bougatsos, C., (2005) *Genetic Risk Assessment and BRCA Mutation Testing for Breast and Ovarian Cancer Susceptibility*. Rockville (MD): Agency for Healthcare Research and Quality (US).

Olbricht, I. (2002) *Brustansichten: Selbstverständnis, Gesundheit und Symbolik eines weiblichen Organs*, 1. Aufl., Berlin: Orlanda.

Pelters, B. (2012) *Doing Health in der Gemeinschaft. Brustkrebsgene zwischen gesellschaftlicher, familiärer und individueller Gesundheitsnorm*. Bielefeld: transcript.

Schilt, K. and Westbrook, L. (2009) 'Doing gender, doing heteronormativity: "gender normals", transgender people, and the social maintenance of heterosexuality', *Gender and Society*, 23, 4: 440–64.

Steinberg, D.L. (1996) 'Languages of risk: genetic encryptions of the female body', *Women: A Cultural Review*, 7: 259–70.

Sulik, G.A. (2011) *Pink Ribbon Blues: How Breast Cancer Culture Undermines Women's Health*. New York: Oxford University Press.

Tuider, E. 'Zur Hybridisierung der Sexualität. Eine sexulapädagogische Standortbestimmung im Zeitlater der Postismen', paper presented at the conference 'Sexualitäten und Lebenszeiten', Gesellschaft für Sexualpädagogik, Hannover, 25 September, 2004.

Unukovych, D., Sandelin, K., Liljegren, A. et al. (2012) 'Contralateral prophylactic mastectomy in breast cancer patients with a family history: A prospective 2-years follow-up study of health related quality of life, sexuality and body image', *European Journal of Cancer*, 11 June.

Vadaparampil, S.T., Miree, C.A., Wilson, C. and Jacobsen, P.B. (2006/2007) 'Psychosocial and behavioral impact of genetic counseling and testing', *Breast Disease*, 27: 97–108.

Wilchins, R. (2004) *Queer Theory, Gender Theory: An Instant Primer.* Los Angeles: Alyson Publications.

Wolf, N. (2002) *The Beauty Myth. How Images of Beauty Are Used Against Women*. New York: Harper Collins.

Young, I.M. (1990) T*hrowing Like a Girl and Other Feminist Philosophy and Social Theory.* Bloomington/Indianapolis: Indiana University Press.

6 It takes a particular world to produce and enact BRCA testing

The US had it, Italy had another

Deborah R. Gordon

> World is . . . so self evident, so much a matter of course, that we are completely oblivious of it.
>
> (Heidegger 1975: 165)

> Disengagement demands that we stop simply living in the body or within our traditions or habits, and by remaking them as objects for us, subject them to radical scrutiny and remaking.
>
> (Charles Taylor 1988: 310)

Prologue to the question

It was the mid-90s and I was trafficking between Tuscany, Italy, where I lived and worked as an anthropologist, and the United States, my country of origin, education and continued academic affiliation.[1] The US, I noticed, was abuzz with excitement, hope and worry over a new 'revolution' in the making: the human genome project and the first mapping of human DNA. The book of life could finally divulge the real truth about who we are and what we are made of. The promise did not stop there; this grail would lead us to understand and eventually cure at long last our most common and elusive maladies like cancer, heart disease and Alzheimer's.

This buzz was not only felt by the scientists as they feverishly raced to identify the culprit genes that caused our common illnesses. Nor was it restricted to the many varieties of clinicians, ethicists and policymakers, anticipating how to handle the new truths that our science and technology could now reveal. It was the stuff of public dissemination, discussion and debate in the popular and specialized media. A new icon, the gene, was produced, and it gathered together in one symbol the wide range of human aspirations and achievements in cracking nature's mysteries.

I returned to Italy, looking for signs I may have missed of this coming revolution. In fact, the American excitement and anticipation found little echo in Italy in the mid-90s, including at the Cancer Prevention Centre where I worked in Tuscany,[2] known in Europe for being on the cutting edge of breast cancer prevention and treatment. While it was initially at the very forefront of the Human Genome Project, Italy's participation ended in 1995 due to lack of funding. Thus, Italy did not participate in the sequencing stage of the project (Dulbecco 1997; Dulbecco and Vezzoni 1998, Pierluigi 1995). Beyond the scientists involved, there appeared to be minimal interest, much less fascination, from a range of professionals and laypersons. 'Italians already know who they are,' I thought. 'They don't need the human genome to tell them.' And besides, DNA in Italy was not a familiar figure, much less an icon with mystique, and it held little claim to truth. The promise of a new technology to light up the future with hope and progress was nothing unusual in the US; just as the relative hesitancy and cynicism in Italy reflected a deep grounding in the past and a hard-earned wariness toward an unknown and potentially ominous future.

While in ways less extreme than in the US, other countries in Western Europe, particularly the UK, also buzzed with scientific and clinical developments, public expectations, national action and financial investments (Gibbon 2008; Hodgson *et al.* 1999; Parthasarathy 2007). BRCA1 and 2 were eventually sequenced in 1995 and 1996, respectively, with Myriad Genetics Inc. winning the patents for both.[3] In fact, although it offered much greater precision, the introduction of BRCA testing in the US and the UK was not entirely novel, as women had long been designated as being at 'high risk' for breast cancer, and familial breast cancer had been a topic of intense research and development for a number of years (Parthasarathy 2007). In contrast, save a few exceptions (e.g., Ottini *et al.* 1999; Pasini and Pierotti 1999), few such linkage studies or risk designations had been institutionalized in practice in Italy, and taking down family histories of breast cancer patients was reportedly an uncommon practice in these early years.

Given the relative dearth of genetic testing activities in Italy, I turned to the European School of Genetics in Italy and from 1996 to 1998 followed the European Union (EU) Demonstration Project on Familial and Hereditary Breast and Ovarian Cancer, which gathered together scientific and clinical leaders from the UK and five other countries (including one person from Italy) (Møller *et al.* 1999; Hodgson *et al.* 1999; Gordon 1999).[4] Simultaneously and intermittently I continued to follow developments in Italy and the US through 2003.[5] Unaware that anyone was being tested in Italy during these early years, I focused primarily on professionals, policymakers and an informal sampling of laypersons, documents and public and professional media.

Some of the unenthusiastic response to these new developments in Italy was aimed at the specific knowledge produced by the new genetic technology and bioscience – genetics was a relatively marginal profession in Italy. Many professionals and laypersons I spoke with questioned whether reliable prediction was in fact possible or credible, and they were less convinced of the power of genes to cause breast cancer. Furthermore, many immediately asked, to what purpose and advantage would knowing one's genetic predisposition serve? There was really nothing to do with that knowledge; there was no real evidence of effective interventions and in any case, a life of worry and intense surveillance is not a life. And prophylactic mastectomy (PM) – carried out in the US since the 1980s (Gifford 1986) and used in the late 90s with 40 per cent BRCA carriers at one centre in Manchester, UK, and another centre in Rotterdam, Netherlands – appeared to be basically unthinkable and ethically unmentionable for many Italian (and French) policymakers and laypersons (Pasini and Pierotti 1999; Eisenger *et al.* 1998; Evans *et al.* 1999; Löwy 2010; Löwy and Gaudillière 1998).[6,7]

As I explored this topic in Italy, the accounts I heard were surprisingly similar to those that colleagues and I had encountered and analysed in earlier ethnographic and quantitative[8] studies of disclosure practices around cancer diagnosis and prognosis in Italy (Gordon 1989, 1990, 1991, 1994; Gordon *et al.* 1990; Gordon and Paci 1997), particularly in contrast to those described in the US (e.g. DelVecchio Good *et al.* 1990, 1994; Gordon and Paci 1997; Orona *et al.* 1994). They were also similar to our findings from studies of the experiences, prevention and risk of breast cancer (Gordon *et al.* 1991; Gordon 1990; Rosselli del Turco *et al.* 1992) and of the end of life and palliative care (Gordon and Peruselli 2001). These accounts described a habitus (Bourdieu 1977)[9] of not telling and not knowing, and they questioned the value of knowing bad news regarding the future, especially if it was felt that little could be done about it. They also expressed great concern over causing worry and a sense of isolation that knowing one's cancer diagnosis could instil and a sense that, if one knows one's cancer diagnosis/prognosis, 'it's as if it's already over.'

Two paradigmatic approches to BRCA testing

New ideas are thought through old ones, writes anthropologist Marilyn Strathern (1992a: 4). As I explore in this chapter, new practices – in this case BRCA testing – are encountered through existing social and cultural backgrounds and habitus. I use the initial encounter with BRCA testing in the mid- to late 1990s in Italy and the US – when impressions were more knee-jerk spontaneous and less meditated, calculated or reasoned than they would become over time – as a point of departure to explore what older shared cultural backgrounds were likely operative and being reproduced in the respective approaches to BRCA testing and prophylactic mastectomy. While the practice of BRCA testing has certainly increased in Italy in the interim years, the relative differences in approaches to future health and life between the US and Italy appear to remain relevant. In this way, I focus less on the emergence of the new genetics – and how they challenged taken-for-granted assumptions before becoming eventually adopted and adapted – and more on how they may enact and reproduce *older* understandings and ways of being (Gibbon and Novas 2008: 4). Thus, while new technologies often challenge older temporalities, they can also produce continuity.

Building on these years of ethnographic research, I explore here the *conditions of possibility* in which the practice of BRCA testing, so important and so awaited in the US, found *relatively* little place in Italian institutionalized medical practices, particularly in the beginning years.[10] I do so by offering a generalized interpretation of one paradigmatic, naturalized logic and response (among others) in Italian practices *in dialogue* with one paradigmatic logic (among others) embedded in the production and enactment of BRCA testing in US institutionalized medical practices. These different logics are grounded in different 'worlds' of background understandings and practices, different ontologies, different habitus and different ways of being-in-the-world. As much as these backgrounds still remain operative in more contemporary approaches to future health and life, even with the greater use of BRCA testing in Italy, I write about these in the present tense.

This dialogue was produced by my tacking back and forth between the two contexts, physically and analytically. This means the two paradigmatic logics are inherently constructed in relation to each other. The goal is to make implicit understandings more visible, not to promote national generalizations. Thus, for narrative purposes, I construct this dialogue *as if* the realities were monolithic, black and white and static, rather than the heterogeneous, interactive, nuanced and diversified realities that they are. Note also that, particularly in the US (Löwy 2010: 180, Dumit 2012: 10), but also to some extent in Italy, these approaches most represent the middle class and above. Finally, while BRCA testing was substantially produced in the US, the actual uptake by individuals and some institutions during the initial period was relatively smaller than expected, albeit often for different reasons than in Italy. To be clear, my focus here is on the institutionalized rather than the individual 'no thanks' to BRCA testing and PM in Italy.

A theoretical framework for describing, interpreting and comparing cultural worlds

The routine description of modern developed societies as 'risk societies' (Beck 1992), in which chance has been tamed, obscures the variation in the prominence of risk discourse and practices in medical and everyday life in the US and Italy as well as in other 'Western' societies. Similarly, the important distinction of women's risk of breast cancer as 'embodied risk' (e.g. Kavanagh and Broom 1998; Lock and Nguyen 2010; Löwy 2010; Lupton 1995; Robertson 2000) can also obscure the different ways that the possibility of developing breast cancer is or is not, in fact, 'embodied', *how* it is 'embodied' and *if* it is understood or experienced in terms of risk.

The interpretive phenomenology of Heidegger (1962, 1975) and Merleau-Ponty (1962), as interpreted by Dreyfus (1991), Taylor (1985, 1988) and Benner (Benner and Wrubel 1989), offers several useful tools to describe and understand such different ways of living the possibility of developing breast cancer, genetic testing and the follow-up options offered. The interpretive phenomenological approach challenges the prevailing Cartesian notion of what it means to be a person as a dichotomy between the world 'out there', the objective world, and the subject who tries to know that world through his or her mind. Seeking a way out of this separation between person and world, Heidegger (1962) and Merleau-Ponty (1962) affirmed that our *natural* way of everyday existing is not as subjects encountering a separate and objective world 'out there', but rather as a unified 'way of being-in-the-world'. The 'in' here refers to involvement, such as 'being-in-love', rather than a spatial 'in'.

'World,' in Heidegger's phenomenological sense, does not refer to the environment or nature or the universe, but rather to 'the meaningful set of relationships, practices and language that we have by virtue of being born into a cultural world'

(Leonard 1994: 46). Think world of medicine or world of breast cancer. World, according to Heidegger, is not what is out there in front of us to see, *world is already there,* beforehand; it is so self evident that we do not even see it (Heidegger 1975). World consists of normative and legitimized *practices* that are learned and reinforced in everyday and biomedical life as skills and know-how, which themselves embody and enact *common understandings* (meanings). These inculcate and are reproduced through habitual predispositions – habitus – which embody taken-for-granted and often unnoticed assumptions. They also account for what 'shows up', for example, as natural, logical, ethical, beneficial or harmful to us. World allows things like genes and breast cancer risk to show up for us as objects. But world also *limits* what can be seen or even noticed, what is existentially possible and what is even 'thinkable' or unthinkable (Strathern 1992b: 33). Thinkability refers to being able to *imagine* doing something, even if one does not actually do it (Dumit 2012: 21), and is thus a useful concept for transcultural comparison.

It takes a lot of 'world' to produce and make sense of BRCA testing. BRCA testing presents a subject's health and future in terms of probability statistics based on a calculation of the subject as a number within a population. This information is abstract and objective, and it proposes a particular way of being-in-the-world – what philosopher Charles Taylor calls 'disengagement' (1988).[11] Disengagement is the basis of objectification – of one's health, one's life, one's future, one's body, one's self – and is becoming a dominant habitus in the US and elsewhere in the world through medical practices such as BRCA testing.[12] It is this disengaged stance that BRCA testing enacts and reproduces. Although once more restricted to science and medicine – we have often distinguished between the 'biomedical' view of cancer and the patient's/layperson's 'common sense view' (e.g. Löwy 2010) – this objective, disengaged stance has been creeping into everyday life and common sense, particularly stimulated by the use of technology and patients' increased role in decision-making. Italian practices support this stance significantly less, as may also be the case with practices that are more commonly found among minority peoples and contexts in the US and elsewhere in the world (e.g. Gibbon *et al.* 2010; Kampriani 2009).

Basic to the different responses to BRCA testing in the US and Italy, I argue, is the relative primacy in everyday and health-related life of these particular ways of being-in-the-world. I am specifically speaking of living one's present and future health more as an objective, anticipatory project to control – in what I am calling a *disengaged-objective-control* approach – as enacted in many medical practices in the US, as opposed to living it more as a relatively embodied, actual situation to adapt to – in what I am calling an *engaged-embodied-adaptation* approach – as appears to be more common in many Italian medical and health practices. These two approaches form part of the *conditions of possibility* for BRCA testing to show up in the particular ways it does.

In fact, the Italy/US dialogue offers a useful glimpse into some naturalized assumptions in biomedicine and social life. Italy presents a good foil for the US for several reasons, including the relative dominance of the Roman Catholic and Protestant religions (both of whose influence awaits serious investigation), a social order influenced by Marxism and weighted more toward collectivity (e.g. a national health care system and a traditionally strong welfare state; Ginsborg 2003; Krause 2005; Molé 2012; Muehlebach 2012), rather than the radical individualism and emphasis on free market neoliberalism and meritocracy in the US, the relative influence of patriarchy vis-à-vis feminism and a significantly smaller economic and social investment in science, biotechnology and genomics in sharp contrast to the political economy of hope offered by new biotechnology in the US (DelVecchio Good *et al.* 1990). However, space limits my focus here to the practices and understandings themselves, and not to the cultural politics of these important contextual influences.

Some conditions of possibility for collective support, or lack of support, for BRCA testing

Below I spotlight and compare a few aspects of the respective worlds embedded in dominant institutionalized approaches in the US and Italy that likely contributed, and continue to contribute, to the respective responses to BRCA testing. Of course, there are not only two worlds operative here. Every institution's descriptor below can be found everywhere, co-existing among people, families, geographies, nations. Many, like the expectations and experiences of control by self and others, are particularly class-biased. I base these interpretations on years of ethnographic studies of my own and by colleagues (e.g. publications by Gordon, Gordon *et al.*, Manca 2006 and Manca *et al.* 2010) in Italy and in the US (e.g. DelVecchio Good *et al.* 1990, 1994; Dumit 2012; Finkler 2000; Haraway 1998; Jain 2013; Kaufman 2010; Löwy 2010; Parthasarathy 2007; Press *et al.* 2000), which will not be restated here.

Condition 1: belief in hereditary breast cancer

Much is made of differences in, and the need for, genetic and medical 'literacy', which are questions of knowledge, of *epistemology*. I propose, however, that perhaps more primary are the differences in the *ontology* of genes, breast cancer risk and hereditary breast cancer that distinguish the US from the Italian medical systems and popular cultures.[13] The enormous investment of US effort and money in technology and bioscience for mapping the human genome, identifying the genes related to breast cancer and designing tests to identify them and interventions to reduce risk have together produced an indubitable sense of the *realness* of hereditary breast cancer. In fact, not just real: as then Director of the Human Genome Project, Francis Collins, explicitly proposed, the dominant model of disease is biological reductionism in which the foundational, ultimately determinative level of truth is biological, in this case molecular (Collins 2010). Furthermore, genes are also proposed as foundational to identity and for defining who *we* are – 'Genes R Us' – who *one* is, and in turn, the basis of biosociality (Rabinow 1992).[14] Parallel to what Gibbon (2008) found in the UK, hereditary breast cancer was of iconic importance.

In contrast to this ultimate material world in the US, many practices and skills in Italy grant the social and immaterial worlds more claim on truth and bottom-line reality. The medical system is more pluralistic, while biomedicine is less hegemonic (Romanucci-Ross 1997; Whitaker 2003). Greater recognition is given to the health impact of social conditions – for example, alienation of labour in the Fordist economy was considered to cause 'social death', and today, 'mobbing' (bullying) in the work place is legally recognized as causing ill health through 'existential damages' (Molé 2012). Furthermore, many practices around ill health and dying use the social context to create and affirm a different social reality than the medically defined one, while others aim at avoiding 'social death' by withholding medical diagnoses and prognoses (Gordon 1990; Gordon and Paci 1997). Finally, identity in Italy is generally defined more in terms of history, residence and family (Krause 2005, Gordon and Manca 2007) than biology, genes and biosociality, as appears to be more common in the US and the UK (e.g. Gibbon and Novas 2008).

Biomedicine also coexists with the power of the church and the *supernatural*, often recognized as an important player in determining reality and truth and thus a limit on how much humans can actually predict what will happen. One hears this in expressions such as 'one never knows' in which the supernatural operates as a type of X-factor, or unpredictable wildcard, and of course in frequent references to God or religion.

One consequence of these different practices and technological biomedical worlds is that, particularly in the early years, hereditary breast cancer had much less reality in Italy. This of course is a two-way process: the lack of material and human resources and infrastructure both reflect and contribute to the concept's not being more fully embraced and accepted as really real and true. Recognizing familial breast cancer may also have been avoided because it locates pathology in the family lineage (Finkler 2000), which, like in France, is central and sacred in Italian life (Rabinow 1999).

Condition 2: risk discourse, ontology and the production of risky bodies

Hereditary breast cancer continues the trend of disembodied definitions of disease.[15] But rather than diagnosing an earlier stage of *disease*, BRCA testing can only 'diagnose' the *probability* of developing the disease within a period of time – as inferred from a genetic mutation – not the *actual* existence of the disease itself. This extends the ubiquitous risk apparatus in the US discourse and practices – an apparatus that constitutes and enacts not only a realness about statistical risk, but often a reification in which risk appears to take on a distinct materiality. Like currency, it is calculated, added, reduced, traded and manipulated; and while proposing only *probabilities*, these too are often concretized, referred to and acted upon as *actualities* or *eventualities*. Furthermore, like in capitalism, time is of the essence and also has a materiality. Finding and acting earlier is considered an unqualified benefit, as is living longer.

As anthropologist Gifford has described it, population and collective risk of breast cancer is typically first individualized, located in a medicalized body and then treated (Gifford 1986). One of the first prescriptions for prevention has always been 'be aware!' – a challenge to an engaged and embodied way of living one's body and health in favour of a disengaged, self-conscious stance. A certain degree of worry and fear is considered necessary and optimal in order for women to monitor themselves (Dumit 2012; Jain 2013), while 'feeling too secure' after a negative test for BRCA, for example, raises concern of complacency. Risk definitions also imply responsibility and accountability (Douglas 1994; Luhmann 1993), and in the US case, this belongs to the individual woman.

This intense focus on the fear of breast cancer and risk in the body threatens to reduce bodies to carriers of pathology, mutations, or faulty genes, in essence, to be inherently ill (Dumit 2012; Fosket 2010; Lock and Nguyen 2010).[16] One exaggerated version is referring to a woman's breasts as 'time bombs' ready to go off (Gifford 1986; Löwy 2010; Parthasarathy 2007) and thus a reason for choosing prophylactic mastectomies. First-hand experience of the deaths of close relatives from breast cancer alone cannot account for women experiencing their breasts this way. Rather, this experience appears to be distinctly, locally and culturally produced (Eisenger *et al.* 1998, 2000; Evans *et al.* 1999; Julian-Reynier *et al.* 2001; Löwy and Gaudillière 1998), and while also not common in the US and the UK, I have never heard similar expressions reported in Italy.[17]

Such risk framing has been practised significantly less in Italy. If risk and probability analyses tame chance, as Hacking famously described (1990), then much chance in Italy remains untamed. Comparatively speaking, risk discourse had not been a familiar or an often used language in clinics, much less in popular media. There was no 'one in nine women' mantra, no litany of 'risk factors' for breast cancer;[18] there was little designation of women as 'low', 'medium' or 'high' risk for breast cancer or 'at risk' for familial breast cancer. Soon after the development of BRCA testing, a national breast cancer professional organization in Italy recommended *against* categorizing women as high risk for breast cancer out of concern for the potential harm such designation could bring – such as the worry on the part of the women involved and the singling out those women as different – without any known benefit (FONCAM 2002). Some breast cancer specialists also expressed concern that learning that one was predisposed to a genetic disease could in fact negatively influence the timing and course of the disease itself – a concern rarely, if ever, heard or seen among US professionals.

Women themselves have expressed strong resentment when being referred to as a 'number' – 'not all people are alike!' (Gordon 1989) – and treatments based on anonymous, objective terms are easily experienced as impersonal and untrustworthy. Not surprisingly, risk – *qua* statistical risk, risk measurements and differentiations – has been, and continues to be, of relatively little interest to many women (and physicians) and of little relevance to their experience (Manca 2013; Manca *et al.* 2009, 2013).

Talking about risk, mentioning it, enunciating it often generates concern that saying so will make it so. This echoed prior concern with communicating a cancer diagnosis and prognosis (Gordon 1990, 1994; Gordon and Paci 1997). Risk, proposed an Italian ethnopsychiatrist, is not just lived by many as a neutral, descriptive statistic that can be manipulated and reduced, but is strongly associated with death (Beneduce 2013).

Encouraging fear is also avoided. In planning publicity for a mammographic screening programme, for example, personnel at the Cancer Centre deliberately proposed having a mammogram as 'doing something good for yourself', while they carefully avoided inciting more fear of breast cancer than the large amount already there. They also did not strongly promote self-monitoring through breast self exams (BSE)[19] or early and frequent mammograms, as has been the enduring US practice (Löwy 2010; Orenstein 2013).

Thus, relative to US practices, the body, and certainly the breasts of Italian women, are less medicalized and 'riskified'. Beauty and seduction are not important 'optionals' for women, nor are they restricted to the young (Crotti 1998, Gundle 2007). They remain fundamental to women's ways of being-in-the-world and to their identity as women for themselves and certainly for men. It is no accident that conservative breast treatment by lumpectomy became standard practice in Italy well before that was the case in the US (Löwy 2010; Veronesi and Zurrida 2009). Also, reportedly, even women who have an operation on a second breast usually have conservative treatment, rather than a mastectomy as is common in the US (Pasini and Pierotti 1999, Tuttle *et al.* 2007, The Hereditary Breast Cancer Clinical Study Group 2008).

Condition 3: temporalities: objectified future versus lived present

Clearly the US and Italy represent very different relations to the past, present and future. Medical and health practices in the US – BRCA testing being exemplary – have typically been directed toward the future. They have been used to anticipate hypothetical scenarios of future risks by probabilistic thinking before taking pre-emptive action to avoid a potential outcome. Such practices present time as linear and as a series of objective 'nows' (Heidegger 1962) rather than as lived time, which is cumulative. Like capitalism, genomics represents an investment in the future (Haraway 1998), fuelled by great hope and expectation of progress.

This hypothetical – this 'what if' and preparing for the worst case scenario – approach in US biomedical practices is found much less in Italy, where worry about what negative things *could* happen is often discouraged: 'Ti fasci la testa prima di romperla!!' ('You bandage your head before you break it!!'). Serenity is highly valued, and worry is considered quite noxious. Thus, one finds an economy of worry. This reflects, on the one hand, an assumption that one need not *look* for problems, they will find you! On the other hand, many feel that we truly do not know what will happen, and that being in a *real* situation is very different from imagining it. We often find resources and possibilities in real situations – situated possibilities (Benner and Wrubel 1989) – that were previously imperceptible and unexpected. 'Aspetta e vedra, tutto andrà bene!' ('Wait, you'll see, things will work out!') is one of many common everyday expressions. Because the other side of the unpredictability of life is that good things can also happen – 'non si sa mai!' ('you never know!'). Miracles do happen, so why ruin the present in anticipation of something that may never happen or will happen no matter what you do? Meet life where it is!

Condition 4: habitus for dealing with future ill health and life

Of the highest priority in this dominant US habitus is that the individual be informed and monitor his or her situation. More knowledge, it is commonly assumed, will reduce uncertainty and bring clarity, empower, offer rational choice and, most importantly, provide the means for controlling the situation. One attraction of BRCA testing for women at high risk, particularly at the beginning, was that it would offer more precise knowledge of their situation, which, even if it entailed bad news, would at least eliminate the uncertainty that many found unlivable. In actuality, such uncertainties were often replaced by others (Lock 1998). Naming, measuring and knowing – through preventive surveillance via frequent exams and monitoring – in themselves seem to offer hope and security but are simultaneously fuelled by the production of fear and the common assumption that knowledge is power and control (Dumit 2012; Jain 2013). In turn, knowing – especially when time is considered to be of the essence – calls for proactive action, epitomized by BRCA testing and PM. Finally, being informed is morally essential for 'taking responsibility for one's health' (Lock 1998; Robertson 2000).

In contrast to this habitus of worry, surveillance, knowledge and proactive action, the more dominant habitus in Italy includes minimizing the situation, not knowing and not telling, conducting exams only when needed, and the frequent use of 'wait and see'. Verbally minimizing a problem and calming someone down has traditionally taken preference to informing them in order to solve a problem. Phrases such as 'non preoccuparti!' ('don't worry!'), 'stai calma!', ('calm down!'), 'Vedrai, non è niente!' ('You'll see, it's nothing!') are automatic, caring responses to someone who has received bad news, but they are also an authority's common response to a person's request for more information. On the other hand, many people say 'meno so, meglio sto' ('the less I know, the better I am') and that they and or family members prefer to 'fare lo struzzo!' ('bury their head in the sand') rather than face difficult realities before they have to (Gordon 1989; Gordon *et al.* 1991). Far from empowering, knowing bad news, such as being a carrier of a genetic mutation, is frequently considered disempowering and unnecessarily harmful by 'taking away hope', especially when 'nothing can be done' (Gordon 1990; Gordon and Paci 1997). The important thing is not so much being informed, but having a health provider you can trust, who knows you and knows what to do for you, as well as having a supportive family (Manca 2013).

Concluding thoughts

Ways of living future health and life: disengaged-objective-control approach versus engaged-embodied-adaptation approach

Is knowing whether one is genetically predisposed to breast cancer better than not knowing, even when nothing can be done about it? Is reducing one's risk of breast cancer through years of intense surveillance compatible with a livable life? Is prophylactic mastectomy, on the one hand, or waiting and seeing, on the other, even thinkable? Part of the answers depend on a person's and a collective's ontology, on their 'natural', habitual ways of being-in-their-worlds – with emphasis on both *ways-of-being* and on *worlds*.

In the paradigmatic US approach, the world, particularly nature and the universe, show up as fundamentally lawful, limitlessly knowable and ultimately controllable (Gordon 1988). Life is full of risks, but they are not inevitable or inherent, and they can and should be identified, explained, reduced or eliminated. We humans can indeed control our individual destinies. The key to this control is to see the world objectively: step out of it, be aware of it, know it and make rational decisions to direct it. This entails disengagement. This belief in our control and in progress provides an implicit background of hope.

Health is health of the body, which is defined by scientifically based, objective abstract notions of 'normal' and 'abnormal'. Health is not a taken for granted, embodied given, it is achieved. It is a project that we are all individually responsible for realizing. Information, surveillance and action are the means for maximizing health and banishing disease. This requires a future orientation that the concept of risk offers. Risk traps chance and danger; probability statistics tame them. To see the world and one's health through risk means to turn objective 'disengaged eyes' onto oneself, one's body and one's future health and see oneself as a statistic. In addition, given the increased identification of new not-yet-but-could-be diseases and processes in our bodies – including BRCA genes – there is always much to monitor.

Many biomedical practices in the US also present future health and life through disengaged lens as something to project, cultivate and author, even by choosing our own longevity (Kaufman 2010). The implicit promise is that, if we follow all the rules, live a 'healthy lifestyle' and fight with great will and courage, we should be able to stave off disease and prolong our lives indefinitely. We expect control, we expect a guarantee.

Different stories, different worlds, different ways of being in the world dominate in Italy. First, nature is orderly, to be sure, but it is not so law-like or very predictable. In fact, life is basically 'an unpredictable stream of events' (Gordon and Paci 1997), and while one may control one thing, another will pop up. For example, upon hearing about prophylactic mastectomies, the director of the Department of Cytology at a major public hospital in Tuscany imagined a woman having a double prophylactic mastectomy then walking out of the hospital and getting hit by a truck!

In fact, it is hubris to think that with our science we humans are capable of completely knowing or predicting, much less controlling, the future. And the idea of the individual, *alone,* controlling one's own destiny – one's life, one's body, one's health – is profoundly foreign. There are always elements of 'predestination' above and beyond science and medicine – not only God, but also networks of family, friends, and alliances – that structure one's choices and ability to cure oneself (Manca 2013).

Furthermore, life presents inherent, non-negotiable limits: at some point we are all going to get sick and we are all going to die. This finitude is not a vague 'maybe' or an abstract truth or a negotiable fact; it is lived as a certainty, grounded in collective and individual histories. In phenomenological terms, it is lived in the background. Knowing that the story ends with death, the space for negotiation lies within that frame, and not precisely knowing one's future and assuming that we cannot know allows that space.

The stance of aggressive surveillance and control, epitomized by proactive management of risk through 'preemptive strikes' such as PMs (Löwy 2010), contrasts with a greater acceptance and cohabitation with uncertainty, risk and death in Italian practices (Paci 2013). Life is to be lived and enjoyed – *engaged* – not managed or problem-solved – *disengaged.* It is more about *dwelling in* life, about *arrangiarsi* ('making do'), than *controlling it,* and these are indeed different phenomenological stances. We need to *care* for our bodies and our health, and we need to *care* for our families and social obligations – take vacations during the summer and days off on the weekend and not be slaves to work and stress – *that's* bad for your health![20] The good life is not translated in the biological; it is not necessarily about living longer. The *kind* and *quality* of future life are fundamental.

Here, the future is not projected as the beacon of hope that is more common in the US (think: The American Dream). It is more about a *practice* of hope that one works at (Mattingly 2010), where hope is a moral requirement to maintain faith. In the final analysis, hope is in social embeddedness and in the security and protection of the family and community (Gordon and Paci 1997). Receiving a diagnosis of cancer, or being told you are at elevated risk, much less a 'carrier of a genetic mutation' – these are not simply technical words that refer to you. Like language in general, these words are lived (Haraway 1998). They invoke, they are embodied and they affect who and how you are. They also have social consequences. They can mark you as different from the rest, even from your family.

* * *

The story I have presented here could have been written in different ways. Instead, I constructed it as a dialogue between two generalized paradigmatic approaches to living future health and life, *as if* they were monolithic and opposites. I did so strategically, because Italy and the US present two extreme positions that make more visible the respective myths, assumptions and possibilities provided within the two worlds.

Even if life is in fact *ultimately* unpredictable, the lack of planning and control practices in Italy produce less control, more unpredictability and more of a 'can't-do' world than is necessary. On the other hand, the many skills and practices aimed at presenting life as truly lawful, knowable and controllable in the US often produce an illusion of control (Finkler 2003) and a tremendous burden on the individual, making illness and death show up not as the inevitable parts of life that they are, but as someone's fault or as a bewildering surprise.

The prevalent biomedical colonialism favours the diffusion of these American biomedical practices and ways of living future health and life through increasingly abstract definitions that depend on technology. As definitions of health and ill health move ever farther away from any embodied sense of health and backward in time to pre-conception, pre-natal, post-natal, pre-disposed, more and more of our lives are being framed in terms of risk and risk reduction. The terrain is very literally endless. There must be resistance to this march against health, and the natural disinclination to join in this march embodied in many Italian professional and popular practices calls for recognition and reflection.

Notes

1. I offer very grateful thanks to the many people who participated in my studies cited here: to my Italian friends/colleagues – Maria-Cristina Manca, Cristiana Giordano, Silvia Camporesi, Roberto Beneduce, Allaman Allamani and Eugenio Paci – who offered insightful answers to my endless questions; to Cristiana and Patricia Benner for their emotional and editorial support; to the organizers and participants of the terrific workshop where this was first presented and discussed; and to the extraordinary editors – Galen Joseph, Sahra Gibbon, and Jessica Mozersky – whose kind support and brilliant editing helped me tame and contain this material.
2. A pseudonym; hereafter referred to as 'the Cancer Centre'.
3. See van Zimmeren *et al.* in this volume.
4. This 'demonstration' project was tasked with developing guidelines and practices for services in the EU (e.g. Møller *et al.* 1999). I attended their biannual meetings, visited clinics and labs and conducted over 20 informal and semi-structured interviews with members and other leaders, participating in five international conferences.
5. From 1996 to 2003 I conducted intermittent and opportunistic observations and interviews in Italy (23) and the US (17) with personnel and laypersons in a range of institutional settings, professional groups, national and international breast cancer meetings, labs and clinics and working groups that directly or indirectly addressed the question of breast cancer risk and genetic testing for breast and ovarian cancer (Gordon 1997, 2000). With a few exceptions, these did not include observations of counselling sessions.
6. Pasini and Pierotti (1999) reported that, as of 1999, no prophylactic surgery appeared to have been performed. To most Italian women, it appeared to be 'over-treatment'.
7. The French in particular expressed resistance to some of these practices (see Eisenger *et al.* 2000, Julian-Reynier *et al.* 2001, Löwy 2010, Löwy and Gaudillière 1998).
8. See Gordon and Paci 1997.
9. Habitual, embodied predispositions.
10. By 1999, genetic counselling on familial breast and ovarian cancer on a research basis had been established in five centres, with another seven in progress (Pasini and Pierotti 1999).
11. Heidegger articulated different ways of being-in-the world. He distinguished between practical, engaged activity, which he considered to be primary ('ready-to-hand' which I call here the *engaged mode*), and a detached and objective mode he considered to be derivative ('present-at-hand' which I call here the *disengaged* mode) (Dreyfus 1991).
12. Disengagement here refers to objectification, not to lack of emotion or caring.
13. Ontology is the study of that which determines entities as entities (Taylor 1988).
14. More recent research has questioned this dominance of the gene (Lock and Nguyen 2010).
15. As opposed to 'embodied' definitions based on patient symptoms and how a person feels.

16. And it begins early: young girls are encouraged to begin BSE after the onset of menstruation (Orenstein 2013).
17. Angelina Jolie's recent piece on prophylactic mastectomy, however, generated pages and pages of discussion in the public media and will likely have an effect (Jolie 2013; Paci 2013).
18. Risk factors explain so little, reasoned the breast cancer specialists at the Cancer Centre.
19. This was based on there being no evidence of the efficacy of BSE, which, in fact, turned out to be the case. A French oncologist told me that BSE was not encouraged in France in order not to put the responsibility on women.
20. Like most of the developed world, Italy has 33 paid vacation/holiday days; the US is the only country with none. Workers in the US reportedly work 260 hours more per year than British workers and 499 more than French workers (Miller 2010).

References

Beck, U. (1992) *Risk Society: Towards a New Modernity.* London: Sage.

Beneduce, R. (2013) *Personal Communication.* University of California, Berkeley: May.

Benner, P. and Wrubel, J. (1989) *The Primacy of Caring: Stress and Coping in Health and Illness.* Reading, MA: Addison-Wesley.

Bourdieu, P. (1977) *An Outline of a Theory of Practice.* Cambridge: Cambridge UP.

Collins, F. (2010) *The Language of Life: DNA and the Revolution in Personalized Medicine.* New York: HarperCollins.

Crotti, N. (1998) *Cancro: Percorsi di cura* (Cancer: Paths to Cure). Rome: Meltemi.

DelVecchio Good, M. J., Good, B. J., Schaffer, C. and Lind, S. E. (1990) 'American oncology and the discourse of hope', *Culture, Medicine, Psychiatry,* 14: 59–78.

DelVecchio Good, M. J., Munakata, T., Kobayashi, Y., Mattingly, C. and Good, B. J. (1994) 'On narrative time', *Social Science and Medicine,* 38, 6: 855–62.

Douglas, M. (1994) *Risk and Blame: Essays in Cultural Theory.* London: Routledge.

Dreyfus, H. (1991) *Being-in-the-World: A Commentary on Heidegger's 'Being and Time, Division I.* Cambridge: MIT Press.

Dulbecco, R. (1997) 'Human Genome Project: Italian contribution. Future directions', *Journal of Cellular Physiology,* 173: 140–3.

Dulbecco R. and Vezzoni P. (1998) 'Il progetto genoma umano', *Le Scienze,* Quaderni-Dossier, Marzo.

Dumit, J. (2012) *Drugs for Life: How Pharmaceutical Companies Define Our Health.* Durham: Duke University Press.

Eisenger, F., Julian-Reynier, C., Sobel, H. et al.(2000) 'Acceptability of prophylactic mastectomy in cancer-prone women', *JAMA,* 283: 202–3.

Eisenger, F., Julian-Reynier, C., Stoppa-Lyonnet, D. et al. (1998) 'Breast and ovarian cancer prone women and prophylactic surgery temptation', *Journal of Clinical Oncology,* 98, 16: 2573–4.

Evans, D.G.R., Anderson, E., Lalloo, F. et al. (1999) 'Utilisation of prophylactic mastectomy in 10 European centres', *Disease Markers,* 15, 1–3: 148–51.

Finkler, K. (2000) *Experiencing the New Genetics: Family and Kinship on the Medical Frontier.* Philadelphia: University of Pennsylvania Press.

———. (2003) 'Illusions of controlling the future: risk and genetic inheritance', *Anthropology and Medicine* 10, 1: 51–70.

FONCAM (Forza Operativa Nazionale sul Carcinoma Mammario) (2002) 'Linee guida: carcinoma eredo-familiare'. www.senologia.it/images/pdf/carcinoma%20eredo-familiare.pdf

Fosket, J.R. (2010) 'Breast cancer risk as disease: biomedicalizing risk'. In Clarke, A.E., Mamo, L., Fosket, J.R., Fishman, J.R. and Shim, J.K. (eds) *Biomedicalization: Technoscience, Health and Illness in the U.S.* Durham: Duke University Press.

Gibbon, S. (2008) 'Charity, breast cancer activism and the iconic figure of the BRCA carrier'. In Gibbon, S. and Novas, C. (eds) *Biosocialities, Genetics, and the Social Sciences: Making Biologies and Identities.* London: Routledge.

Gibbon, S., Kampriani, E. and zur Nieden, A. (2010) 'BRCA patients in Cuba, Greece, and Germany: comparative perspectives of public health, the state, and the partial reproduction of 'neoliberal' subjects', *Biosocieties,* 5: 440–66.

Gibbon, S. and Novas, C. (eds) (2008) *Biosocialities, Genetics, and the Social Sciences: Making Biologies and Identities.* London: Routledge.

Gifford, S. (1986) 'The meaning of lumps'. In Janes, C.R., Stall, R. and Gifford, S.M. (eds) *Anthropology and Epidemiology: Interdisciplinary Approaches to the Study of Health and Disease.* Dordrecht: Reidel Publishers.

Ginsborg, P. (2003) *Italy and Its Discontents: Family, Civil Society, State 1980–2001.* London: Palgrave Macmillan.

Gordon, D.R. (1988) Tenacious Assumptions in Western Medicine. In Lock, M. and Gordon, D.R. (eds) *Biomedicine Examined.* Dordrecht: Reidel Publishing.

———. (1989) '"Vivendo questa nostra storia": la voce delle donne' ('"Living this story of ours": the voice of the women'). In Paci, E. and Venturini, A. (eds) *Dall'esperienza di Malattia Una Nuova Cultura* (*From the Experience of Illness a New Culture).* Florence: La Comune di Firenze e Lega Italiana Contro i Tumori.

———. (1990) 'Embodying illness, embodying cancer', *Culture, Medicine and Psychiatry,* 14: 273–95.

———. (1991) 'Culture, cancer, and communication in Italy'. In Pfleiderer, B. and Bibeau, G. (eds) *Anthropologies of Medicine: A Colloquium on West European and North American Perspectives,* Special Edition of *Curare,* 7: 137–56.

———. (1994) 'The ethics of ambiguity and concealment around cancer: Interpretations through an Italian world'. In Benner, P. (ed.) *Interpretive Phenomenology: Embodiment, Caring, and Ethics in Health and Illness.* London: Sage.

———. (1997) 'Culturally predisposed to testing for genetic predisposition to breast cancer: The role of cultural context', paper prepared for the Stanford White Paper on Genetic Testing for Breast and Ovarian Cancer, Stanford University Center for Bioethics, Program in Genomics, Ethics, and Society.

———. (1999) 'Cultural contexts and familial breast cancer: considerations for non-target populations', paper presented at the conference Familial Breast Cancer: The Problems and the Solutions, Heidelberg, Germany, 27–29 May.

———. (2000) 'Interrogating cross-national differences in prophylactic mastectomy use for women at high risk', American Anthropology Association Annual Meeting, San Francisco, November.

Gordon, D.R. and Paci, E. (1997) 'Disclosure practices and cultural narratives: understanding concealment and silence around cancer in Tuscany, Italy', *Social Science and Medicine,* 44: 1433–52.

Gordon, D.R., Belloni, L. and Allamani, A. (1990) *La Comunicazione con Pazienti con Neoplasia* (Communication with Patients with Cancer). Florence: Regione Toscana.

Gordon, D.R. and Manca, M.C. (2007) 'Producing ethical blood: Encounters of an American apparatus in Tuscany, Italy', paper presented at Genomics and Justice Workshop, Session 1. New Forms of Participation, University of California, Santa Cruz, CA, May.

Gordon, D. and Peruselli, C. (2001) *Narrazione e Fine della Vita: Qualita' della Vita e della Morte* (Narrative and End of Life: Quality of Life and Death). Milan: Franco Angeli.

Gordon, D.R., Venturini, A., Rosselli del Turco, M., Palli, D. and Paci, E. (1991) 'What healthy women in Italy think, feel and do about the prevention of breast cancer', *European Journal of Cancer,* 27: 913–17.

Gundle, S. (2007) *Bellissima: Feminine Beauty and the Idea of Italy.* New Haven: Yale University Press.

Hacking, I. (1990) *The Taming of Chance.* Cambridge: Cambridge University Press.

Haraway, D.J. (1998) *How Like a Leaf: An Interview with Thyrza Nichols Goodeve.* London: Routledge.

Heidegger, M. (1962) *Being and Time, Division I.*, translation by J. Macquarrie and E. Robinson, New York: Harper and Row. (Original work published 1927.)

———. (1975) *The Basic Problems of Phenomenology,* translated by A. Hofstadter, Bloomington: Indiana University Press.

The Hereditary Breast Cancer Clinical Study Group (2008) 'Predictors of contralateral prophylactic mastectomy in women with a BRCA1 or BRCA2 mutation', *Journal of Clinical Oncology,* 26, 7: 1093–97.

Hodgson, S., Milner, B., Brown, I. et al. (1999) 'Cancer genetics services in Europe', *Disease Markers,* 1–3: 3–13.

Jain, S.L. (2013) *Malignant. How Cancer Becomes Us.* Berkeley: University of California Press.

Jolie, A. (2013) 'My medical choice', op-ed in the *New York Times,* 14 May.

Julian-Reynier, C.M., Bouchard, L.J., Evans, D.G. et al. (2001) 'Women's attitudes toward preventive strategies for hereditary breast or ovarian carcinoma differ from one country to another: differences among English, French, and Canadian women', *Cancer,* 92, 4: 959–68.

Kampriani, E. (2009) 'Between religious philanthropy and the individual: situating inherited breast cancer risk in Greece', *Anthropology and Medicine,* 16, 2: 165–78.

Kaufman, S. (2010) 'Time, clinic technologies, and the making of reflexive longevity: the cultural work of "time left" in an aging society', *Sociology of Health and Illness,* 32: 225–37.

Kavanagh, A.M. and Broom, D.H. (1998) 'Embodied risk: my body, myself?', *Social Science and Medicine,* 46, 3: 437–44.

Krause, E. (2005) *A Crisis of Births: Population Politics and Family-Making in Italy.* Belmont, CA: Wadsworth/Thomson Learning.

Leonard, V. (1994) 'A Heideggerian concept of person'. In Benner, P. (ed.) *Interpretive Phenomenology: Embodiment, Caring, and Ethics in Health and Illness.* London: Sage.

Lock, M. (1998) 'Breast cancer: reading the omens', *Anthropology Today,* 14, 4: 7–16.

Lock, M. and Nguyen, V.K. (2010) *An Anthropology of Biomedicine.* London: Blackwell Pub.

Löwy, I. (2010) *Preventive Strikes: Women, Precancer and Prophylactic Surgery.* Baltimore: Johns Hopkins Press.

Löwy, I. and Gaudillière, J.P. (1998) 'Localizing the global: testing for hereditary risks of breast cancer', *Science, Technology and Human Values,* 33: 299–325.

Luhmann, N. (1993) *Risk: A Sociological Theory.* New York: Aldine de Gruyter.

Lupton, D. (1995) *The Imperative of Health: Public Health and the Regulated Body.* London: Sage.

Manca, M.C. (2006) *La Parola Riconosciuta. Storie di Malattia di Donne Operate per Tumore al Seno* (The Recognized Word: Illness Stories of Women Operated for Breast Cancer), Un DVD del Centro Studio Prevenzione Oncologica racconta l'esperienza di 13 donne, *La Nostra Salute,* anno XXIII, Marzo.

———. (2010) *Lingue e linguaggi della prevenzione,* Osservatorio Nazionale Screening, ISPO, USL 4 Prato, Ass. Stenone, LILT, ASF, ITT, Ass. Mediamente, Ass. Mondincontro.

———. (2013) Personal communication.

Manca M. C, Miccinesi G., Susini N. and Paci E. (2013) 'La gestione del follow-up per il tumore al seno' ('The management of follow-up for breast cancer'), *Salute e Territorio,* anno XXXIV, Gennaio-Marzo, 196: 2–8.

Manca, M.C., Susini, N., Miccinesi, G. and Paci, E. (2009) 'La parola riconosciuta. Storie di malattia di donne operate per tumore al seno. Uso e validità del prodotto multimediale' ('The recognized word. Illness stories of women operated for breast cancer: the use and validity of a multi-media product'), *Salute e Territorio,* anno XXX, Maggio-Giugno: 143–46.

Mattingly, C. (2010) *The Paradox of Hope: Journeys Through a Clinical Borderland.* Berkeley: University of California Press.

Merleau-Ponty, M. (1962) *Phenomenology of Perception.* New York: Simon and Schuster.

Miller, G.E. (2010) 'The U.S. is the most overworked developed nation in the world – when do we draw the line?' *20something Finance,* 12 October. Accessed 22 July, 2013. http://20somethingfinance.com/american-hours-worked-productivity-vacation/

Molé, N.J. (2012) *Labor Disorders in Neoliberal Italy: Mobbing, Well-Being, and the Workplace.* Bloomington: University of Indiana Press.

Møller, P., Evans, G., Haites, N. et al. (1999) 'Guidelines for follow-up of women at high risk for inherited breast cancer: consensus statement from the Biomed 2 Demonstration Programme on Inherited Breast Cancer', *Disease Markers,* 15, 1–3: 207–11.

Muehlebach, A. (2012) *The Moral Neoliberal: Welfare and Citizenship in Italy.* Chicago: University of Chicago Press.

Orenstein, P. (2013) 'Our feel-good war on breast cancer', *New York Times Magazine,* 25 April.

Orona, C.J., Koenig, B.A. and Davis, A.J. (1994) 'Cultural aspects of nondisclosure', *Cambridge Quarterly of Healthcare Ethics,* 3, 3: 338–46.

Ottini, L., D'Amico, C., Noviello, C. et al. (1999) 'BRCA1 and BRCA2 gene mutations in Breast/ovarian cancer patients from central and southern Italy', *Disease Markers,* 15, 1–3: 96.

Paci, E. (2013). 'Commenti sull'effetto Jolie' ('Comment on the Jolie effect').

Parthasarathy, S. (2007) *Building Genetic Medicine: Breast Cancer, Technology, and the Comparative Politics of Health Care.* Cambridge: MIT Press.

Pasini, B. and Pierotti, M.A. (1999) 'Familial breast and ovarian cancer: genetic counseling and clinical management in Italy', *Disease Markers,* 15, 1–3: 41–43.

Pierluigi, P. (1995) 'Dulbecco: senza fondi, addio progetto Genoma' ('Dulbecco: without funds, goodbye to the Genome Project'), *Corriere della Sera,* September 9: 10.

Press, N., Fishman, J.R. and Koenig, B.A. (2000) 'Collective fear, individualized risk: the social and cultural context of genetic testing for breast cancer', *Nursing Ethics,* 7, 3: 237–49.

Rabinow, P. (1992) 'Artificiality and enlightenment: From sociobiology to biosociality'. In *Essays on the Anthropology of Reason.* Princeton: Princeton University Press.

———. (1999) *French DNA: Trouble in Purgatory*, Chicago: University of Chicago Press.

Robertson, A. (2000) 'Embodying risk, embodying political rationality: women's accounts of risks for breast cancer', *Health, Risk and Society*, 2, 2: 219–35.

Romanucci-Ross, L. (1997) 'Creativity in illness: methodological linkages to logic and language of science in folk pursuit of Central Italy'. In Moerman, D. and Romanucci-Ross, L. (eds) *The Anthropology of Medicine: From Culture to Method.* Westport, CT: Bergin and Garvey.

Rosselli del Turco, M., Gordon, D. and Venturini, A. (1992) 'Fattori del rischio per tumore al seno: punto di vista delle donne' ('Risk factors for breast cancer: women's perspectives'). In Napoli, R. (ed.) *Ricerca sul Tumore al Seno.* Milan: Masson.

Strathern, M. (1992a) *After Nature: English Kinship in the Late Twentieth Century.* Cambridge: Cambridge University Press.

———. (1992b) *Reproducing the Future: Essays on Anthropology, Kinship, and the New Reproductive Technologies.* New York: Routledge.

Taylor, C. (1985) *Philosophy and the Human Sciences: Philosophical Papers*, vol. 2. Cambridge, UK: Cambridge University Press.

———. (1988) 'A moral topography of the self'. In Messer, S.B., Sass, L.A. and Woolfolk, R.L. (eds) *Hermeneutics and Psychological Theory: Interpretive Perspectives on Personality, Psychotherapy, and Psychopathology.* New Brunswick, N.J.: Rutgers University Press.

Tuttle, T.M., Habermann, E.B., Grund, E.H., Morris, T.J. and Virnig, B.A. (2007) 'Increasing use of contralateral prophylactic mastectomy for breast cancer patients: a trend toward more aggressive surgical treatment', *Journal of Clinical Oncology*, 25, 33: 5203–9.

Veronesi, U. and Zurrida, S. (2009) 'Preserving life and conserving the breast', *The Lancet Oncology*, 10, 7: 736.

Whitaker, E. (2003) 'The idea of health: history, medical pluralism, and the management of the body in Emilia-Romagna, Italy', *Medical Anthropology Quarterly*, 17, 3: 348–75.

Middleword II

Pushing the boundaries

Nina Hallowell

These days, I have less and less time to think. Indeed, I rarely do more than review papers, grants or books, or process emails and memos and attend to other bits of administrative twaddle. For this reason, being asked to read the chapters in this book and to actually think about and comment on them is not only an honour, but also a luxury. So how do these pieces fit together for me? On one very obvious level, the research reported here very clearly and elegantly illustrates the increasing reach of genetics in the twenty-first century. The different chapters describe how genetic testing has come to cut across cultural and national boundaries and, in the process, is changing the ways in which we think about our bodies, identity, health, illness, risk, causation and so forth. At the same time, the contributors to this volume demonstrate how social research on genetic approaches to breast cancer (BRCA genetics) cuts across a number of intellectual and disciplinary boundaries. This is indeed a multidisciplinary collection. However, for me, the most important thing about this book is how the authors play (directly and indirectly) with the notion of categorization. This collection demonstrates not only how different cultural contexts have come to alter the ways in which BRCA identities are taken up or played out, but also how the practices of breast cancer genetics are problematizing some discrete categories and, as a result, are eroding or blurring some relatively entrenched dichotomies, such as traditional and modern (Macdonald, this volume), social and material (Pelters, this volume), individual and group (Mozersky and Gibbon, this volume), research and care (Lee, this volume), genetic and nongenetic (Bourret, Keating and Cambrosio, this volume).

In this commentary, or middleword, I will reflect on the extent to which having a family history of cancer and/or carrying a gene mutation has come to level and define individuals and groups during the early twenty-first century. I will concentrate my comments on Sections I and II, because many of the chapters in these sections can be read as primarily focusing on the impact of BRCA genetics on identity. These contributions focus on the intersection between material and social bodies and demonstrate how social identity may (or may not) be understood as forged in, and by, the identification and management of material risks that emanate within the body (genome). In addition, these contributions emphasize the temporal nature of genetics, showing us the ways in which material risks in the molecular present are mobilized to make identity claims about the genealogical past and/or the future person.

Genealogical practices

Pelters' contribution demonstrates how the adoption of a BRCA identity can be experienced as empowering, because it allows women to challenge heterosexist assumptions about the nature of femininity. She argues that BRCA risk-management practices – risk-reducing mastectomy and oophorectomy – are consistently portrayed in a negative light within the biomedical literature. According to Pelters, biomedicine depicts oophorectomized or mastectomized women as incomplete – hence, the existence of a number of replacement technologies – breast reconstruction, oestrogen replacement therapy, IVF, oocyte freezing – all of which, if deployed, enable women to re-create or rebuild themselves as a 'proper' woman.

Drawing on a small number of case studies of BRCA-positive women, Pelters demonstrates that women's identities are impacted in complex ways by the identification of BRCA risk status and subsequent risk management. However, in contrast to biomedical discourses, she shows that risk-reducing surgery can be experienced positively – as liberating women from their material bodies, and as enabling them to challenge and redefine gendered norms. BRCA risk management, it is argued, provides women with (a feeling of) agency; rather than risk-reducing surgery being experienced as necessarily resulting in a loss of femininity, it enables women to gain control of their bodies and actively participate in the construction of an alternative (gendered) identity. Thus, for Pelters, the management of material risks can be experienced as existentially liberating, for it enables gene carriers to engage in positive identity management.

MacDonald's ethnography of breast cancer patient activist groups in Mumbai paints a much more negative picture of the adoption of an at-risk identity. She notes that, although there is an emphasis on preventative medicine in India, familial cancer services and opportunities to access BRCA testing are limited. However, while the uptake of BRCA testing may not be widespread, knowledge about breast cancer risks, in a more generic sense, is extensive. MacDonald describes how lay knowledge of cancer is underpinned by a lay epidemiology in which a number of causes of breast cancer are identified – including familial, but not necessarily genetic, transmission. She argues that these aetiological explanations not only impact the uptake of BRCA testing, but also on the ways in which cancer risks are, or can be, incorporated into identity. To be confirmed as at risk of breast cancer is not seen as liberating (see Pelters) in this case, but as deeply problematic, because being identified as belonging to a family that contains breast cancer in this cultural context is potentially stigmatizing. Cancer spoils family identity and thus family members' social possibilities. Bearing this in mind, it is suggested that the adoption of an at-risk identity can be actively resisted.

While aetiological explanations that situate risks within the familial body may be resisted in India, lifestyle explanations of breast cancer risk, in contrast, are actively propagated. Macdonald argues that that the emphasis on breast cancer prevention and lifestyle risks (including hormonal and reproductive risks, diet and lack of exercise) can be seen as part of an ongoing commentary about the nature of women's changing role within Indian society. Framing breast cancer risk in this way locates breast cancer as a disease of modernity – a disease that is associated with urban/modern rather than rural/traditional lifestyles. Prevention discourses construct urban migration and the adoption of an urban lifestyle as risky. Risk, according to this narrative, derives from the adoption of a modern lifestyle or the relinquishing of traditional gender roles within Indian society.

Pelters's and MacDonald's research shows how the material body affords the possibility of different social identities. Their work also beautifully illustrates the context-dependent nature of the construction of different at-risk identities. For Pelters, the management of bodily risks results in existential liberation – the chance to adopt a BRCA identity that challenges oppressive social constraints. In contrast, MacDonald shows how the increasing modernization in India has meant that women's social mobility is seen as threatening the status quo, with the result that their lifestyle is reconstructed as the catalyst for personal material decline. That the uptake of particular BRCA identities is influenced by political, cultural and social factors is explored further in Section II, which focuses on research that looks at the interplay between molecular genetics and group identity.

Practices of population

Genetics transcends time by exposing origins, defining existence and revealing potentialities. The social meanings of genetic testing in terms of the interplay between past, present and future and individual and collective identities is very elegantly demonstrated in this section in the juxtaposition of Joseph's, Mozersky and Gibbon's and zur Neiden's contributions.

Joseph's chapter focuses on a public health initiative for African American women in the US, the Family History Project (FHP), which has been set up to tackle health inequalities and disparities in the uptake of BRCA testing. One of the official aims of the FHP is to more effectively target technology by identifying at-risk women who meet the criteria for BRCA testing/counselling – women who currently have little or no access to these forms of healthcare. To achieve this, the FHP runs education workshops in African American churches that help women to learn to analyse their family history, so that they may come to identify themselves as at risk of breast cancer. The project therefore starts from a premise that risk management involves self-management, and Joseph notes that this process of biosocialization is underpinned by discourses of responsibility and empowerment.

The FHP is, as its name suggests, oriented toward the past. This historical focus is, of course, typical of the approach adopted in clinical genetics, which constructs at-risk identity on the basis of historical excavations of the molecular past as inscribed in medical records, familial memory or the ordering of base pairs. However, as Joseph notes, the adoption of a historical focus in the FHP is not just confined to biology, but is interpreted more widely by workshop participants.

She observed that the real-life case studies and materials used in the training workshops were frequently interpreted as examples of discriminatory practices in health care. Indeed, social discrimination often became the focus of discussion. The FHP workshops, it would appear, are not just raising awareness of the importance of individuals' molecular history, but are also highlighting the socio-political past of this ethnic group.

The influence of social history on genetic explanations is also the focus of zur Neiden's chapter, in which she discusses the influence of political history on the practice of clinical genetics in modern Germany. She argues that the molecular past is not so much an unknown territory within the German clinic, but a forbidden one. BRCA genes in Germany exist in the present, revealing individuals' futures; and while the genealogical past may indeed be important in predicting the genetic future, it remains off limits.

Mozersky and Gibbon, in contrast, emphasize the importance of the genealogical past for the practice of cancer genetics in the UK and Brazil. They demonstrate the roles played by the historical narratives of ethnic group membership or migration patterns in the practice and/or development of genetics in these locations. Thus, in the UK, Ashkenazi Jewish ethnicity is used as a surrogate genetic marker or risk factor for carrying particular types of BRCA mutations – thus, Jewish ethnicity is used to determine access to particular types of BRCA tests. In this case, social identity can be seen as channelling, or defining, the strategy for uncovering material risks. However, this relationship is not exactly linear, for, as Mozersky notes, although social identity and material identity are elided within the discourse of the clinic in the sense that ethnicity is reduced to the probability of carrying material risks, the actual identification of these risks through molecular testing is itself used to reconfirm and thus essentialize a socio-historical narrative or identity. In other words, ethnicity becomes 'biologized' by BRCA testing, and cancer risk, as defined by the presence of particular mutations, in turn becomes socialized.

Gibbon demonstrates that BRCA testing plays a similar, but contrasting, role within Brazilian clinics. She shows how, in an effort to expedite cost-effective BRCA testing, the search for founder BRCA mutations in Brazil has impacted the social identity of patients with a family history of breast cancer. In contrast to clinics in the UK, it is not ethnicity, or migration narratives, that drive the excavation of material risks in the Brazilian clinic; rather, the identification of particular BRCA mutations – i.e. the identification of material risk – is interpreted as evidence of a particular social history. Thus, in Brazil, genetic testing, or the identification of a particular material form, gives rise to a particular social identity, or at least provides the conditions for the construction of particular identities and migration narratives.

Reflections on BRCA research and medical practices

The chapters contained in the first two sections of this book illustrate the complex relationship that exists between the material and social body and emphasize the fluid and dynamic nature of these categories. This emphasis on fluidity, on pushing the categorical boundaries, is carried forward in the final section, which demonstrates that some of our most cherished boundaries, such as the boundary between research and clinical care, or genotype and phenotype, are less relevant when confronted by developments in genetics and genomics. However, for me, the real issue emerging from my reading of this book is not the dynamic and fluid nature of the ways in which we categorize the world, but its complexity. In order to contextualize this statement, I am going to finish my commentary with some personal reflections.

Reading this book has reminded me of when I gave my first-ever conference paper nearly twenty years ago. The time was 1996, the place Johannesburg. The weather was hot, the country full of hope, the city exciting, if a little bit scary. The people who attended the conference were great. We had, as you often do at conferences, a bit of a wild time. The intellectual focus of the proceedings was postmodern approaches to the body, and I had submitted a paper discussing risk management for hereditary breast and ovarian cancer – more specifically, the perceived impact of risk-reducing surgery on women's lives. I wanted to draw attention to the complexities of living with and managing genetic risk – as I saw them, and as the women I interviewed experienced them. I was, in reality, on a mission to defend gender identity, to protect women's healthy bodies from over-medicalization and to interrogate the intersection between material and social bodies. I had the most perfect opportunity to do this in front of a very sympathetic audience – the planets seemed perfectly aligned for my first foray into paper-giving. But as I took to the stage at Wits University, slightly trembling, I became acutely aware of the topic of my research and where I was standing. Here I was about to talk about the impact of high-technology medicine – breast cancer genetics – in a country where clean running water was a luxury, where many girls died long before they developed breasts and where most women could not access breast screening, let alone DNA screening. Standing there, in post-apartheid South Africa, I realized that the battle I had opted to fight did not rate as even a minor skirmish in the war against disease that existed in Africa at that time, and indeed is still being waged today. I stood there feeling uncomfortably embarrassed, thinking: why am I talking about this subject, in this place, at this time? Twenty years later, I am still acutely aware that only the very privileged few can hope to access BRCA testing. However, after reading this book, I am more convinced of the importance of social research in this area, for, as this collection of papers demonstrates, the development and use of genetic technologies over the last two decades in very different corners of the globe raises a number of important and challenging questions about the nature of our world and our place within it. But that is enough from me, for Section III beckons.

Section III

Shifting terrains of BRCA knowledge and practices

7 ‘Empowerment’ and the rendering of biocapital in direct-to-consumer personal genomics

Sandra Soo-Jin Lee

For over a decade, since the completion of the Human Genome Project, the scientific community has predicted an imminent era of personalized medicine.[1] In 2008, LeRoy Hood, a well known systems biology scientist involved in the discovery and commercialization of automated gene sequencing techniques, predicted that ‘a paradigm shift in medicine will take place, replacing the current approach, which is predominantly *reactive,* to one that can increasingly predict and prevent cellular dysfunction and disease’ (Hood and Galas 2008). The emphasis here is on knowledge as a powerful form of intervention – eradicating a disease before it has become one. Hood and his colleagues asserted that the next 10–15 years will be characterized by ‘a predictive medicine capable of determining a probabilistic, individualized future health history.’ Personalized medicine would become ‘P4 medicine’: ‘predictive’, ‘personalized’, ‘preemptive’ and ‘participatory’ (Hood and Galas 2008).

While the first three P’s focus on the clinical promises of personalized medicine, the fourth P, ‘participatory’, suggests a new biomedical regime characterized by a reconfiguration of stakeholders into new social formations around scientific discovery and translation. Hood and Gallas (2008) predict this shift will ‘empower and activate patients’ and ‘shift behaviour from “system” to “individual responsibility” ’. With the explicit goal of making the US the healthiest nation in the world, a participatory turn reflects the need for ‘systematic coordination among key stakeholders’ in ‘optimizing the interactions of the complex network of interacting healthcare constituents’ (Hood and Gallas 2008: 3). Making plain the convergence of high-throughput technology and gene sequencing, ubiquitous Internet connectivity and the corporatization of wellness in the US, Hood and Gallas frame the realization of personalized medicine in moral terms of individual action and social problem-solving that relies on the labour and the self-disciplining practices of individual citizens (Heath *et al.* 2004; Rose 2007). Such framings have contributed to the commodification of genetic risk as intricately tethered to not only one’s management of health, but also to one’s participation in research.

The discovery of and efforts to capitalize on BRCA mutations is an informative case study for understanding how evolving social relations around genetics are imbricated with concepts of individual responsibility, scientific efficiency and the centrality of the market. This chapter probes the coalescence of relationships around BRCA mutations in order to understand the construction of personalized medicine and its impact on the role of key stakeholders in the genome research pipeline. The focus is on the tropes of freedom and empowerment, which are emblematic of the direct-to-consumer (DTC) personal genomics marketplace in the US and the simultaneous elision of individual labour in the development of personalized medicine. I discuss the increasingly explicit reframing of patients into consumers in the targeted commercialization of genetic testing and sequencing. This shift asserts that individual freedom is realized through the act of consumption and the expectations that the public will incorporate information into workable knowledge in managing one's health (Henneman *et al.* 2004). Genetic testing for BRCA mutations is born of the 'knowledge economy' (Brown 2003: 5, Delvecchio Good *et al.* 1990) that builds on expectations that are loaded with value and are tradable. The basis of exchange relationships among consumers who congregate virtually and otherwise become 'communities of promise' reflects the inherent asymmetries between individuals and groups in their access to information. DTC genomics is only possible within this landscape of expectations and biocapital.

In this chapter, I draw on a four-year ethnographic study of personal genomic testing to describe the shift toward the idea of 'participatory' that defines new biosocial alignments between social actors in harnessing and transforming genomic data into biocapital. This study included in-depth, open-ended interviews with consumers and producers of DTC personal genomic testing services, extensive literature research and participant observation of meetings, hearings and online exchanges. Drawing on these data, this chapter discusses how these new alignments render the boundaries separating the categories of patients, consumers and research participants increasingly porous, blurring burdens of responsibility – specifically the responsibility owed to individual actors whose consumption of, donation to and trust in the promise of bioscience fuels the ever-imminent, ever-elusive era of personalized medicine. DTC personal genetic testing is an inevitable outgrowth of the race toward personalized medicine, putting in even more uncertain terms the ambiguous relationship between the individual and biomedical enterprise. As Helmreich's taxonomy of theories on biocapital suggests (2008), the biocapitalization of genetic data through genetic testing decouples the individual from her DNA through an ironic exercise of individual 'freedom'. Consumption and production become entangled, as individual biomaterial is transformed or rendered into biocapital. In describing the current historical context of regulatory struggles over gene patents and the elision of value attributed to individual DNA as necessary capital in the personal genomics marketplace, this chapter engages with the promissory framing of DTC personal genomics while accessing the meaning of 'participatory' in personalized medicine in the US.

Patents, promises and regulatory practice

In triumphant language, *New York Times* science writer Natalie Angier reported a major development in research on breast cancer nearly two decades ago. She wrote: 'Capturing a genetic trophy so ferociously coveted and loudly heralded that it had taken on a near-mythic aura, a collaborative team of researchers has announced the discovery of a gene whose mutation causes hereditary breast cancer' (Angier 1994: 1). The motif of the 'race' has been a hallmark of the history of the genome sciences ever since, beginning with the victory officially bestowed to James Watson and Francis Crick for their discovery of the double helical structure of DNA in 1953 to the more recent race to complete the Human Genome Project between the publicly funded National Institutes of Health's (NIH) scientific team and private efforts led by Craig Venter at Celera Genomics, Inc. The race to discover BRCA mutations continues this tradition, but it also reflects an emerging model of networked science that has been deemed necessary for population genomics research. Led by a team of 45 scientists from the University of Utah; the National Institute of Environmental Health Sciences in North Carolina's Research Triangle Park; Myriad Genetics, Inc in Salt Lake City and several other institutions, the discovery of BRCA mutations and its translation into diagnostic tools could only occur through a complex network of public and private collaborations.

The initial discovery of BRCA1 involved the investigation of the genetic patterns of inheritance in large families, mostly Mormon families in Utah, in which many relatives suffered from breast and/or ovarian cancer. One of the leading scientists in the discovery of both the BRCA1 and BRCA2 genes, Mark Skolnick, founded Myriad Genetics, a biopharmaceutical and genomics company, to develop a diagnostic test for the mutations. His company applied for, and was granted, patents for how the genes could be used. The broad language of these patents gave Myriad tight control over how, and whether, researchers and clinical practitioners could study and test patients for the mutations. Until recently, Myriad has vigorously and successfully enforced its patent rights on BRCA genes in the US. The result is that all hospitals and health insurance plans have been required to purchase Myriad's test as a means of its establishing the company's complete control of the US BRCA testing market (Borger 1999, Murray 1999).

The result of the Myriad patents is that competition has been stifled and Myriad has been allowed to effectively set the price for its test without market pressure. In 1996, Arupa Ganguly, a researcher at the University of Pennsylvania who had developed a test for mutations associated with breast cancer that was funded and approved by the National Cancer Institute (NCI), received a cease-and-desist letter from Myriad for patent infringement. Deterred by the high cost of bringing the case to court, the university's lawyers decided not to challenge the claims, although Myriad's patents had been overturned in Europe and several legal experts had argued that they failed to stand up on appeal. After Ganguly's incident, the NIH signed a licensing agreement with Myriad, allowing NCI to continue genetic testing, but requiring the institute's researchers to send all test samples to Myriad's Utah lab for analysis. Women who would have been charged \$1,600 by Ganguly's lab were immediately forced by Myriad to pay approximately \$2,400. Currently, the test costs more than \$3,000.

In her detailed comparative analysis, Parthasarathy (2011) discusses how BRCA diagnostic testing has unfolded differently in the American and British contexts. She argues that patent protection has allowed Myriad to dominate the market for the genetic testing for the mutations, which has ultimately proved too costly for many women and prevented much needed confirmatory testing. In contrast, Parthasarathy describes how control over access to testing by the National Health Service in the UK has allowed for an integrated approach to counselling, testing and interpreting genetic information, which has resulted in cost-effective, preventive care. Although the comparison between the two countries' approaches can be overstated, the US commercialization of the test has catalyzed a maelstrom of controversy and accusations of corporate profiteering at the expense of women's health.

Recently, the validity of the Myriad patents has come under increasing legal pressure. In 2009, the American Civil Liberties Union (ACLU) filed the lawsuit *Association for Molecular Pathology, et al. v US Patent and Trademark Office, et al.* on behalf of researchers, genetic counsellors, women patients, cancer survivors, breast cancer and women's health groups and scientific associations representing 150,000 geneticists, pathologists and laboratory professionals. The lawsuit charges that patents on human genes violate the First Amendment and patent law because genes are 'products of nature' and therefore cannot be patented.

In 2010, a New York federal court ruled that the patents on the BRCA1 and BRCA2 genes were invalid. The US Court of Appeals for the Federal Circuit heard Myriad's appeal and ruled that companies can obtain patents on the genes, but were prohibited from patenting methods to compare those gene sequences. In March 2012, the US Supreme Court vacated the decision of the appeals court and instructed the court to reconsider the case in light of *Mayo v Prometheus,* a Supreme Court decision unanimously invalidating patents on algorithms and methods for evaluating a patient's drug response. In August 2012, the divided federal appeals court ruled 2–1 for the second time that companies can obtain patents on the genes, but it invalidated patents on methods to compare those gene sequences. In September 2012, the plaintiffs again asked the US Supreme Court to rule on the patentability of genes, and in November 2012, the Supreme Court granted the plaintiffs' cert petition and agreed to hear arguments during the current session on the patentability of human genes.

At the time of writing this chapter, the Supreme Court has heard arguments on April 15, 2013, and a ruling is expected in the summer of 2013. If the court rules in favour of the plaintiffs, BRCA mutation testing could become immediately more widely available at a lower cost, allowing for DTC personal genomics companies like 23andMe to include these tests in services without threat of patent violation. However, Myriad's patents for BRCA tests are set to expire in 2015. As a precedence-setting case, the ruling will determine whether or not genetic diagnostic testing will be patent-protected in the future, which could dramatically impact the commercial strategies for developing services and products for personalized medicine (see van Zimmeren *et al.* in this volume).

Market solutions and the elision of individual capital

In his book *Biocapital: The Constitution of Postgenomic Life,* Rajan (2006) argues that new capitalist practices are emerging from regulatory practices that allow the holding of intellectual property in biological matter and knowledge. The Myriad case is a pivotal one, emblematic of the practices described by Rajan. Even the challenge against Myriad by the ACLU does little to undermine the corporate translation of biomaterial into biocapital. This case reveals a powerful framing of the relationship between genes, disease and access and makes plain the primacy of the market for personalized medicine.

For the ACLU, market monopolization and limited access to the test has become a focal point of critiques aimed at the legitimacy of patenting genes. Under the title and banner of 'Liberate the breast cancer genes' (2010), the ACLU made a short video, describing the stakes of the Myriad lawsuit. In the film, breast cancer patient Lizbeth Ceriani, a European American woman, is filmed in her house where her young daughter skips busily from room to room. She describes her struggle: 'As a single mother, I'd like to see my daughter go off and graduate from college. The government created this monopoly by giving Myriad the patents in the first place. I don't know what they are thinking.' The government, implicated in this video for its role of issuing patents to Myriad, is seen as a barrier to a free market. The argument presented by the ACLU through Ceriani is an unabashedly economic one: that market competition is necessary for public access to genetic testing through competitive pricing. Uncontested by the ACLU is any questioning of the ultimate benefit of genetic testing for consumers such as Ceriani. Recent critiques of recommendations for PSA screening for prostate cancer and the use of mammography for breast cancer question the clinical utility and the potential harm of early risk assessment (Carter *et al.* 2013, Orenstein 2013). The free market solution focuses the discourse on the appropriate role of governmental regulation by protecting the commercial development of genetic data rather than engaging in a debate on the putative common good of the increased availability of genetic testing.

Federal investment in genomic science and translational medicine continues to rise, even in the context of a struggling economy and decreased overall funding of research. The infrastructure for a genomic highway, paved by the integration of electronic medical records and institutional biobanks, is made possible only through private and public partnerships that rely on the commercialization of genetic data. Myriad is an early actor in this triumvirate of government, private industry and the public, and it defends its patent by citing the high cost of development that went into the research of BRCA1 and BRCA2 and the resources needed to create a diagnostic test. In his presentation for the National Academies of Science, William Rusconi, vice president of marketing at Myriad, cited that the development of their genetic test resulted from approximately $7 million in funding. Using the figure below, Rusconi identifies the key stakeholders in the development of their BRCA genetic test as well as the public and private funding streams that support the pipeline. Rusconi uses the diagram to make the point that the production of genomic technologies is dependent on a complex network of academic institutions and companies who provide public and private funding in return for property rights, which are leveraged as future returns dependent on patent licenses.

Missing among the stakeholders listed in the figure is the role of the individual patients who have donated their genetic samples for research. Critical questions,

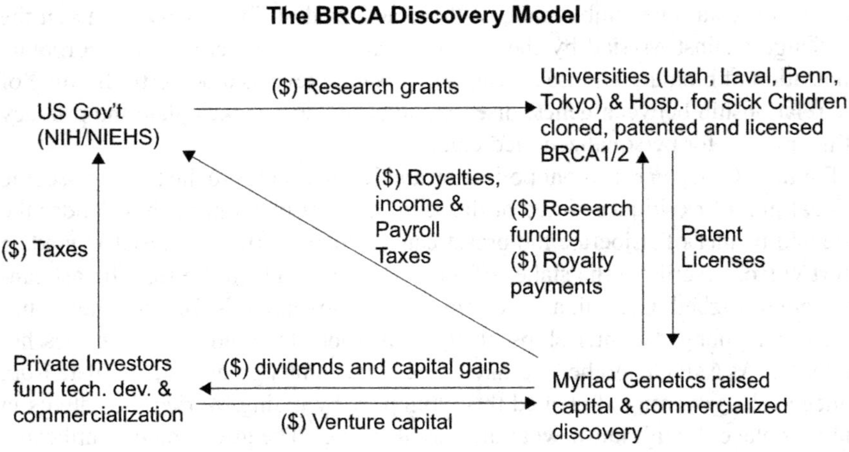

Figure 7.1 BRCA Discovery Model

Source: Rusconi, 11 February, 2005.

such as how does the accumulation of individual DNA create capital for the pipeline of potential therapeutics and diagnostic tools, and how are these contributions accounted for and compensated in the flow of knowledge and benefits, remain unanswered. Biocapital in the form of DNA samples from individual customers may be integral, but it is rendered invisible in the modelling of gene discovery.

Rusconi's claims that the downstream contribution of their test is an increased awareness of genetic services and, ultimately, improved healthcare for the general population seem misplaced in light of testimonials offered by women like Ceriani. Diagnosed with bilateral stage IIA breast cancer in 2008, Ceriani describes not being able to pay for BRCA testing. 'I don't even have a credit card with a limit of $3,000 that I could just charge and have it be done.' The theme of monopolization is resonant throughout the testimonials offered by the ACLU as the basis for the lawsuit against Myriad. Governmental actors and the political economy in which patents on genetic tests function have prevented patients from accessing potentially actionable genetic information. Ceriani explains the constraints of the system, stating:

> My health insurance is MassHealth, a form of Medicaid. The Massachusetts Office of Health and Human Services (MOHHS), which oversees the Medicaid plans in the state, has confirmed in writing that I do have coverage for BRCA genetic testing at 100% with no prior approval *if* the test is performed by a contracted provider. There is only one lab in the country that performs BRCA genetic testing, Myriad Genetic Laboratories in Utah. MOHHS told me that Myriad will not sign a contract with my insurance, because it believes the reimbursement level is too low. The BRAC Analysis test costs $3,225. MassHealth would pay half, $1,599.
>
> (ACLU 2010)

In a system where reimbursement schedules cover only a portion of the price tag for personalized medicine (Kieran *et al.* 2007), Ceriani's plight seems to be evidence of economic disparities that accrue when expensive genomic technologies are out of reach for the majority of the relevant public. These diagnostic interventions are introduced in a landscape where economic disparities map onto health disparities. Deference to the potential of technical innovation and faith in the free market to develop and then make good on investment through patent-regulated bioscience can only foreshadow the further entrenchment of these vital differences. Models for gene discovery build on the biosocial alignment between patients and commercial entities, where DNA is culled without reciprocity and expensive healthcare problems are addressed through market solutions.

The ACLU video describing the case against Myriad attempts to shift the focus toward the individuals who are shut out of these market solutions by making the point that the patents not only prevent access to testing and to the information that would allow women like Ceriani to make a choice, but it also prevents further research that could be helpful to minority populations. The turn toward arguments of social justice is a strategic framing of patents as dampening much needed research and development. Citing that most of the research on BRCA mutations was conducted on white women, the ACLU argues that the variants of BRCA could have unknown significance for minority women. That both BRCA1 and 2 mutations were discovered, in part, by mining the detailed genealogical records of large Mormon (predominantly white) families with a high incidence of breast and ovarian cancer is a result of the historically embedded research practices that have focused on white Americans and the opportunistic sampling strategies that have informed who participates in research. However, the ACLU's suggestion that Myriad's patent licenses prevent research on minority populations is misleading and places greater faith in the market than is warranted. The sampling of minority populations remains a challenge in both publicly and privately funded research, and there are few indications that patents are the major barrier to achieving a greater diversity of samples. There is little evidence that research of minority populations has been more successful for non-patented mutations associated with known diseases. Beyond the arguments presented by the ACLU, the larger question of whether more genetic testing (and the significant investment in research and development it requires) will lead to improved public health remains largely ignored in the assessment of the potential harm of patenting genes.

Selling empowerment through DTC genomics

In 2011, Marsha, a 27-year-old yoga instructor living in Boston, received a text from her older sister Stacey: 'New gene test. Check it out.' Underneath was the URL for the website of 23andMe, a direct-to-consumer (DTC) personal genetic testing company based in Silicon Valley. Marsha recounted that she knew immediately what her sister was suggesting. Their grandmother had died of breast cancer and an aunt had recently been diagnosed with ovarian cancer. The sisters had been worrying together about their risk for the diseases[2] and had even discussed the idea of being tested for the BRCA genetic mutations that their aunt had been discovered carrying. Logging on to the 23andMe website, Marsha was surprised by the simplicity of the process. She was told to send a saliva sample to the company lab and within weeks she would know whether she had the mutations. Marsha described the decision as a 'no brainer': 'No doctors. No medical record. No hassle. It seemed the responsible thing to do. You know, to find out and then I could plan to do something.' She explained, 'I just don't want to have to keep wondering. And, the test – what $99? – that was cheap. I could even afford that.' Marsha purchased the 23andMe test, and 10 days later she logged on to her account to see her results. She recalled being surprised at the sheer number of results – over two hundred – and quickly scanned over the list in search of her breast cancer risk results. She clicked through to get past the series of questions intended to ensure she really wanted to know her results. Holding her breath, she was relieved to find the following statement at the bottom of her technical report page: 'No copies of the three early-onset breast and ovarian cancer mutations identifiable by 23andMe.' Marsha remembered the moment of relief, saying: 'If this is personalized medicine, then definitely sign me up.'

The first wave of DTC genetic testing companies was launched in 2007 and 2008 to much fanfare, offering consumers personal genetic information related to ancestry, disease risk, carrier status and drug response. At a time when political forums in the US are dominated by debates about the need to reform the healthcare system, companies are promoting their genomic products by building on the hype of revolutionary advances in medical care (Williams-Jones 2006, Williams-Jones and Burgess 2006). Unlike Myriad, companies like 23andMe challenge the traditional flow of medical information and question the role of physicians and other healthcare providers as gatekeepers to genetic information. In fact, the DTC genetic testing model departs from professional guidelines, such as those offered by the American Society of Clinical Oncology (ASCO) (U.S. Preventive Services Task Force 2005; Statement of the American Society of Clinical Oncology 1996), which recommends that cancer predisposition testing be offered only in cases when: 1) the person has a strong family history of cancer or very early age of onset of disease, 2) the test can be adequately interpreted and 3) the results will influence the medical management of the patient or family member. Products offered by DTC genetic testing companies challenge any need to provide elevated risk information as justification for genetic analysis. Instead, companies assert that genetic information should be freely available to individuals as a matter of principle.

Concerns about the potential for psychological harm have been levied by critics of the DTC personal genomic industry. The impact of genetic testing of known disease mutations is unclear. However, given the practice of prophylactic mastectomy and oophorectomy, BRCA testing presents unique challenges. In a study conducted by Lynch *et al.* (2006) on the psychological impact on women who underwent BRCA diagnostic testing, they reported that 23 per cent of women with a positive family history but without genetic results underwent prophylactic bilateral mastectomy, oophorectomy or both. Of these, 53 per cent were subsequently found to be mutation-negative on confirmation. In comparison, none of the women who had a history of breast cancer in their family and tested negative for the mutations underwent prophylactic surgeries. Psychologically, a significantly higher percentage of carriers, regardless of their cancer status, felt guilt compared with non-carriers without cancer about passing a mutation on to their children and worried about developing cancer or their children developing cancer.

Acknowledging the seriousness of these concerns, 23andMe conducted their own in-house study of their customers and published the results in an article entitled 'Dealing with the unexpected: consumer responses to direct-access BRCA mutation testing' (2013). The small qualitative study reports that 11 women and 14 men without a known family history of breast cancer received positive results of having BRCA1 or BRCA2 mutations. The study stated that most carriers engaged in further testing and over 60 per cent of the women had elected or planned to have prophylactic mastectomy and oophorectomy procedures.

Despite the broad range of reactions and decisions made by their customers in response to their mutation test results, the authors conclude that none of their participants reported extreme anxiety, and only four experienced moderate anxiety that was transitory. The authors emphasize that five women and six men described their response as 'neutral', although they offer little explanation of what neutral means. Instead, the company emphasizes that the direct access model allows customers to exercise a fundamental individual right to genetic information and personal liberty in controlling one's genetic data:

> 23andMe believes people have the right to access their personal genetic information. Genetic information is a fundamental element of a person's body, identity and individuality. As such, the rights that people enjoy with regard to financial, medical and other forms of personal information should apply to genetic information as well.
>
> (Harmon 2007)

The charge that individuals should exercise their personal liberty in controlling their genetic data suggests that companies like 23andMe are somehow liberating that which has been taken away from them, or at least made inaccessible. The question of what this newfound freedom is and perhaps, more importantly, what it offers remains unanswered. Francke *et al.* states that only one person reported a negative impact from learning of his BRCA mutations. The study participant, a mutation-positive man with a family history of breast cancer, is reported to state that the 'emotional cost' was too great and that he would prefer not to know his mutation status:

> I would not do it again, because it is really not information I need to know. I don't think the cost in dollars was important, I think the emotional cost is more. The impact of the results to a greater extent was negative. It's just basically knowing that I have it, I might pass it on. And that's the main thing. Sometimes ignorance is better.
>
> (Francke *et al.* 2013: 15)

The trope of empowerment forbids the right *not* to know, and assumes genetic knowledge is an unqualified good. Furthermore, the trope of empowerment demands a level of genetic literacy that may be too high for what interested and invested individual consumers can bring. Marsha, like several 23andMe customers I interviewed, was initially under the incorrect impression that the 23andMe test would provide information on the same BRCA1 and 2 mutations offered by Myriad. Only after Marsha had paid for the service online and had sent in her saliva sample did she begin to probe 23andMe's information on their breast cancer risk assessments more carefully. After realizing the BRCA mutations identified by the company were not the same and were mainly found in women who identified as Ashkenazi Jewish,[3] Marsha said she was initially disappointed, then in a subsequent interview, she stated that she was still glad that she had purchased the testing. This complicated process of understanding exactly what she had signed up for is discussed in further detail in a forthcoming article. However, it is important to note here that Marsha's misunderstanding reveals the limits of the putative empowerment that the company asserts, as individual consumers are expected to comprehend the significance of the different mutations associated with disease. The trope of freedom and the assumption that providing genetic data in the form of uncertain, highly contingent risk information as a source of empowerment begs further consideration.

Participation and the hunt for big data

Helmreich (2008) and others have emphasized that the units of analysis for biocapital are no longer individuals and populations, but also cells, molecules, genomes and genes. Biomaterial, as separated from subjective corporeality, has become the object of capitalist speculation (Waldby 2000). Companies like 23andMe have had strong precursors – web-based community groups focused on health that provide a platform for communities of patients, health professionals and organizations in an effort to build a consumer-based biobank of genetic samples. In establishing these collaborations, companies like 23andMe attempt to address a major problem in population-based genomics research: the challenge of garnering sufficient power to detect genes of modest effect (Hunter *et al.* 2008). DTC genomic companies engage this challenge by creating their own large databases in order to more efficiently 'scale up' for population-based research. Going a step further toward 'accelerating genomic research', 23andMe unveiled its research arm, 23andWe, in the spring of 2008. Stating that '23andMe isn't just about you', the company advertised 23andWe as a new model of actively engaging with their consumers in research by giving 'customers the opportunity to leverage their data by contributing it to studies of genetics'. Announcing this as a 'new paradigm for genetic research', the company emphasizes to would-be participants that:

> 23andWe is a new, more efficient way of doing genetic research. Even though new technologies have made it possible to link genes to diseases, traits and conditions more effectively than ever before, collecting the data for this

> research can be a costly, time-consuming and logistically difficult process. Progress is hindered by the fact that these studies require both genetic and personal information from thousands – sometimes tens of thousands – of people.[4]

Under this theme of generating 'enough data' to yield results that would 'benefit us all',[5] 23andWe participants are asked to complete surveys that query customers on health and environmental information that might be used in conjunction with their genotypic information in future research.

Building on the research objectives of the company, in March 2012, 23andMe announced another 'opportunity to participate in genetics research' made possible through a partnership with Genentech, the biotechnology drug development company owned by Roche Pharmaceuticals. In a pilot clinical trial to test the feasibility of using the DTC model to collect patient-reported genetic data and outcomes for genome wide association research, the companies launched the 'InVite Study'. This study aimed to recruit 1,000 metastatic breast cancer patients who had been treated with Genentech's drug Avastin, generically known as bevacizumab. The study came on the heels of the FDA decision in 2011 to revoke approval of the breast cancer indication for Avastin, after concluding that the drug had not been shown to be safe and effective for that use.[6] Aiming to identify the subset of women who might benefit from Avastin, Genentech collaborated with 23andMe to recruit patients to identify mutations associated with a positive drug response.

Touting the benefits of the ongoing clinical trial, 23andMe asserts that, as InVite Study participants, patients would not only learn more about their health by receiving genetic information on their risk for health conditions and genetic ancestry, but that it would be possible to 'take a direct role in research that may benefit you and other patients with advanced breast cancer'.[7] The study uses active advertising among patient advocacy groups, such as the Avon Foundation for Women, Facing Our Risk of Cancer Empowered (FORCE), and Triple Negative Breast Cancer Foundation, all of which have signed on as official partners with 23andMe. The diversity of partners in the study reflects the biosociality that Rabinow (1996) and Rose and Novas (2005) have described in which the body, as constituted by genetics, coalesces patient advocacy groups toward research objectives. Through this partnership, the organizations' members receive heavily discounted 23andMe services, and member samples are deposited into the company biobank and made available for company research.

The study emerges at a particularly interesting time – not only because of the developments with the Myriad patents, but also concerning the increasing ambiguity as to how personal genomics companies like 23andMe will engage with the patent protection of their internal research activity. From its inception, the company has taken a strong stand on 'individual rights' to their genome, stating explicitly:

> We believe patents should not be used to obstruct research or prevent individuals from knowing what's in their genome. We believe that everyone has a right to know their genomes – their sequence of As, Ts, Cs, and Gs – and

> should be able to access them should they want to. This has been our guiding principle since day one, and 23andMe has pioneered the ability for individuals to have unfettered access to their genomes.[8]

However, over time, the company's position against patents has become confusing. The limits of the right to an unfettered genome have become open to debate. A sticking point among 23andMe consumers has been the company's waffling on its position regarding the proprietary nature of mutations identified in association with Parkinson's disease, on which the company's scientists published a study in 2011 (Do *et al.* 2012). Following up on the discovery of the correlation, the company announced its first patent to its customer base on May 2012. The patent was for the discovery of the variant in the SGK1 gene, which the company reported as protective against Parkinson's disease in individuals who carry the rare risk-associated LRRK2 G2019S mutation.

Emphasizing the potential translation of their discovery into therapeutics, 23andMe framed their application as consistent with their stated core beliefs, attempting to decouple their interests in ownership from patents. Amidst public outcry among consumers that 23andMe had betrayed their trust by taking out a patent, the company's president and co-founder Anne Wojcicki wrote an addendum in June 2012. In defending the company's patent application, Wojcicki alluded to the company's 'core values', arguing that patents actually protected 23andMe customers, stating:

> Patents give organizations researching and developing new drugs confidence that their significant investments will be commercially viable. Developing new drugs and treatments costs time and money. A lot of time and money. Often the only way a company will even think about pursuing a drug lead is if they have assurance that they can recoup their investment. Having patent protection over the entire line of discovery gives a company confidence to invest in this resource-intensive process. . . . Our ultimate goal is to make discoveries that will benefit everyone.[9]

The company capitalizes off of what Brown (2005) has asserted is the centrality of the public imagination in brokering new and highly privatized consumption markets in the biosciences – the most salient in global efforts to store the present for the future through biobanking. However, not all consumers are convinced. Writing on the 23andMe community blog, one consumer shared his sentiment:

> I just can't help but feel that this proclamation of individual rights to know thine own genome is merely a thinly veiled smokescreen for the pursuit of profits. Not that there is anything wrong with profits, and not that there is anything inherently wrong in using the DTC gene sequencing business model, but at least call the spade what it is. All of this talk about gene patenting as being the 'high road' taken for patient and consumer benefit just does not ring true to me, and seems at the very least to be very disingenuous.[10]

Marsha, who had so enthusiastically signed up for 23andMe testing in order to find out her BRCA status 'in private', only vaguely remembered reviewing the company's consent form and terms of service agreement. When presented with copies of the agreements, Marsha shrugged with indifference:

> They [sic] are a company and anyone who thinks they aren't going to try to make money . . . that this isn't the reason they are doing this testing is simply naïve. I knew that it was a risk to be tested, but it was a risk I'm willing to take. Maybe if there are lots of companies for consumers to choose from . . . well, we would be better off.

Marsha's turn to the market as a solution to the shortcomings of the current medical system is resonant of the sentiments of salvation inherent to the process of creating biocapital (Fortun 2008). The promise of genetic medicine where value is constituted by the market gives rise to the speculative character of biotechnology, which becomes, according to Rajan (2006), the basis for the postgenomic life. The significance of the biobank for efforts to translate genomic data into clinically useful information has emerged in the case of Myriad, which holds the largest database of genetic mutations related to breast cancer in the world. The change in policy from open access to the now proprietary nature of the database has spurred angry efforts among scientists to ascertain the valuable genetic and medical information for research (Kolata 2013). These scientists have accused Myriad of holding trade secret monopolies from unknowing consumers. Individual genetic information as biomaterial only becomes biocapital in the aggregate that constitutes the database, which is owned and licensed by the corporate entity.

Conclusion

The turn toward DTC personal genomics and the tropes of freedom and empowerment invokes values associated with what it means to be a health-seeking American in the era of ubiquitous sources of self-knowledge. The expectation of individual responsibility, scientific efficiency and the centrality of the market has given rise to DTC genetic testing and has propelled a paradigm shift away from institutional, hierarchical models of the governance of health management toward direct public access to personal genetic data. Regulatory efforts to address questions of who has a right to access individual DNA and how do individual patients *participate* in their own health care have shifted the focus from more fundamental questions regarding the assumed good that is expected to come with personal genetic testing and what value it provides in the lives of individual consumers. Aside from promises to protect the privacy of their customers and to provide unfettered access to genetic risk information, there are few, if any, other tangible benefits that flow to individual consumers, despite the essential value of their genetic samples as biocapital. At stake is the elusive idea of the commons, where resources return to the public via the therapeutic pipeline. Structural inequities of the bioeconomy bear directly on the questions of who ultimately has the power to determine who has access to and benefits from genetic research. The turn to a free market results in a reconfiguration of individuals as patients in need of medical interventions to mere consumers. With risk information in hand, the 'empowered' consumer is left to excavate value and meaning from genetic data and to transform data into usable information. Such struggles leave bare the limits of freedom for individuals exercising their presumed right to their genomes.

The coupling of disease risk information and research participation is a significant dilemma for this era of personalized medicine. Despite companies' emphasis on the role of individual participation in the scale up of genomic research, the model of drug development and the struggle over gene patents renders individual DNA invisible as the necessary capital in the modelling of personalized medicine. The focus on the controversies over the legality of Myriad's patents on BRCA mutations further elides fundamental questions regarding how genetic testing offers value to individuals. The emergence of DTC personal genomic services further troubles the promise of better health by shifting the gaze toward the free market to intervene in ongoing disparities in health care. The trope of individual empowerment has failed to create new pathways for true freedom outside of the patent system. The meaning of 'participatory' in the realization of personalized medicine remains elusive; as responsibilities to individuals are evacuated, they are simultaneously framed as consumers and research participants – and thus left to confront the limits of transformation through personal genomics.

Notes

1. Several terms have been used to describe the focus on genomic science to deliver tailored medicine. These have included individualized medicine, personalized medicine and, more recently, precision medicine. These changes in language are subtle but important shifts in the framing of genomic medicine that are not the focus of this chapter. I use the term 'personalized medicine' to refer to the incorporation of genomic information in the management of individual health.
2. Women have approximately a one-in-eight chance of developing breast cancer and one-in-seventy chance of developing ovarian cancer over the course of their lifetime (American Cancer Society 2007). Also, 5 per cent to 10 per cent of all breast and ovarian cancer is related to an inherited gene mutation. Of these cases, 84 per cent of hereditary breast cancer and more than 90 per cent of hereditary ovarian cancer is caused by mutations in the BRCA1 or BRCA2 gene (Marshall and Solomon 2007).
3. The mutations identified by 23andMe are not those identified by Myriad's screen. 23andMe provides data for only three specific cancer-associated mutations that are found mainly in people with Ashkenazi Jewish ancestry – 185delAG (DD or DI at i4000377) in BRCA1, 5382insC in BRCA1 (II or DI at i4000378) and 6174delT in BRCA2 (DD or DI at i4000379). The mutations identified by 23andMe in their secondary breast cancer report were in or near genes CHEK2, FGFR2, TNRC9, 2q35, CASP8, SLC4A7 and NEK10 and STXBP4, none of which are in the BRCA genes.
4. http://mediacenter.23andme.com/press-releases/23andme-makes-new-discoveries-in-genetics-using-novel-web-based-participant-driven-methods.
5. www.23andme.com/you/23andwe/research/.

6. Avastin remains on the market as an approved treatment for certain types of colon, lung, kidney and brain cancer.
7. www.23andme.com/invite-study/faq/.
8. http://blog.23andme.com/news/announcements/announcing-23andmes-first-patent/.
9. http://blog.23andme.com/news/announcements/announcing-23andmes-first-patent/.
10. http://blog.23andme.com/news/announcements/announcing-23andmes-first-patent/.

References

American Cancer Society (2007) *Cancer Facts and Figures 2007,* American Cancer Society, Inc. Accessed 20 February, 2013. www.cancer.org

American Civil Liberties Union (2010) 'Liberate the breast cancer genes'. Accessed 20 February, 2013. www.aclu.org/free-speech_womens-rights/liberate-breast-cancer-genes

Angier, N. (1994) 'Vexing pursuit of breast cancer gene'. *New York Times.* Accessed 1 December, 2013. www.nytimes.com/1994/07/12/science/vexing-pursuit-of-breast-cancer-gene.html?pagewanted=all&src=pm

Borger, J. (1999) 'Rush to patent genes stalls cures for disease'. *The Guardian.* Accessed 1 December, 2013. www.theguardian.com/science/1999/dec/15/medicalresearch.genetics

Brown, N. (2003) 'Hope against hype – accountability in biopasts, presents and futures', *Science Studies,* 16, 2: 3–21.

———. (2005) 'Shifting tenses: reconnecting regimes of truth and hope', *Configurations,* 13, 3: 331–55

Carter, H. B., Albertsen, P.C., Barry M. J. et al. (2013) *Early Detection of Prostate Cancer: AUA Guideline,* American Urological Association Education and Research, Inc.

DelVecchio Good, M. J., Good, B.J., Schaffer, C. and Lind, S.E. (1990) 'American oncology and the discourse on hope', *Culture, Medicine and Psychiatry,* 14: 59–79.

Do, C. B., Tung, J.Y., Dorfman, E. et al. (2012) 'Web-based genome-wide association study identifies two novel loci and a substantial genetic component for Parkinson's disease', *PLoS Genetics,* 7, 6: e1002141.

Fortun, M. (2008) *Promising Genomics: Iceland and deCODE Genetics in a World of Speculation.* Berkeley: University of California Press.

Francke, U., Dijamco, C., Kiefer, A. K. et al. (2013) 'Dealing with the unexpected: consumer responses to direct-access *BRCA* mutation testing', *PeerJ,* 1: e8. http://dx.doi.org/10.7717/peerj.8

Harmon, A. (2007). 'My genome, myself: seeking clues in DNA', *The New York Times,* 17 November. Accessed 20 February, 2013. www.nytimes.com/2007/11/17/us/17dna.html

Heath, D., Rapp, R. and Taussig, K. S. (2004) 'Genetic citizenship'. In Nugent, D. and Vincent, J. (eds) *A Companion to the Anthropology of Politics.* Malden, MA: Blackwell.

Helmreich, Stefan (2008) Species of Biocapital. *Science as Culture.* 17, 4: 463–478.

Henneman, L., Timmermans, D.R.M. and van der Wal, G. (2004) 'Public experiences, knowledge and expectations about medical genetics and the use of genetic information', *Community Genet* 7: 33–43.

Hood, L. and Galas, D. (2008) 'P4 medicine: personalized, predictive, preventive, participatory. A change of view that changes everything', Version 6: 12 December. Accessed 1 November, 2013. www.cra.org/ccc/resources/ccc-led-white-papers

Hunter, D.J., Altshuler, D. and Rader, D.J. (2008) 'From Darwin's finches to canaries in the coal mine: mining the genome for new biology', *New England Journal of Medicine*, 358, 26: 2760–3.

Kieran, S., Loescher, L. J. and Lim, K. H. (2007) 'The role of financial factors in acceptance of clinical *BRCA* genetic testing', *Genetic Testing,* 11, 1: 101–10.

Kolata, G. (2013) 'DNA project aims to make public a company's data on cancer genes', *New York Times,* 12 April. Accessed 1 May, 2013. www.nytimes.com/2013/04/13/health/dna-project-aims-to-make-companys-data-public.html?pagewanted=1&_r=2&hp

Lynch, H.T., Snyder, C., Lynch, J.F. et al. (2006) 'Patient responses to the disclosure of BRCA mutation tests in hereditary breast-ovarian cancer families', *Cancer Genet Cytogenet,* 165: 91–7.

Marshall, M. and Solomon, S. (2007) 'Hereditary breast–ovarian cancer: clinical findings and medical management', *Plastic Surgical Nursing,* 27, 3: 124–7.

Murray, J. (1999) 'Owning genes: Disputes involving DNA sequence patents.' *Chicago-Kent Law Review.* 75: 231–257.

Orenstein, P. (2013) 'Our feel-good war on breast cancer', *New York Times Magazine,* 25 April.

Parthasarathy, S. (2011) *Building Genetic Medicine: Breast Cancer, Technology, and the Comparative Politics of Health Care.* Cambridge: MIT Press

Rabinow, P. (1996). 'Artificiality and enlightenment: from sociobiology to biosociality', *Essays on the Anthropology of Reason.* Princeton, NJ: Princeton University Press.

Rajan, K. S. (2006) *Biocapital: The Constitution of Postgenomic Life.* Chapel Hill, NC: Duke University Press.

Rose, N. (2007) *The Politics of Life Itself: Biomedicine, Power, and Subjectivity in the Twenty-First Century.* Princeton, NJ: Princeton University Press.

Rose, N. and Novas, C. (2005) 'Biological citizenship'. In Ong, A. and Collier, S. (eds) *Global Assemblages: Technology, Politics, and Ethics as Anthropoligical Problems.* Malden, MA: Blackwell.

Rusconi, W. E. (2005) 'Patenting and licensing of the breast cancer susceptibility genes – *BRCA1* and *BRCA2*', presentation at the National Academies, Washington, DC, 11 February. Accessed 20 February, 2013. www.genome.duke.edu/centers/cpg/case-histories/clinical-genetic-testing/documents/NAS%20Patents%20and%20BRCA%20 2–11–2005%20%282%29.pdf

'Statement of the American Society of Clinical Oncology: genetic testing for cancer susceptibility, adopted on February 20, 1996', *Journal of Clinical Oncology,* 14, 5:1730–6; discussion 1737–40.

Waldby, C. (2000) *The Visible Human Project: Informatic Bodies and Posthuman Medicine.* London: Routledge.

Williams-Jones, B. (2006) '"Be ready against cancer, now": Direct-to-consumer advertising for genetic testing', *New Genetics and Society,* 25, 1: 89–107.

Williams-Jones, B. and Burgess, M. M. (2006) 'Democratising access to genetic services', *Familial Cancer,* 5: 117–21.

U.S. Preventive Services Task Force (2005) 'Genetic risk assessment and BRCA mutation testing for breast and ovarian cancer susceptibility: recommendation statement', *Annals of Internal Medicine,* 143, 5: 355–61.

8 The BRCA patent controversies

An international review of patent disputes[1]

Esther van Zimmeren, Dianne Nicol, Richard Gold, Julia Carbone, Subhashini Chandrasekharan, A. Lane Baldwin and Robert Cook-Deegan

1 Introduction

A book focusing on transnational perspectives on BRCA would certainly be incomplete without a chapter on the international uproar regarding patents on the BRCA gene sequences and testing methods. BRCA 'gene patents' have been the focus of intense controversy for decades and – more recently – the subject of court battles in the US and Australia. Most conspicuously, the US Supreme Court handed down its ruling on whether human genes are patentable subject matter on 13 June, 2013 (*AMP v. Myriad* [2013]).

General patentability criteria are globally uniform and technology-neutral (requiring that the invention is new, involves an inventive step and is capable of industrial application).[2] National patent systems show considerable variation, however, in how each criterion is applied, either through patent legislation or as developed through case law. As with any other field of technology, biological materials are, in principle, capable of fulfilling these criteria. In all jurisdictions, however, a question of threshold must be addressed before these patentability criteria are applied. This question concerns whether or not the invention constitutes patentable subject matter. Although not traditionally viewed as satisfying this threshold requirement, many kinds of living matter are now considered to be eligible, and as a consequence patents have intruded on the field of human genetics as well. This intrusion has not gone unnoticed and has led to a 'policy storm' (Gold and Carbone 2010) surrounding the desirability of human gene patents since the late 1980s.

At the centre of this storm is Myriad Genetics Inc (hereinafter Myriad). Myriad is a biotech spin-off from the Center for Genetic Epidemiology at the University of Utah. It is not the only owner of patents related to human genes, mutations and diagnostic methods with respect to the BRCA1 and BRCA2 genes. However, it has been singled out in the policy storm largely because of the way in which it chose to use its patent rights. Myriad accumulated sufficient patent rights to create a service monopoly in the US, but it did not achieve that level of dominance in any other jurisdiction. It also made a number of commercialization decisions that did not sit well within the research community (Baldwin and Cook-Deegan 2013, Gold and Carbone 2010, Parthasarathy 2007).

Efforts to identify the BRCA genes started with the International Breast Cancer Linkage Consortium with researchers from all over the world. Mary-Claire King's discovery of chromosome 17 linkage to a risk susceptibility locus for breast cancer (Hall *et al.* 1990) set off a furious competition to find the actual gene by comparing DNA from those who developed cancer to others who did not develop cancer within family pedigrees in search of DNA changes correlating with developing cancer (Davies and White 1996, Marshall 1997). The race to be the first to isolate and sequence the genes (and to be the first at the patent office) was fierce. Over the course of this race to uncover these enigmatic 'breast cancer genes', several research teams published the gene sequences and filed for patents.[3] The race to BRCA1 on chromosome 17 was won in 1994 by Mark Skolnick and his colleagues at the University of Utah, also affiliated with Myriad Genetics, who identified mutations in BRCA1 and cloned and sequenced the gene (Davies and White 1996, Miki *et al.* 1994). There were more doubts about which team had actually 'won' the race to BRCA2 on chromosome 13, with the team affiliated with Michael Stratton in the UK publishing first and securing a UK patent, but with Myriad having filed a patent application just days before that publication after 'getting wind' of Stratton's progress. The patent race led to a complex international patent landscape and often to errors in the filed sequences, which were later employed to challenge some of the BRCA patents in Europe (see Section 2 of this chapter).

In addition to the intense patent race, Myriad's stringent enforcement and licensing practices also contributed to its negative public image (Gold and Carbone 2010). In the US, once Myriad had obtained its patents, it attempted to eliminate the BRCA testing by competing laboratories. Until the Supreme Court ruling, Myriad was successful in 'clearing the market' of US competitors. Outside the US, Myriad applied a different strategy. In each country or region, Myriad identified an exclusive licensee for single-mutation tests (once a mutation had been identified in a family), while it intended to perform the more expensive first-line sequence-based proband testing at its own laboratory in Utah, obliging clinicians to send samples to the US (Gold and Carbone 2010).

In Europe, each country has its own health care and laboratory system, meaning Myriad had to engage in country-by-country licensing negotiations. With respect to the UK and Ireland, Myriad established a strategic alliance with Rosgen Ltd for BRCA testing. Rosgen then negotiated an agreement with the UK's Department of Health that would allow the national health authority, the National Health Service (NHS), to perform the testing. Cancer Research UK (CRUK), which held a BRCA2 patent in the UK (see Section 2.2), licensed its patent to OncorMed with the stipulation that the NHS could continue to provide testing services for free. Rosgen soon went bankrupt, which effectively ended Myriad's agreement with the NHS. Myriad and the NHS did not agree on a replacement license (Llewelyn 2003, Parthasarathy 2007). However, Myriad found another private company, Lab21, which was willing to sign a licence agreement for the BRCA test. For the Swiss, German and Austrian markets, Myriad licensed Bioscientia to market its test for proband testing and provide the follow-on testing to family members for single mutations. When it became illegal in France to send blood samples out of the country, Myriad claimed that it would be willing to allow local laboratories to perform proband sequencing. However, in practice, no laboratory in France was ever licensed to perform the testing (Gold and Carbone 2010). In 2012, Myriad opened its own laboratory in Germany and offices in four European countries (see below).

In Canada, Myriad awarded the private company MDS Laboratories (MDS) the exclusive right to market the BRCA tests. Myriad performed proband sequencing in Utah, but MDS arranged for individual mutation testing within its 'network of physicians and hospitals' (Gold and Carbone 2010). In Australia, Myriad entered into a strategic licensing agreement with Genetic Technologies Ltd (GTG), a Melbourne-based biotechnology company. The alliance resulted from Myriad's alleged infringement of GTG's patents claiming rights to intron sequence analysis and genomic mapping, the so-called 'junk DNA' patents (Nicol 2005). As a result of the agreement, GTG became Myriad's exclusive licensee in Australia and New Zealand for a number of its products, including its breast and ovarian cancer tests. The CEO of GTG indicated in 2003 that he had no intention of enforcing the BRCA patents on behalf of Myriad, but that rather they were 'GTG's gift to Australia'. When GTG announced its plans to take back that gift in 2008, a firestorm erupted, and the company backed down.

In response to Myriad's restrictive licensing practices, at least nine US laboratories stopped offering BRCA testing (Cho *et al.* 2003). These licensing practices led to patent litigation in the US (see Section 4.2) and Australia (see Section 5.2) as well as opposition procedures at the European Patent Office (EPO) (see Section 2.2) and various legislative proposals and policy measures in Europe, Canada, the US and Australia (see Sections 2.3, 3.2, 4.3 and 5.3). Moreover, many clinicians simply ignored the enforcement practices and offered testing quietly under the radar.

The research, legal and policy contexts in which these decisions were made have been described in several case studies (Gold and Carbone 2010, Parthasarathy 2007, Williams-Jones 2002). This chapter reviews these case studies and draws on a number of formal and informal interviews with stakeholders as well as workshops and conference presentations by key players (i.e. Gold and Carbone 2010, Van Overwalle 2007). It also provides an update of recent developments in litigation, policy and decision-making processes. The chapter has two objectives: first, to highlight features that distinguish the Myriad case from other patent cases; and second, to explain how BRCA patent disputes have unfolded very differently in Europe, Canada, the US and Australia with different roles of institutional actors in diverse legal and legislative fora and the use of alternative solutions.

In the following sections, we describe – more or less chronologically – how BRCA gene patent controversies have travelled around the world. In Section 2, we start off in Europe in the 1990s with a short description of the particularities of the European 'multilevel' patent regime, followed by a sketch of the procedures against the BRCA patents at the European Patent Office (EPO). Contrary to the European story, no formal means were used to contest Myriad's patent rights in

Canada: the Ontario Ministry of Health took the lead using informal pressure to steer Myriad away from its restrictive licensing practices (Section 3). We move to the US in Section 4, where we learn that, in the early 2000s after Myriad settled lawsuits with OncorMed and the University of Pennsylvania, for a few years the gene patent debate was mainly a topic for academics and advisory committees. This quickly changed when the American Civil Liberties Union (ACLU) and the Public Patent Foundation (PPF) challenged Myriad's patents at the New York City federal district court, where Judge Sweet decided that 'isolated' nucleic acid molecules could not be considered patent-eligible subject matter. Whereas Sweet's decision was initially reversed by the Court of Appeals of the Federal Circuit (CAFC), in June 2013 the US Supreme Court confirmed Sweet's conclusion regarding 'isolated' DNA sequences. In contrast, in Australia, Judge Nicholas reached the opposite conclusion, ruling that 'isolated' nucleic acids *are* patentable subject matter (Section 5). However, as the appeal in the Australian case remains to be decided, the patentable subject matter requirement may still converge. After a brief analysis of positions on gene patents in emerging economies and at the international level (Section 6), we conclude with an inventory of the available toolkit for contesting patents and licensing practices and some closing remarks on the potential impact of the recent case law on the new generation of sequencing technologies (Section 7).

2 Europe

2.1 Background

In order to fully comprehend how the Myriad case proceeded in Europe, it is important to have a basic understanding of the structure and distinctive features of the European patent system. The European patent system is a complex, multilevel system:[4] in addition to the national patent offices that grant patents that are valid only within each country, the European Patent Office (EPO) can grant so-called 'European patents'.[5] Once European patents have been granted, they become a 'bundle' of national patents, which means that the patents need to be translated and validated in the designated countries and can only be litigated in each country's courts in case of a dispute. This can lead to high litigation costs, and these costs deter patent litigation in Europe. Fortunately, the EPO offers some alternative routes for challenging patents, such as the so-called 'post-grant opposition procedure', which is an internal administrative procedure within the EPO.

The EU and EPO have adopted a uniform approach to gene patents. Because the EU wanted to harmonize patent law between the member states with respect to biotechnology, it thus approved a directive on the legal protection of biotechnological inventions (EU Biotechnology Directive) (Council and European Parliament 1998, Gold and Gallochat 2001). This directive stipulates conditions for patenting biotechnological processes and products, including materials of human origin. The EPO incorporated the directive as part of its implementing regulations (Brody 2007, Gold and Gallochat 2001). The European baseline is that discoveries are not patentable, but a 'technical' or useful application of a discovery may be patentable. The simple discovery of one of its elements, including DNA sequences or partial sequences, cannot constitute patentable inventions. However, elements 'isolated' from the human body or otherwise produced by means of a technical process may constitute a patentable invention, even if the structure of those elements is identical to natural elements.[6] Despite this, a mere DNA sequence without indication of a function does not contain any 'technical information' and is therefore not a patentable invention (Council and European Parliament 1998, para. 23). Typically, the EPO has awarded patents for DNA sequences by treating them in the same way as other chemical substances without much reference to the information that DNA encodes.

2.2 Opposition and appeal at the EPO

The European story of Myriad's patents shows the importance of a well-timed and accurate disclosure of the invention at the patent office. Filing dates of applications are extremely important. Delays or errors may have a disastrous impact on patent prosecution (the process for getting a patent granted by a patent office). In August 1995, Myriad and its co-applicants (e.g. the University of Utah Research Foundation) filed four separate patent applications at the EPO for the sequences, mutations and diagnostic tests regarding the BRCA1 and BRCA2 genes. In 2001, the EPO granted EP699754 for a diagnostic method for breast and ovarian cancer, EP705903 for 34 mutations in the BRCA1 gene and methods for detecting the mutations and EP705902 for the BRCA1 gene itself and for several applications. In November 1995, Cancer Research UK (CRUK), led by Mike Stratton, first applied for patent protection in the UK (national patent) based on the BRCA2 sequence and several diagnostic methods. This UK application was followed by an EPO application in November 1996, claiming priority[7] on the basis of the UK applications. The EPO granted patent EP858467, sometimes referred to as the Stratton patent, in 2003. Myriad applied for protection in December 1996 for a variant of the BRCA2 gene, several mutations and a range of diagnostic applications. Patent EP785216 was granted in 2002. Myriad opposed the Stratton patent on the BRCA2 gene. One of the deficiencies of the Stratton patent, the filing of incomplete sequences, was the consequence of the 'race to the patent office'. The opposition division allowed the rectification of the claims, but on appeal the Stratton patent was revoked (T902/07, 2010). CRUK thus has a UK BRCA2 patent but no EPO patent.

A number of scientists and clinical geneticists, including Mary-Claire King and Dominique Stoppa-Lyonnet, expressed concern about the potential impact of the patents on their research and access to health services. They spoke out against the 'Myriad patents', asserting that they would prevent scientists from assessing the quality of Myriad's tests, developing more comprehensive or accurate BRCA tests (Puget *et al.* 1999) and developing treatments (Benowitz 2003, Lecrubier 2002). Fuelled by these concerns, a French association of research institutes and hospitals and an informal coalition of the Belgian, Dutch, British, Danish and

German genetic societies opposed the first BRCA1 patent (EP699754).[8] The number of opponents accumulated with later opposition procedures (Matthijs and Halley 2002).

The opposition and appeal procedures did not result in the revocation of all the patents, but they were quite successful in limiting their scope.[9] For instance, for patent EP785216 the claims were restricted to a particular sub-population of Ashkenazi descent. Despite the criticism on this discriminatory limitation (Abbott 2005), the amendment was ultimately accepted. The opponents tried to raise broader policy concerns about the eligibility of gene sequences for patent protection, their impact on research and health services and their compatibility with 'public order and morality',[10] but success in narrowing patent claims was mainly due to arguments based on 'traditional' patentability criteria regarding novelty, inventive step, industrial applicability and disclosure.[11] Those procedures took place within the EPO, and no litigation has raised issues of patent eligibility.

As a result of narrowing the patent claims through the various EPO procedures, fears within the European BRCA community about the patents have diminished significantly. By curbing the scope of the patents, the EPO has decreased their clinical relevance for genetic diagnostics. For the most part, the patents have been ignored and will begin to expire in late 2014. Moreover, the patent owners have allowed their patents to lapse in several countries, which is possible in Europe, as the patents are considered a 'bundle of national patents' that must be maintained (including the payment of fees) on the national level. Testing by laboratories located in those particular countries thus no longer entails any risk of patent infringement liability.[12] In view of the expansion of Myriad's activities in Europe, this situation has become quite important. In the past, Bioscientia was Myriad's exclusive licensee in Europe (see Section 1). Nonetheless, BRCA testing has persisted in many European laboratories. To date, Myriad has refrained from aggressive patent enforcement in Europe. To do this, it would first have to start infringement procedures before national judges in all the relevant countries, which would be expensive and time-consuming. However, Myriad did open a molecular diagnostic laboratory in 2012 in Munich, where they will carry out BRAC*Analysis*™. It also established sales and marketing offices in Munich, Paris, Milan, Madrid and Zurich (Myriad 2013). It remains to be seen whether this expansion will entail changes with respect to Myriad's enforcement strategies.

2.3 Policy and law reform

Several national advisory bodies have weighed in on the debate about the patent eligibility of gene sequences. For instance, the Nuffield Council of Bioethics in the UK noted that DNA sequences should be regarded as 'just genetic information', distinguishing them from other patentable chemical compounds, and they recommended that patentability requirements (novelty, inventive step, industrial applicability) be applied more stringently to DNA patents (Nuffield Council 2002). Two years later, the Danish Council of Bioethics echoed these arguments based on the 'information content' of gene sequences in its report *Patenting Human Genes and Stem Cells* (Danish Council of Bioethics 2004). The Danish Council argued that, while the informational nature of DNA would not be a reason to preclude patents entirely, it may be a reason to limit the effects of DNA patents, such as through the granting of compulsory licences for public interest reasons, allowing users to apply the patented invention without the consent of the patent owner with fair compensation (Danish Council of Bioethics 2004). Moreover, several geneticists who had been active as opponents of Myriad patents at the EPO formed a working group under the umbrella of the European Society of Human Genetics (ESHG) and issued recommendations, ranging from a limitation of patentable subject matter to a higher bar for patentability requirements, the introduction of compulsory licences for public health and the use of alternative licensing models, such as patent pools and clearinghouses (ESHG Working Party on Patenting and Licensing 2008).

For the EU Biotechnology Directive to take effect, legislatures in the EU member states needed to transpose it into national law. In the process of doing so, some countries decided to go beyond the rules imposed by the directive and added provisions, creating new tools for judges or governments when dealing with restrictive licensing practices. The BRCA patent situation was the main driver for these initiatives. France and Belgium created mandatory licensing regimes for diagnostic testing in the interest of public health, enabling the French and Belgian government to put a regime into place that allows the use of a particular patented invention without the authorization of the patent owner (Debrulle *et al.* 2007, van Zimmeren and Van Overwalle 2011, van Zimmeren and Requena 2007). To our knowledge, these licensing regimes for public health have never been invoked, but their existence effectively limits the enforceability of diagnostic patents and is a tool for persuading patent owners to collaborate. In addition, the Belgian legislature also modified the research exception, extending its scope from 'research on' to 'research with' the patented invention, enabling further BRCA research without the risk of patent infringement (Van Overwalle and van Zimmeren 2006).

3 Canada

3.1 Background

The storm surrounding Myriad and its patents played out very differently in Canada than in Europe. Rather than being led by clinicians, patients or civil society, health departments responsible for the public health care system took the lead. The Canadian story began in 2000, after Myriad and its Canadian exclusive licensee, MDS Laboratories, met with provincial health care procurement officers. At the time, the Ontario Ministry of Health and Long-Term Care had already begun considering genetic testing and its implications for the health care system. During the six months that the Ontario Health Ministry was contemplating its response, Myriad and MDS issued so-called 'cease-and-desist letters' to several provincial governments, including Ontario, in May and June 2001. This surprised ministry officials and led the Minister of Health to state that the government had not violated any valid patent. In response, the Republican senator from Utah, Orrin Hatch, threatened to put Canada on the 'watch list' for international trade violations, and the Biotechnology Industry Organization (BIO) threatened to move its annual meeting from Toronto. This reflected a complete misunderstanding of what the province was doing and resulted in an intensification of the policy storm (Gold and Carbone 2010).

3.2 Policy and law reform

While the Myriad storm in Canada may have been turbulent, it did not lead to any legislative reform at either the federal level (with jurisdiction over patent law) or the provincial level (with jurisdiction over the provincial health care systems). A federal parliamentary committee, the Standing Committee on Health, briefly discussed the topic of gene patents in 2001 in the course of examining a bill on assisted reproduction, but it wrongly stated that genes could not be patented in Canada (Standing Committee on Health 2001). Instead, Canadian provincial governments adopted a simple strategy using the leverage of their procurement power, since they regularly purchase patented goods (i.e. medicines, equipment, diagnostic kits). The provinces focused on creating a united front so as to send a signal not only to Myriad, but to the entire diagnostics industry that they needed to adopt a flexible approach to licensing in Canada.

What concerned the provinces most was not the fact that Myriad had a patent on a gene, but that Myriad was interfering with the efficiency of the administration of their health care system. As Myriad attempted to use its patents to require that samples be sent to its Salt Lake City laboratories, provinces were left with no flexibility regarding how to screen their populations (using less expensive tests together with family histories to identify who ought to receive the expensive test). Moreover, if Myriad's model were to prevail, provincial health care systems could never centralize genetic testing so as to build expertise and efficiencies in diagnostics (Gold and Carbone 2010).

The provinces, with the assistance of one federal department, Health Canada, employed soft law measures to demonstrate their opposition to Myriad's business strategy in the form of the organization of an expert policy forum, an inter-provincial report approved by the First Ministers and a reference to a federal expert panel on biotechnology to investigate the issue of gene patents and their effect on the health care system. None of these steps flowed from strict regulatory authority, but they generated pressure to thwart Myriad's monopoly.

Canada's largest province according to population, Ontario, took the lead in dealing with Myriad. It organized a policy forum that brought together industry, health professionals and patent experts in December 2001. The policy forum's objective was to discuss and explore ways for Ontario to deal with Myriad's demands as well as the expected future demands from other firms. The final report, entitled *Genetics, Testing and Gene Patenting: Charting New Territory in Healthcare,* recommended a combination of measures. These included a federal government review to ensure the continuation of clinical genetics research, a review of competition law policy and the introduction of a research exemption into the Canadian Patent Act (Ontario 2002). A month later, all other Canadian provinces agreed with the report's recommendations (Gold and Carbone 2010).

Throughout 2002, Ontario maintained the lead on this issue. However, in the spring of 2003, it was hit by a more immediate health crisis: SARS. All of the government's attention turned to address that virus. Further, the feeling was that Myriad and other firms had received the message that they needed to change their business strategy in Canada. Therefore, the continued work on the Myriad dossier was not viewed as a priority. Then, in October 2003, Ontario elected a new government. This new government was apparently content to let the issue of gene patents rest and considered the united policy response among the provinces sufficient for sending a clear message to industry (Gold and Carbone 2010).

Meanwhile, at the federal level, Health Canada took up the mantle of the debate over gene patents. It engaged Industry Canada, which is responsible for the Canadian Patent Act, in discussions about how to resolve the problem, but Industry Canada and Health Canada could not agree on a solution. Instead, in 2004, they jointly commissioned the Canadian Biotechnology Advisory Committee (CBAC) to examine the issue. In 2006, CBAC issued its report *Human Genetic Materials, Intellectual Property and the Health Sector,* in which it called on the federal government to take proactive measures, such as introducing a research exemption and a targeted compulsory licensing provision for health care (CBAC 2006). The Canadian federal government never responded to the recommendations.

3.3 'Post-Myriad' atmosphere

In the absence of a forcing action such as a lawsuit, policymakers, laboratory directors and hospitals seemed satisfied that, despite a lack of overt federal government action, industry understood that Myriad's business strategy was not acceptable in Canada. This assumption turned out to be incorrect. In 2008, Warnex Inc issued letters to laboratories across Canada informing them – incorrectly as the patent did not issue until 2012 – that it was the exclusive licensee of the patent on the JAK2 gene related to myeloproliferative disorders. The patent application had been filed by a French public laboratory, which had exclusively licensed it to Ipsogen, a diagnostics company in France. Ipsogen had developed a diagnostic kit that it marketed in the US, but it decided to leave the Canadian market to Warnex (Piper and Gold 2008). Warnex proposed to discuss having tests of the JAK2 gene conducted in its laboratory. Laboratory directors saw Warnex's letters as a reprise of the Myriad business model and complained to Health Canada. Given that the patent had not been issued, laboratories and provincial health administrators simply ignored the letters. Nevertheless, laboratory directors began, once again, to worry.

Following Warnex, further concerns began when the Canadian patents over the Long QT genes, related to a fatal heart condition, were issued. While there were no formal threats, the authors have been told that several laboratories either stopped working on the development of a test for Long QT, or they never began to develop a test. Efforts to develop comprehensive cancer gene panels have also been reported to the authors to have been hampered by fears over issued gene patents, including the patents related to the BRCA1 and BRCA2 genes. Canadian laboratories and hospitals have thus been left with great uncertainty. With the absence of any litigation or legislative proposal, they remain frustrated at the lack of clarity as evidenced by their calls that genes should not be considered patentable subject matter in Canada (Richer *et al.* 2012).

4 United States

4.1 Background

The BRCA patent landscape in the US is relatively muddled.[13] The most significant are 24 patents assigned or licensed exclusively to Myriad Genetics. Fifteen claims in seven patents were challenged in *Association for Molecular Pathology et al. v. Myriad Genetics et al.* (*AMP v. Myriad*). The background behind these patents and the ensuing litigation is complicated. A company named OncorMed licensed a University of California patent on Mary-Claire King's BRCA1 discoveries regarding the inherited risk of breast and ovarian cancer (Marshall 1997). While the Myriad team is credited with winning the race to the BRCA1 gene itself, the first BRCA1 patent was granted to OncorMed. US patent 5,654,155 was issued on 5 August, 1997, on a 'consensus sequence of BRCA1' (Murphy *et al.* 1997). Several other patents were initially licensed to OncorMed.

As patents were granted by the US Patent and Trademark Office (USPTO), a complex patent landscape with dispersed patent ownership emerged in the US. OncorMed owned the rights to some mutations, while Myriad owned the rights to others. Both companies had claims on the entire BRCA1 gene. This may be puzzling to those not familiar with patents, but it is not uncommon for patents to overlap, because there are different patent examiners handling different applications, and there is no systematic way to coordinate the separate examination processes. With ownership divided and overlapping, several solutions existed: ignoring the patents, sorting out legitimate inventorship by way of an administrative procedure (called interference) at USPTO, aggregating patent rights and knocking other companies out of the market, cross-licensing and competing or litigating. The choice was to litigate, and it was initiated by OncorMed.

4.2 Litigation

OncorMed filed suit against Myriad on 17 November, 1997. Myriad counter-sued on 2 December, after receiving its first of many BRCA1 patents (US 5,693,473) (Shattuck-Eidens *et al.* 1997).[14] Before the case went to trial, OncorMed and Myriad settled out of court with the BRCA patent rights conveyed to Myriad. In a second case, *Myriad v University of Pennsylvania,* Myriad had sent several notification and cease-and-desist letters to, and eventually filed suit against, the University of Pennsylvania (Penn) for offering BRCA testing. Penn had been proposed as a clinical testing core for a cluster of federal grants studying the use of genetic testing in clinical practice. The case was settled when Penn agreed not to perform testing for other institutions.

AMP v. Myriad[15] is the only diagnostic gene patent case that has proceeded far enough to address the merits of patent claims. The two lawsuits between Myriad, OncorMed and Penn were settled before they went to trial under terms known only to the parties directly involved. *AMP v. Myriad* was filed by the ACLU and PPF on 12 May, 2009. As with the European oppositions, it involved many plaintiffs, including women who wanted to be tested, physicians who wanted to order tests, three laboratory directors who had received enforcement letters from Myriad as well as organizations representing those constituencies (in total more than 20 plaintiffs).

AMP v. Myriad became by far the most important and conspicuous case over gene patents. There have been 11 previous cases that centred on gene patents decided by the Court of Appeals for the Federal Circuit (CAFC), which hears patent appeals from all 94 US federal district courts. Those cases, however, concerned ownership and control of patent rights for therapeutic proteins, not whether patents should be granted in the first place (indeed, in previous cases, all the parties wanted such rights to exist). *AMP v. Myriad,* in contrast, was much more about changing the law than divvying up the profits. It was a public interest lawsuit rather than litigation among competitors, and as such, it drew in constituencies not generally party to patent suits.

In March 2010, Judge Robert Sweet of the New York federal district court stunned the patent world by ruling that all challenged patent claims were invalid. In his 156-page decision, he reasoned that DNA is 'the embodiment of genetic information'. Furthermore, Judge Sweet argued that the claimed isolated DNA was not 'markedly different' (standard derived from the famous *Chakrabarty* case) from DNA, as it exists in nature and could not be considered patent-eligible subject matter. Furthermore, the general method claims were also not considered patent-eligible. All the challenged claims were thus held invalid. The case was appealed to the CAFC, which decided in July 2011 that the general method patents were indeed invalid (affirming Judge Sweet), but it reversed Judge Sweet's judgment that 'isolated' DNA molecules cover patent-ineligible products of nature. Judge Bryson dissented, saying such DNA molecules were not 'markedly different' from their naturally occurring counterparts and were not patentable subject matter.

The case was further appealed to the US Supreme Court. The Supreme Court then remanded the case to the CAFC for reconsideration in light of its decision in *Mayo v. Prometheus* (2012), a case about diagnostic methods in general, not genetic diagnostics, and about methods not molecules. The CAFC reaffirmed its decision in *AMP v. Myriad* in August 2012. That decision was appealed, and the Supreme Court finally agreed to address the question: 'Are human genes patentable?' In June 2013, the Supreme Court ruled that a naturally occurring DNA sequence is a product of nature and therefore not patent-eligible simply because it has been 'isolated'. The core rationale for this holding was that Myriad did not create a composition of matter 'with markedly different characteristics from anything found in nature' in line with Judge Bryson's dissent. However, the Court also held that cDNA is patent-eligible, because it is not naturally occurring (in other words, cDNA is sufficiently man-made).

4.3 Policy and law reform

Conflict in the US over gene patents has not been restricted to litigation; it has also played out in administrative procedures and in proposed legislation. It all started with a highly contentious debate within the National Institutes of Health (NIH) about patenting human gene fragments focusing on 'expressed sequence tags' (ESTs). ESTs were considered great scientific tools for identifying genes for further characterization. NIH filed several EST patent applications, which triggered a vigorous debate within NIH about the propriety of applying for such patents. In 1994, the new NIH director, Harold Varmus, decided to abandon the NIH EST patent applications. The EST patent controversy was just beginning to die down when the BRCA1 gene was discovered in 1994.

As indicated above, not only questions of patenting but also questions as to how patents on genetic and genomic inventions should be licensed prompted the gene patent policy storm. Because of the degree of uncertainty and controversy surrounding DNA technologies, the NIH Office of Technology Transfer developed 'best practices' as to when, and whether, to patent DNA-based inventions and how to license such inventions for use (NIH 2004). In addition, in 2007 a group of academic institutions published a paper, later endorsed by the Association of University Technology Managers (AUTM), proposing 'Nine Points to Consider' when licensing university-generated intellectual property (Stanford 2007). Point 2 argues that patents on diagnostics should be pursued with an eye to avoiding patent logjams, taking care to preserve broad access and to avoid constraints on research.

The controversies over gene patents and their impact on access to genetic testing have bred several US initiatives for statutory reform ranging from the creation of an exemption from infringement liability for diagnostic use (2002) to a declaration that DNA sequences and products derived from them would be patent-ineligible subject matter (2007). These bills were, however, never subject of a hearing or put to a vote. A report from 2006 by the National Research Council (NRC) recommended establishing an exemption to patent infringement liability to allow independent verification of test results (Merrill and Mazza 2006). A federal advisory committee, the Secretary's Advisory Committee on Genetics Health and Society (SACGHS), also recommended the inclusion of a statutory exemption tailored to diagnostics that was not confined to verification testing but covered all diagnostic use (SACGHS 2010). It also recommended the adoption of a research exemption. In 2011, as bills that became the America Invents Act were moving through Congress, a use exemption for verification genetic testing was proposed along the lines of the 2006 NRC report, but it was withdrawn in the face of intense controversy. Those embroiled in *AMP v. Myriad* were concerned about how a legislative measure might colour the court decisions. In its place, Section 27 of the America Invents Act called for USPTO to submit a study of verification genetic testing, a report still pending release to Congress.

5 Australia

5.1 Background

The BRCA patent landscape is much less cluttered in Australia than in the US.[16] Despite this, there has been wide-ranging activity in Australia in the contexts of patent litigation, policy and law reform. This frenetic activity can in no small part be attributed to concerns about the risk that Myriad might start enforcing its BRCA patents and the likely impact that this might have on breast cancer research and diagnostic testing services.

5.2 Litigation

Proceedings challenging the validity of Myriad's foundational BRCA1 patent in Australia were commenced on 26 November, 2010, on the sole ground that isolated gene sequences are not patentable subject matter. Questions relating to the patentability of diagnostic methods and satisfaction of the general patentability criteria were not raised. The first instance decision in *Cancer Voices Australia v. Myriad Genetics* was handed down on 15 February, 2013. Judge Nicholas upheld the validity of the patent on the basis that '[i]solated nucleic acid is the product of human intervention involving the extraction and purification of the nucleic acid found in the cell', thus satisfying the Australian requirement for patentable subject matter of an 'artificially created state of affairs' (*National Research and Development Corporation v Commissioner of Patents* 1959). The decision has been appealed and was heard in August 2013.

The *Cancer Voices* case is unusual, not only because the limited nature of the challenge to the Myriad patent, but also because of the parties to the case. Public interest litigation is rare in Australia. The case was initiated by Cancer Voices Australia, a national network of state-based organizations representing cancer sufferers. The other applicant is a breast cancer sufferer, Yvonne D'Arcy. In practical terms, the final decision in this case is unlikely to impact BRCA testing for two reasons: first, the patent is not being enforced in Australia, but is a 'gift' to the Australian people; second, even if the sequence claims are ultimately held to be invalid, the method claims (which are not subject to challenge in this case) are still likely to be infringed by conventional BRCA testing should GTG decide to enforce the patent in the future. It remains to be seen whether the final decision in this case will have broader legal implications for the patentability of genes in Australia and to what extent the Australian courts will follow the lead from the US Supreme Court, if at all.

5.3 Policy and law reform

In 2003, the Australian Law Reform Commission (ALRC) was given a reference by the Australian government to inquire into the impact of gene patents on human health. The final report of the gene patent inquiry, *Genes and Ingenuity* (ALRC 2004), illustrates that BRCA patents were a key focal point for discussion. Despite concerns about the BRCA patents, the ALRC decided not to recommend excluding genes from the patent system but rather supported more nuanced amendments to patent law, including changes to the requirements for patentability (particularly inventive step and utility), limitations on the scope of patent claims, the introduction of an exception from infringement for research purposes and changes to the laws allowing compulsory licensing and Crown use (use for government purposes without prior authorization from the patent owner). The ALRC also called for granting agencies to provide guidelines on how patented inventions resulting from publicly funded research should be used.

Following the ALRC report, the Advisory Council on Intellectual Property (ACIP) was requested to explore the need for a statutory exception from patent infringement for experimental purposes (ACIP 2005). The ACIP recommended an experimental use exception, which largely reflects current industry practice (Nicol and Nielsen 2003). Then, in 2009, the Australian Senate commenced an independent inquiry into gene patents. Many recommendations largely mirrored those of the ALRC (Australian Senate Community Affairs Committee 2010). One of the key recommendations was that the government should respond to the senate inquiry as well as to the ALRC and ACIP inquiries. In November 2011, some seven years after the ALRC completed its report, the Australian federal government finally issued a formal response to that report as well as the ACIP and senate reports. The government largely accepted their recommendations, noting that the recently enacted *Intellectual Property Laws Amendment ('Raising the Bar') Act 2012* (Cth) addressed many of these (Australian Government 2011). The major reform aspects of the Raising the Bar Act included the introduction of an experimental use exception to infringement and modification of the inventive step and utility requirements. While the experimental use exception provides some protection for research use of patented inventions, it may have limited applicability with regard to the use of BRCA and other gene patents for genetic testing purposes because it is limited to 'research on' the patented invention.

In addition to the Raising the Bar Act, two other relevant bills have been introduced into the Australian Parliament over the past few years. The first was introduced in 2010 and sought to exclude genes and other biological materials from patenting. The bill did not proceed to vote because it was not supported by a parliamentary review committee. The reason provided by the committee was that it was considered too blunt an instrument and that it could have more negative than positive consequences (Australian Senate Legal and Constitutional Affairs Legislation Committee 2011). A second government-sponsored bill was introduced into parliament in late May 2013. In addition to a number of other amendments to patent law, this bill was intended to amend the Australian Crown use provisions to clarify that the provision of health services (including genetic testing services) can constitute so-called 'Crown use'. Unfortunately, however, although the bill was passed by the House of Representatives of the Australian Parliament, it was not passed by the Australian Senate before the end of the parliamentary session. As a consequence, the bill has now lapsed and will need to be introduced again following the election of a new parliament towards the end of 2013. Until then, it remains unclear whether Crown use provisions can be relied on by the government to step in when patients are denied reasonable access to health care by the unreasonable act of a patent holder. Nonetheless, the fact that the government has introduced this amendment to the Crown use provisions provides a very clear indication that it is prepared to rely on these whenever the need arises.

6 Emerging economies and international perspective

To our knowledge, Myriad's patent enforcement activities have mainly occurred within these developed countries. However, this does not mean that developing countries are immune from the risks associated with gene patent enforcement. Obviously, the extent of the risk facing each of these countries will vary, depending on a range of factors. First, companies may decide not to take out patents on DNA sequences in developing countries because the market in those countries does not warrant patent protection. Second, there is a wide diversity in scientific capacity and infrastructure to support health research and health care delivery. Third, the extent of patentability of DNA sequences differs (WHO 2005).

Brazil, China and India[17] are, however, becoming increasingly active in gene-based research and its applications. At the same time, their patent policies with respect to patent eligibility of DNA sequences diverge. The Brazilian Patent Act and Biotechnology Examination Guidelines do not consider isolated biological material an invention. Nevertheless, claims on DNA sequences are not excluded in cases where they would fit within the interpretation of a 'chemical compound'.[18] This approach is ambiguous (WHO 2005) and seems to be somewhere between the European and the (recently modified) US approach. The Indian guidelines from March 2013 appear to be compatible with the decision of the US Supreme Court, as they state that DNA sequences that are 'directly isolated from nature' are not patentable subject matter.[19] In contrast, the approach taken in the Chinese guidelines seems to be more closely aligned with the EPO policy, providing that DNA sequences, including those isolated from the human body as well as those obtained by other means, are a 'chemical substance', which is patentable.[20] While the Myriad controversy has not spread into these emerging economies, there may have been some spill-over effects from the policy storm in the other jurisdictions. Time will tell whether the decision of the US Supreme Court will lead to changes in the approaches to patentability in these jurisdictions.

There has been surprisingly little debate and guidance in this area at the international level, except for the initiatives of the Organization for Economic Cooperation and Development (OECD). In comparison to the fierce discussions on the national and European levels, the organizations most responsible for regulating intellectual property (IP) law at the international level, including the World Intellectual Property Organization (WIPO) and the World Trade Organization (WTO), have generally stayed out of the limelight. The OECD filled the gap left by WIPO and the WTO with its report *Genetic Inventions, IPR and Licensing Practices* (OECD 2002) and with licensing guidelines (OECD 2006). In the report, a number of potential remedies were examined in line with the proposals by national advisory committees described above, such as 'raising the bar' for the patentability requirements as well as research or experimental use exceptions, compulsory licences, licensing guidelines, patent pools and clearinghouses and the role of competition law (OECD 2002).

7 Concluding remarks

Increasingly, patent cases are going global and are featuring on the front pages of our newspapers (see for instance *Apple v. Samsung*). The debate surrounding Myriad's patents on BRCA1 and BRCA2, however, appears to be unique in its vigour and persistence. This paper's primary objective was to explain what makes this case distinctive. First, litigation in the US and Australia has focused primarily on the fundamental question of whether or not a human gene is patent-eligible subject matter and not on the 'traditional' patentability criteria of novelty, inventive step and industrial applicability (this is different in the opposition procedures in Europe, see Section 2.2). Typically, patent cases tend to concentrate on which of the contending parties will secure exclusive rights; but BRCA cases have challenged whether genes can be patented at all. This underlines the fundamental nature of the dispute. Second, the Myriad case has occupied the minds of patients, scientists, clinical geneticists, medical doctors, patent attorneys, lawyers, academics, business people, investors, analysts, economists, journalists, politicians, policymakers, advisors and legislators for more than a decade in several jurisdictions. The case has offered a significant opportunity for new and unexpected constituencies who are not usually interested in the intricacies of patent law (Murray and van Zimmeren 2011) to enter the debate about patents and make their voices heard.

Our second objective was to emphasize the variety of legal and policy responses in Europe, Canada, the US and Australia. The chapter clearly shows the different roles of institutional actors in diverse fora. In some countries (like France and Belgium), legislatures have crafted new tailored regimes in response to Myriad's restrictive licensing practices. Policymakers and advisory committees have proposed a variety of alternative mechanisms. Opposition (and appeal) procedures that already exist at some patent offices are another potential venue to invalidate or limit the scope of patents.

Advisory committees and councils in Europe, Canada, the US and Australia and the OECD have repeatedly issued reports questioning the rationale behind the patenting of genes and raised concerns about their implications. Notably, however, there has been little indication of a desire to create an absolute bar on the patenting of (isolated) DNA sequences in any of these reports. Rather, the reports

Table 8.1 Spectrum of 'tools'

	Europe	*Canada*	*US*	*Australia*
Post-grant opposition/review	yes (at EPO inter partes)	no	yes (after AIA at USPTO inter partes)	no
Litigation	yes (national)[1]	yes	yes	yes
Compulsory licence for public health (esp. diagnostics)	yes (national)	yes (but not specific to diagnostics	no	in process of implementation (crown use)
Research exception/exemption, experimental use doctrine	yes (national research exceptions)	yes (judicially created)	yes (judicially created, but very limited)	yes (but limited to 'research on')
Diagnostic exemption	no (but, very broad Belgian research exception)	no	no	no

[1] This will change as soon as the unitary patents and the unified patent court are operational.

have focused on rethinking the full spectrum of 'tools' for contesting undesirable patents and licensing practices (see Table 8.1). Some of these tools could be invoked in an early stage of the procedure at the patent office (i.e. third party submissions, re-examinations, oppositions), while others have appeared after the grant of the patent, allowing the use of the invention without the authorization of the patent owner in particular circumstances (i.e. research or diagnostic exceptions or exemptions) – with compulsory licences as a last resort mechanism. In particular, new provisions allowing compulsory licensing for diagnostic use have been incorporated into several national patent laws in Europe (including in France and Belgium) in response to the Myriad case and are in the process of being incorporated into the Crown use provisions in Australia. Similar proposals have also been floated in the US and Canada in the academic legal literature, but have not been formally incorporated into law.

The judgment of the US Supreme Court has invalidated patents on isolated DNA sequences, which may render some of the earlier proposals unnecessary. However, the Myriad storm has not fully dissipated, and it remains uncertain whether and when it might fully subside. In the months following the Supreme Court judgement, Myriad has sued various companies – Ambry, Gene by Gene, Quest, GeneDx, InVitae and LabCorp – for patent infringement. Several companies have also counter-sued or petitioned for declaratory judgment of non-infringement in separate court procedures. As this chapter was going to press, that litigation was still pending. Depending on their outcome, those cases may begin to develop case law about gene patents.

Moreover, the US Supreme Court decision has reinvigorated global discussions about gene patents, and although the US court has made it clear that DNA is not rendered patentable by merely being isolated, isolated DNA sequences are still patentable in many other jurisdictions, including Europe, Canada and Australia. In Europe, the European Commission must meet annual reporting obligations with regard to the development and implications of patent law in the field of biotechnology and genetic engineering through the Biotechnology Directive. In December 2012, the Commission decided to set up an expert group that will assist it in preparing its report. This may provide an opportunity to reconsider the issue of patent-eligible subject matter. Given the similarities between US and Canadian patent law, the fact that the US Supreme Court has held claims over isolated genomic DNA to be invalid will cast doubt on the validity of the same claims in Canada. In Australia, Judge Nicholas made a brief analysis of EU policy and US case law in his judgment (up until the CAFC decision, as the US Supreme Court decision was not yet available) before stating that Australian law is different and concluding that isolated sequences are patent-eligible. It remains to be seen to what extent the Australian appeal court will align with his position or follow the US Supreme Court.

Concerns about the Next-Generation Sequencing (NGS) technologies were looming in the background of *AMP v. Myriad,* although there was no clear consensus on whether NGS infringed BRCA1 and BRCA2 patents. Since NGS technologies, such as single-molecule sequencing, do not require amplifying specific exons of genes, tests using such methods may not infringe on genetic diagnostic claims that use PCR. Some experts have indeed interpreted claims on patented diagnostic methods this way, including some claims in Myriad's patents. Scholars have also argued that the composition of matter claims, such as those on BRCA1 and BRCA2 cDNA sequences, are not infringed on by NGS (Holman 2012, Price 2012). Whether Whole-Genome Sequencing (WGS) and Whole-Exome Sequencing (WES) infringed on BRCA1/2 and other gene patents has also been an area of considerable debate. While some have raised concerns that clinical WGS and WES applications face a patent thicket (SACGHS 2010) others have suggested that the problem is not so severe (Holman 2012). Additional uncertainty has also stemmed from evolving business models for clinical WGS/WES in which actual sequencing and clinical interpretation are uncoupled. This 'uncoupling' has complicated the assessment of infringement liability, because – at least in the US – infringement of most patents occurs only in cases when all steps of an alleged act of infringement are performed by a single entity (*Akamai and McKesson* [2012]). This would mean that if sequencing analysis and other steps (e.g. diagnosis or interpretation) are separated, infringement is 'split,' and no one party may be held liable.

Concerns about patent infringement have clearly deterred some providers, such as Ambry Genetics, from including BRCA in NGS breast cancer panels,[21] and until recently no US providers would offer testing for BRCA1/2 using NGS platforms. The fear that a legacy of claims on individual genes could impede WGS has motivated much of the opposition among the leaders at the NIH, and they – with support from the Department of Justice – have successfully argued that executive branch policy should change three decades of practice granting claims on isolated DNA at the USPTO. This proved persuasive to the US Supreme Court.

The outcome of *AMP v. Myriad* has encouraged many providers to enter the market quickly with competitive NGS tests for BRCA1/2 and to include these in multigene cancer risk panels.[22] However, in light of recent (*AMP v. Myriad* [2013], *Mayo v. Prometheus* [2012]) and anticipated case law (*Akamai and McKesson,* which appears to be moving up to the Supreme Court), some degree of uncertainty will likely persist, especially for diagnostic method claims. Moreover, a thorough freedom to operate analysis will be necessary for each specific test to assess the risk of patent infringement. For tests with large numbers of genes, such as cancer panels with one hundred or more genes, a freedom to operate analysis will often be quite expensive. Business practices such as bundling patent licenses through patent pools or clearinghouses (van Zimmeren *et al.* 2011) and sharing clinical data could reduce patent-related uncertainty and facilitate the development of the next generation of breast cancer diagnostics.

This opens the door for a new generation of patenting and licensing strategies, tailored to the changing diagnostic testing environment unencumbered by expensive opposition and litigation procedures. Technology is moving quickly, while courts, policymakers and legislators are trailing behind. Therefore, valuable, alternative market-based measures, such as patent pools and clearinghouses (van Zimmeren *et al.*, 2011; Nicol, 2010; OECD, 2006) that may facilitate patent licensing in the biomedical sector and that could serve as a sustainable, international model for diagnostic testing, should be welcomed more openly by legislators, industry, academia, patient advocates, professional societies and funders.

Notes

1. A longer version of this chapter will likely be published in *Biotechnology Law Report.*
2. For reasons of uniformity, the wording of Article 27(1) of the *Agreement on Trade-Related Aspects of Intellectual Property Rights* (TRIPs 1994) is used here. The terms 'inventive step' and 'capable of industrial application' are generally deemed to be synonymous with the terms 'non-obvious' and 'useful' of US patent law.
3. Deciding on the right time to file a patent application is notoriously difficult, in particular in competitive and rapidly developing areas, such as the biomedical sector. Inventors need to take a decision as to whether they want to delay filing in order to gather more data to support the invention risk being outrun by a competitor, or alternatively they may file early to secure a filing date ahead of their competitor, risking that their application contains errors or will be rejected for lacking adequate experimental support (cf. White 2007). Determining the right time is especially challenging in jurisdictions that operate a first-to-file rather than a first-to-invent system. In a first-to-file system, the right to the grant of a patent for a given invention lies with the first person to file a patent application for protection of that invention, regardless of the date of the actual invention. In contrast, in a first-to-invent system, the date of the actual invention is decisive. Nowadays, the first-to-file system rules. In the past, Canada and the US had a first-to-invent system. Under this system, when two people claimed the same invention, such a dispute could be solved by way of an 'interference proceeding' between them to review evidence of conception, reduction to practise and diligence. In March 2013, the US shifted toward what has been called a first-inventor-to file system.
4. We note that the European patent system will soon become even more complex. After more than 40 years of negotiations, the EU institutions have finally agreed on

the establishment of a 'patent with a unitary effect' and a specialized patent court (van Zimmeren, forthcoming). The patent is called 'unitary patent' or 'patent with unitary effects', because not all EU member states will participate. Spain and Italy did not agree with the translation arrangements associated with the unitary patent.

5. Please note that European patents are not EU patents; the membership of the EPO goes beyond the membership of the EU.
6. Article 5 of the EU Biotechnology Directive.
7. A patent application may claim priority from another application that was filed prior to it in order to take advantage of the filing date of information disclosed in that earlier application. Claiming priority is advantageous, because the earlier effective filing date reduces the number of prior art disclosures that need to be taken into account in the examination of the application (novelty and inventive step). This therefore increases the likelihood of obtaining a patent. The priority system, based on an international treaty (the Paris Convention), is useful in filing patent applications in many countries, as the costs of some of the filings can be delayed up to a year, and the earlier applications for the same invention will not be taken into account against the later applications.
8. According to Article 99 EPC (1973):

   > [w]ithin nine months of the publication of the mention of the grant of the European patent in the European Patent Bulletin, *any person* may give notice to the European Patent Office of opposition to that patent, in accordance with the Implementing Regulations' (emphasis added). 'Opposition may only be filed on the grounds that: (a) the subject-matter of the European patent is not patentable under Articles 52 to 57; (b) the European patent does not disclose the invention in a manner sufficiently clear and complete for it to be carried out by a person skilled in the art; (c) the subject-matter of the European patent extends beyond the content of the application as filed, or, if the patent was granted on a divisional application or on a new application filed under Article 61, beyond the content of the earlier application as filed. (Article 100 EPC)

9. We note that, around the time the opposition procedures were launched, the patents were assigned to the University of Utah Research Foundation.
10. In Europe, 'public order and morality' is regarded as an exception to patentability: 'European patents shall not be granted in respect of: (a) inventions the commercial exploitation of which would be contrary to "ordre public" or morality; such exploitation shall not be deemed to be so contrary merely because it is prohibited by law or regulation in some or all of the Contracting States.'
11. The patent application should disclose the invention in a manner sufficiently clear and complete for it to be carried out by a person skilled in the art (Art. 83 EPC). Moreover, the patent claims shall define the matter for which protection is being sought. They shall be clear and concise and be supported by the description (Art. 84 EPC). Applications or patents may be amended in proceedings before the EPO, and applicants will be given at least one opportunity to voluntarily amend the application, but amended claims may not contain subject-matter which extends the scope beyond the content of the application as filed.
12. Another loophole identified in the past was the lack of patent protection in Malta. A Maltese biotechnology firm, Synergene, offered a 'legitimate' alternative for Myriad for BRCA testing (Check 2002).
13. In a search done in March 2013 of US patents and patent applications that include the terms 'BRCA1' or 'BRCA2' in their claims, 598 results were found, of which 143 were granted patents.
14. Myriad's broadest BRCA1 patents were granted the following year: US patent 5,747,282 claimed 'isolated' BRCA1 DNA molecules and variants and fragments with BRCA1 sequences (that is the molecules themselves); US patent 5,753,441

claimed methods for detecting differences between a BRCA1 sequence from a person's sample and the disclosed BRCA1 reference sequence.

15. The suit initially included the USPTO as a defendant, but legal grounds under dispute were narrowed on appeal, and the USPTO was dropped as a defendant. The case name thus also changed from *Association for Molecular Pathology, et al. v. US Patent and Trademark et al. (AMP v. USPTO)* to Myriad as the defendant (*AMP v. Myriad*).
16. A search in March 2013 on the Auspat database (www.ipaustralia.gov.au/auspat/index.htm) for Australian patents and patent applications that included the term 'BRCA' revealed five lapsed applications. There were 20 results for 'BRCA1', with one granted patent (777341), three live applications and the remainder being lapsed or ceased applications. There were 10 results for 'BRCA2', with one repeat from the 'BRCA1' search, one live application, one refused application and the remainder lapsed or ceased.
17. In India, since (at least) 2008, the Molecular Medicine Group of Reliance Life Sciences has been offering a diagnostic test sequencing the entire BRCA1 and BRCA2 genes (for more information, see www.rellife.com/molecular_medicine.html). We are not aware of other commercial sources in India, or in Brazil and China, at this time.
18. Article 18 (III) of the Brazilian Industrial Property Law states that living beings, in whole or in part, are not considered patentable. Article 10 (IX) states that natural living beings, in whole or in part, and biological material encountered in nature or isolated including the genome or germplasm of any natural living being are not considered to be inventions. The law does, however, allow for the patenting of chemical products, provided they fulfil the patentability criteria. As far as DNA sequences are regarded as chemical products and the claims are written in accordance with the guidelines, they may be patentable. For more information, see Industrial Property Law No.9.279 of 14 May, 1996, available at www.wipo.int/wipolex/en/text.jsp?file_id=125397, and 'Diretrizes de Exame de Patentes nas Áreas de Biotecnologia e Farmacêutica', available at www.inpi.gov.br/images/stories/Diretrizes_Farmaceutica_e_Biotec.pdf (31 December, 1994, under revision).
19. According to Section 11 of India's Biotechnology Examination Guidelines (2013), Section 3 (c) of the Indian Patents Act prescribes that the mere discovery of a scientific principle or the formulation of an abstract theory or discovery of any living thing or nonliving substance occurring in nature is not a patentable invention. Products such as microorganisms, nucleic acid sequences, proteins, enzymes, compounds, etc., which are directly isolated from nature, are not patentable subject matter. However, processes of isolation of these products can be considered subject to requirements of Section 2 (1) (j) of the Act. For more information, see: http://nbaindia.org/uploaded/Biodiversityindia/Legal/14.%20The%20Patents%20Act,%201970.pdf and www.ipindia.nic.in/whats_new/biotech_Guidelines_25March2013.pdf.
20. Section 9.1.2.2 of China's State Intellectual Property Office (SIPO) Examination Guidelines (2010), Part II, Chapter 10 provides: 'No matter it is a gene or a DNA fragment, it is, in substance, a chemical substance. The said gene or DNA fragment includes those isolated from microorganism, plant, animal or human body, as well as those obtained by other means. As stated in Section 2.1 of this Chapter, a gene or DNA fragment found in the nature and existing in its natural state is merely a discovery. It falls into "scientific discoveries" as provided for in Article 25.1 and is unpatentable. However, a gene or a DNA fragment per se and the process to obtain it are subject matters of patent protection if it is isolated or extracted for the first time from the nature, its base sequence is unknown in the prior art and can be definitely characterized, and it can be exploited industrially.' For more information, see: http://english.sipo.gov.cn/laws/lawsregulations/201101/t20110119_566244.html and www.sipo.gov.cn/zlsqzn/sczn2010eng.pdf

21. www.pbs.org/wgbh/nova/next/body/gene-patents-and-personalized-medicine/.
22. www.genomeweb.com/sequencing/competition-myriad-heats-us-testing-labs-launch-brca-tests-hereditary-cancer-pan.

References

Abbott, A. (2005) 'Genetic patent singles out Jewish women', *Nature,* 436: 12.

ACIP (2005) *Patents and Experimental Use.* www.acip.gov.au/reviews_completed.html

Akamai Technologies v. Limelight Networks, Inc. and McKesson Technologies, Inc. v. Epic Systems Corp, (Fed. Cir. 2012) (en banc).

ALRC (2004) *Genes and Ingenuity: Gene Patenting and Human Health,* Report No. 99. www.alrc.gov.au/publications/report-99

AMP v. Myriad, 569 U.S. (2013).

AMP v. USPTO, 653 F.3d 1329 (Fed. Cir. 2011).

AMP v. USPTO, 702 F. Supp. 2d 181 (S.D.N.Y. 2010).

Australian Government (2011) *Response to Senate Community Affairs References Committee Gene Patents Report.* www.ipaustralia.gov.au/about-us/what-we-do/gene-patents-response

Australian Senate Community Affairs Committee (2010) *Report on Gene Patents.* www.aph.gov.au/senate/committee/clac_ctte/gene_patents_43/report/index.htm

Australian Senate Legal and Constitutional Affairs Legislation Committee (2011) *Report on the Patent Amendment (Human Genes and Biological Materials) Bill 2010.* www.aph.gov.au/senate/committee/legcon_ctte/patent_amendment/report/index.htm

Baldwin, A. L. and Cook-Deegan, R. (2013) 'Constructing narratives of heroism and villainy: a case study of Myriad's BRACAnalysis and Genentech's Herceptin', *Genome Medicine,* 5.

Benowitz, S. (2003) 'European groups oppose Myriad's latest patent on *BRCA1*', *Journal of the National Cancer Institute,* 95: 8–9.

Brody, B. (2007) 'Intellectual property and biotechnology: the European debate', *Kennedy Institute of Ethics Journal,* 17: 69–110.

Canadian Biotechnology Advisory Committee (2006) *Human Genetic Materials, Intellectual Property and the Health Sector.* Ottawa: CBAC.

Cancer Voices Australia v. Myriad Genetics, Inc. [2013] FCA 63.

Check, E. (2002) 'Malta provides loophole for breast-cancer screen', *Nature,* 419: 767.

Cho, M.K., Illangasekare, S., Weaver, M.A., Leonard, D.G.B., Merz, J.F. (2003) 'Effects of patents and licenses on the provision of clinical genetic testing services', *Journal of Molecular Diagnostics*, 5: 3–8.

Council and European Parliament (1998) *Directive 98/44 of the European Parliament and of the Council of 6 July 1998 on the Legal Protection of Biotechnological Inventions, OJ* L2013/13.

Danish Council of Bioethics (2004) *Patenting Human Genes and Stem Cells.* Copenhagen: Danish Council of Bioethics.

Davies, J. and White, M. (1996) *Breakthrough: The Race to Find the Breast Cancer Gene.* USA: Wiley and Sons.

Debrulle, J., De Cort, L. and Petit M. (2007) 'La licence obligatoire belge pour raisons de santé publique'. In Van Overwalle, G. (ed.) *Gene Patents and Public Health.* Brussels: Bruylant.

EPC (1973) *Convention on the Grant of European Patents* (European Patent Convention) of 5 October, 1973, as revised by the Act revising Article 63 EPC of 17 December, 1991, and the Act revising the EPC of 29 November, 2000, Decision Administrative Council of the European Patent Organisation of 28 June, 2001, OJ EPO 2001, Special edition 4: 55.

ESHG Working Party on Patenting and Licensing (2008) 'Patenting and licensing in genetic testing – recommendations of the European Society of Human Genetics', *European Journal of Human Genetics,* 16: S3–S9.

Gold, E. G. and Carbone, J. (2010) 'Myriad Genetics: in the eye of the policy storm', *Genetics in Medicine,* 12, 4 Suppl.: S39–S70.

Gold, E. G. and Gallochat, A. (2001) 'The European biotech directive: past as prologue', *European Law Journal,* 7: 331–66.

Hall, J. M., Lee, M. K., Newman, B. et al. (1990) 'Linkage of early-onset familial breast cancer to chromosome 17q21', *Science,* 250: 1684–1689.

Holman, C. M. (2012) 'Debunking the myth that whole-genome sequencing infringes thousands of gene patents', *Nature Biotechnology,* 30: 240–44.

Lecrubier, A. (2002) 'European institutions are challenging Myriad Genetics patent monopoly on the *BRCA* gene', *EMBO Reports,* 3: 1120–22.

Llewelyn M. (2003) *Implications of Intellectual Property Rights on Public Healthcare: The UK as Case Study,* ATRIP Annual Congress, Tokyo, 4–6 August.

Marshall, E. (1997)'The battle over BRCA1 goes to court, BRCA2 may be next', *Science,* 278: 1874.

Matthijs, G. and Halley, D. (2002) 'European-wide opposition against the breast cancer gene patents', *European Journal of Human Genetics,* 10: 783–84.

Mayo v. Prometheus, 132 S.Ct. 1289 (2012).

Merrill, S.A. and Mazza, A-M. (eds.) (2006) *Reaping the Benefits of Genomic and Proteomic Research: Intellectual Property Rights, Innovation, and Public Health,* Washington, D.C., National Academies Press

Miki, Y., Swensen, J., Shattuck-Eidens, D. et al. (1994) 'A strong candidate for the breast and ovarian cancer susceptibility gene BRCA1', *Science,* 266: 66–71.

Murphy, P.D., Allen A.C., Alvares C.P. et al. (1997) *Consensus Sequence of the Human BRCA1 Gene,* United States patent application, 5 August.

Murray, K. and van Zimmeren, E. (2011) 'Dynamic patent governance in Europe and the United States: the Myriad example', *Cardozo Journal of International and Comparative Law,* 19: 287–342.

Myriad Genetics, Inc. (2013) *2012 Annual Report,* Salt Lake City.

National Research and Development Corporation v. Commissioner of Patents (1959) 102 CLR 252.

Nicol, D. (2005) 'Balancing innovation and access to healthcare through the patent system – an Australian perspective', *Community Genetics,* 8: 228–34.

———. (2010) 'Collaborative licensing in biotechnology: a survey of knowledge, experience and attitudes in Australia', *Biotechnology Law Report,* 29: 465–83.

Nicol, D. and Nielsen, J. (2003) *Patents and Medical Biotechnology: An Empirical Analysis of Issues Facing the Australian Industry.* Hobart: Centre for Law and Genetics Occasional Paper No. 6.

NIH (2004) 'Best practices for the licensing of genomic inventions', *Federal Register* 69.

Nuffield Council of Bioethics (2002) *The Ethics of Patenting DNA.* London: Nuffield Council of Bioethics.

OECD (2002) *Genetic Inventions, IPR and Licensing Practices.* Paris: OECD.

OECD (2006) *Guidelines for the Licensing of Genetic Inventions.* Paris: OECD.

Ontario Ministry of Health and Long-Term Care (2002) *Genetics, Testing and Gene Patenting: Charting New Territory in Healthcare.* Ontario: Ontario Ministry of Health and Long-Term Care.

Parathasarathy, S. (2007) *Building Genetic Medicine: Breast Cancer, Technology, and the Comparative Politics of Health Care.* Cambridge: MIT Press.

Piper, T. and Gold, E. R. (2008) *Practices, Policies and Possibilities in Licensing in Human Genetics.* Report for Health Canada, Montreal, Canada: The Innovation Partnership. www.theinnovationpartnership.org/data/documents/00000015–1.pdf

Price, W. N. (2012) 'Unblocked future: why gene patents won't hinder whole genome sequencing and personalized medicine', *Cardozo Law Review*, 33: 1601–32.

Puget, N., Stoppa-Lyonnet, D., Sinilnikova, O. et al. (1999) 'Screening for germ-line rearrangements and regulatory mutations in BRCA1 led to the identification of four new deletions', *Cancer Research,* 59: 455–61.

Richer, J., Nelson, T. N., Evans, J. Armstrong, L. Lauzon, J. and McGillivray, B. (2012) 'CCMG statement on gene patents', *Clinical Genetics,* 82: 405.

SACGHS (2010) *Gene Patents and Licensing Practices and Their Impact on Patient Access to Genetic Tests.* http://oba.od.nih.gov/oba/sacghs/reports/SACGHS_patents_report_2010.pdf

Shattuck-Eidens, D. M., Simard, J., Durocher, F., Emi, M. and Nakamura, Y. (1997) *Linked Breast And Ovarian Cancer Susceptibility Gene,* United States patent application, 2 December.

Standing Committee on Health, Parliament of Canada (2001) *Assisted Human Reproduction: Building Families.* Ottawa, Canada: Standing Committee on Health Parliament of Canada.

Stanford University (2007) 'In the public interest: nine points to consider in licensing university technology'. http://otl.stanford.edu/documents/whitepaper-10.pdf

TRIPs (1994) *Agreement on Trade-related Aspects of Intellectual Property Rights* (TRIPs-Agreement). Annex 1C to the Marrakesh Agreement establishing the World Trade Organization (Marrakesh, Morocco, 15 April, 1994).

UC v. Lilly, 119 F.3d 1559 (1997).

Van Overwalle, G. (ed.) (2007) *Gene Patents and Public Health.* Brussels: Bruylant.

Van Overwalle, G. and van Zimmeren, E. (2006) 'Reshaping Belgian patent law: the revision of the research exemption and the introduction of a compulsory license for public health', *IIP Forum,* 64: 42–49.

van Zimmeren, E. (forthcoming) 'European patent reform: transforming the governance network and enhancing innovation?'. In E. Sorensen, A. K. Hagedorn, B. Damgaard and A. Agger (eds) *Public Innovation in Europe.* Bentham Science.

van Zimmeren, E. and Requena, G. (2007) 'Ex-officio licensing in the medical sector: the French model'. In: Van Overwalle, G. (ed.) *Gene Patents and Public Health.* Brussels: Bruylant, 123–47.

van Zimmeren, E., Vanneste, S., Matthijs, G., Vanhaverbeke, W., Van Overwalle, G. (2011) 'Patent pools and clearinghouses in the Life Sciences', *Trends in Biotechnology*, 29: 569–76.

van Zimmeren, E. and Van Overwalle, G. (2011) 'A paper tiger? Compulsory license regimes for public health in Europe', *IIC,* 42: 4–40.

White, N. L. (2007) 'Time waits for no man: deciding when to file a patent application in Europe', *Nature Biotechnology,* 25: 639–41.

WHO (2005) *Genetics, Genomics and the Patenting of DNA: Review of Potential Implications for Health in Developing Countries.* Geneva. www.who.int/genomics/FullReport.pdf

Williams-Jones, B. (2002) 'History of a gene patent: tracing the development and application of commercial BRCA testing', *Health Law Journal,* 10: 123–46.

9 From BRCA to BRCAness

Tales of translational research

Pascale Bourret, Peter Keating and Alberto Cambrosio

At some point one has to pass from explanation to mere description.

Wittgenstein, *On Certainty* § 189

The roots of this chapter[1] lie in an unexpected event – unexpected, that is, for social science observers. We are referring to the decisive and recent turn in BRCA research and related clinical activities. Previously confined largely to *hereditary* breast and ovarian cancer (HBOC), around 2004 the field shifted sharply in the direction of *sporadic* cancers, a transition marked by the coining of the notion of *BRCAness* (Turner *et al.* 2004). There are several reasons why this somewhat esoteric event attracted our attention. The most important is that the discovery of the BRCA susceptibility genes and of their role in the development of HBOC in the 1990s has often been used by science studies scholars as a prototypical illustration of the 'molecularization' of contemporary oncology (and of the life sciences in general), and, even more importantly, as a paradigmatic example of the establishment of a new kind of clinical practice centred on the management of risk rather than actual disease (see Bourret 2005, Gibbon 2007, Löwy and Gaudillière 2008, Parthasarathy 2007). These observations have occasionally been coupled with the critical remark that hereditary forms of breast cancer, which represent only a small percentage of the total number of cases, attracted more than their fair share of funding. This, critics argued, revealed an inherent bias in medical research.[2] The transition from hereditary to sporadic cancers belies or qualifies these traditional lines of argument – first, by vindicating the original investment in BRCA research, insofar as it has obviously led to insights and applications that extend beyond the narrow domain of family mutations; and second, by showing the need to revisit social scientists' focus on risk as the defining characteristic of this new set of practices, since these practices now concern patients who are suffering from the actual disease as opposed to 'asymptomatic' patients with a history of familial risk.[3]

To avoid any misunderstanding, let us clearly state that we do not claim that a concern with translational research has replaced an initial focus on risk – in other words, that in the clinical domain there has been a sharp shift away from risk. These two elements are not mutually incompatible: in the case of BRCA, while early work centred on hereditary risk, it was also performed as part of translational research initiatives (in fact, as mentioned below, it immediately became a poster child of this kind of research), and nowadays risk continues to be an important element of the shifting BRCA landscape (see also Figure 9.5). What we are claiming is that *social scientists* (as contrasted with clinicians and biomedical researchers) have focused their attention on the risk component, thus overlooking the translational research dimension that provides for a more consistent account of the BRCA trajectory and, in particular, its present interest in sporadic cancers. As far as biomedical practitioners are concerned, we can also speak of a transition – namely, the expansion of BRCA clinical activities that used to be mostly confined to the hereditary domain to the sporadic cancer domain. As we will argue in this chapter, however, clinical researchers were investigating the clinical utility of BRCA in the sporadic cancer domain already in the 1990s, albeit with limited success – only managing to establish a robust connection around 2004–2005 via the notion of BRCAness.

How should this crossing over (to use a chromosomal metaphor) from the hereditary to the sporadic domain be described? When we asked clinicians involved in BRCA research, it was their turn to be surprised, since they saw no sharp divide between these two domains. They viewed the field from a more practical stance. Far from operating within two separate, self-contained socio-technical worlds, clinical oncologists have long been confronted with patients affected with both hereditary and sporadic forms of the disease. Work on HBOC has, of course, led to the emergence of a specific form of clinical activity – a 'clinic of mutations' (Bourret 2005, Rabeharisoa and Bourret 2009) – as well as related professional figures (the 'onco-geneticist'), but the oncology ward remains the locus of clinical encounters and exchanges between different types of patients and specialists. This is particularly true in the case of institutions such as Guy's Hospital in London, where local demographics present clinicians with an inordinate number of young black women who suffer from a very aggressive form of breast cancer known as 'triple negative' (more on this below), which has been linked to BRCAness. Basic researchers have a similar perspective – for instance, Laura van't Veer, the lead author of a highly cited paper from 2002 in *Nature* on breast cancer genomics (van't Veer *et al.* 2002, with over 3,700 citations by October 2012). Dr van't Veer has been simultaneously involved in the investigation of BRCA hereditary susceptibility genes and of somatic gene mutations at the Netherlands Cancer Institute and has participated in the hospital's familial breast cancer clinic. In keeping with this trend, we have noted that the term genetics itself has undergone a marked shift in meaning. Previously, it referred to the transmission of hereditary characters, now it refers more broadly to molecular processes, such as DNA transcription and expression, which take place in all somatic cells, and no longer concerns only germline (inherited) cells (Keating and Cambrosio 2001). This is why Dr van't Veer's dual activities, far from creating divided loyalties or a split personality, cohere in a consistent, albeit differentiated, domain of practice.

Wherein lies that domain? To answer this question, we must foreshadow our principal argument, which consists of an alternative account of the BRCA story – one that, as already suggested, defines translational research, not risk, as the central characteristic of this domain. Translational research first emerged in the early 1990s in the course of a series of initiatives funded by the National Cancer Institute in the US. Aimed at reducing the perceived gap between basic research and clinical applications, the original impetus for these initiatives was provided by the characterization of cancer susceptibility genes, in particular BRCA (Brown 2007, Butler 2008, Kohli-Laven *et al.* 2011). More than a mere interface, or bridge, between clinical activities and fundamental research, translational research has morphed into a distinct sphere of activity, albeit one with fuzzy boundaries. The BRCA story, and the sequence of events that has led from the hereditary to the sporadic domain via the emergence of liminal notions such as BRCA-like, BRCA-associated and, especially, BRCAness, illustrates the fact that translational research operates simultaneously on several research fronts.

In our analysis, we draw on Michel Morange's (1997) fruitful suggestion that, in order to understand innovation in the life sciences, one should take into account not only the specific content of scientific practices, but also their temporal dynamics – i.e. the order in which they intersect and assemble. Innovations can fail because they come too early or, arguably, too late – at a moment when alternative configurations have already been stabilized. In the present case, BRCA translational researchers had to juggle with pre-existing and emerging areas of clinical and laboratory research on chemotherapeutic drugs, targeted therapies, molecular oncogenesis pathways, epigenetic mechanisms, pathological and clinical classifications and biomedical instrumentation (to name a few). Moreover, the need to demonstrate the clinical utility of their findings played a key role in this process. BRCA-related activities thus represent, in our view, a paradigmatic instantiation of translational research – one that cannot be reduced to the mechanical interplay of predetermined interests or strategies, given the emergent nature of the opportunities seized by researchers and clinicians.

Setting the stage for BRCAness

In 2004, three British authors from the London-based Breakthrough Breast Cancer Research Centre published a paper entitled 'Hallmarks of "BRCAness" in sporadic cancer' (Turner *et al.* 2004).[4] The article introduced a new notion, BRCAness, which became the rallying point of a number of contributions that set BRCA research on a new laboratory and clinical trajectory. The authors defined BRCAness as a *phenotype* – i.e. as a number of clinical and molecular characteristics – which some sporadic cancers share with cancers occurring in BRCA1/2 germline mutations carriers. Traditionally, the term phenotype refers to the observable characteristics of a given organism, whereas the counterpart notion of genotype refers to the genetic 'instructions' contained in the organism's germline cells. In the present case, the term phenotype was extended to include molecular entities in addition to gross anatomical features: another instance of molecularization. But what struck us as rather peculiar and thus warranting further examination is the choice of uniting BRCA – a gene and its mutations – with the phenotypic characteristics of sporadic cancers by coining the threshold notion of BRCAness.

The history of these developments is relatively complex, and we can only provide a capsule version of the events. In the 1980s and 90s, given the available technologies, a viable option for dissecting the molecular components of cancer – i.e. for identifying genes involved in its aetiology – was to analyse families harbouring several cases of the disease. So-called 'linkage studies' of large families led researchers to the chromosomal locus of susceptibility genes, such as BRCA, opening the door for their subsequent characterization. Although hereditary cancers are relatively rare, the search for inherited mutations was perceived as a shortcut, providing quick and easy access to molecular mechanisms whose understanding could subsequently inform the analysis of somatic mutations. This strategy – resting as it did on the 'ability to generalize knowledge gained from germline mutation carriers' (Maxwell and Domcheck 2012: p. 3) – panned out in several instances, but not in the case of breast cancer. While researchers successfully managed to identify a locus in 1990 and to clone BRCA1, BRCA2 and related mutations in 1994 and 1995, respectively, they failed to find equivalent BRCA mutations in cases of sporadic cancer, despite a significant research effort.[5] As was opined in an editorial from 1995 in *Nature Genetics* (Boyd 1995), 'interesting though these findings are, it remains curious that BRCA1 alterations in sporadic breast cancers have yet to be described, in spite of a mutation search the intensity of which is probably without parallel in cancer molecular genetics.'

As a result, a number of scientists in the 1990s began to look for mechanisms other than mutations that could silence BRCA and thus lead to cancer. Research on an epigenetic mechanism known as DNA methylation led to a series of contrasting results that we cannot go into detail about here. Suffice it to say that studies carried out in cells lines (Rice *et al.* 1998) were first contradicted by studies carried out on breast cancer tissue (Magdinier *et al.* 1998) and then confirmed by other studies (Catteau *et al.* 1999). A close look at these contributions shows that, from the very outset, they confronted the issue of clinical utility by trying to establish correlations between their results and subtypes of breast cancer. Pathologists had long recognized that breast cancer comes in different subtypes, which were initially described via the visual (histopathological) examination of tissues. Starting in the 1980s using first biochemical and then in the 1990s immunohistochemical methods, pathologists introduced a new classification based on the presence or absence of hormonal receptors on tumour cells, in particular the oestrogen (ER) and progesterone (PR) receptors. These were soon joined by a third entity, known as HER2 (Human Epidermal Growth Factor Receptor 2). Beyond its diagnostic and prognostic dimensions, this new categorization directly translated into therapeutic choices: hormone therapy is offered only to patients with positive hormone receptor status, while the new 'revolutionary treatment' trastuzumab (known commercially as Herceptin; Bazell 1998), introduced in 1998, targets HER2-positive patients. While the original study by Magdinier *et al.* (1998) had concluded that no connection existed between methylation status and pathological prognostic factors – thus pointing to a lack of clinical utility – now the study by Catteau *et al.* (1999) pointed to a possible, but unproven correlation between methylation and receptor status. There was, however, an additional question: did methylation in sporadic cancers lead to the inactivation of BRCA function as mutations did in hereditary cancer? A study by Esteller *et al.* (2000) provided indications that this was the case, but its results, marred by uncertainties (Allemani *et al.* 2004), remained tentative.

Thus, to summarize the two main factors of the situation so far: (a) the strategy of looking for the genetic characteristics of cancer in hereditary cases and then transposing the results to sporadic cancers, which was successfully deployed in other instances, was unsuccessful in the case of BRCA mutations; (b) these negative findings produced a search for alternative mechanisms of silencing BRCA functions in sporadic cancers, although initial studies in the second half of the 1990s produced uncertain results that did not pass the test of clinical utility. As we will see below, the situation changed significantly in the new century when novel technologies, notably gene expression profiling (GEP), began to uncover the molecular nature of breast cancer. In particular, GEP changed 'the way breast cancer is perceived . . . breast cancer is now perceived as a heterogeneous group of different diseases characterized by distinct molecular aberrations, rather than one disease with varying histological features and clinical behaviour' (Reis-Filho and Pusztai 2011: p. 1812). How did this lead to BRCAness?

BRCA-associated, BRCA-like and BRCAness

The availability of the new GEP technology did not necessarily simplify our understanding of breast cancer. In fact, one could argue that it made it even more complex, because clinicians and researchers now had to cope with three different ways of framing the disease: (a) GEP studies, (b) immunohistochemical investigations carried out by research pathologists and (c) the line of work initiated by the aforementioned methylation studies postulating the existence of a BRCA phenotype.

The first series of findings appeared in 2000 when Perou *et al.* published an article in *Nature* that introduced their novel GEP-based classification of breast cancers. It has since become a classic (over 4,000 citations by October 2012; see also the follow-up article by Sorlie *et al.* 2001, which has received almost 3,200 citations by the same date). A doctor of philosophy rather than a clinician, Charles Perou embodies the transgressive ethos of translational research, having achieved not only the rank of professor of genetics, but also of pathology and laboratory medicine. Perou's contribution came at a time (in the late 1990s) when BRCA-mutated tumours could not be distinguished clinically from sporadic cancers. Practitioners generally agreed that 'these kinds of family syndromes [HBOC] have no clinical definition' (Essioux and Bonaïti-Pellié 1997: p. 38). Nonetheless, the clinical specificity of these tumours quickly became a burning issue among clinicians in charge of treating patients already affected by the disease, and of implementing chemopreventive strategies for patients at risk of getting the disease. At the turn of the century, it became clear that BRCA tumours are largely ER receptor-negative, and yet practitioners (for instance, in the French Cancer Genetics Group; see Bourret *et al.* 2006) continued to ask: 'are BRCA-negative receptor tumours and sporadic negative receptor tumours identical?' (fieldwork, 22 April, 2003). Perou and his team did not immediately tackle this issue, as they had not included cases of BRCA carriers in the work leading to their 2000 publication. The resulting classification did not feature a specific BRCA category but did, however, comprise a molecular subtype termed 'basal-like tumours' that would later overlap with BRCA. Specifically, a team of researchers that included Perou (Grushko *et al.* 2004) subsequently examined a collection of cases they termed 'BRCA1-associated breast cancers' and concluded that 'the *BRCA1* mutant tumors appear to have a profile that is most consistent with the basal-like subtype' (p. 506), thus connecting sporadic basal-like tumours and BRCA mutant tumours.

In the meantime, at the phenotypic corner of the triangle, an international (US, UK, Sweden) consortium (Hedenfalk *et al.* 2001) had used GEP to compare hereditary and sporadic breast cancers and reached the conclusion that some sporadic and BRCA hereditary cancers might be related at the level of phenotype rather than genotype (Hedenfalk *et al.* 2001). Additional contributions brought partial support for the phenotypic hypothesis: Jazaeri *et al.* (2002) found indications (albeit in ovarian cancer) of the existence of 'BRCA-like' phenotypes in sporadic cancers, while van't Veer *et al.*'s highly cited paper from 2002 also described, albeit in passing, a sporadic tumour that ended up being classified as BRCA, most likely because of a methylation mechanism. Figure 9.1 shows the number of citations received by the early papers connected to the phenotypic hypothesis. As can be seen, the paper by Magdiner *et al.* (1998), which concluded that methylation patterns lacked clinical utility, did not fare as well as the paper by Catteau *et al.*

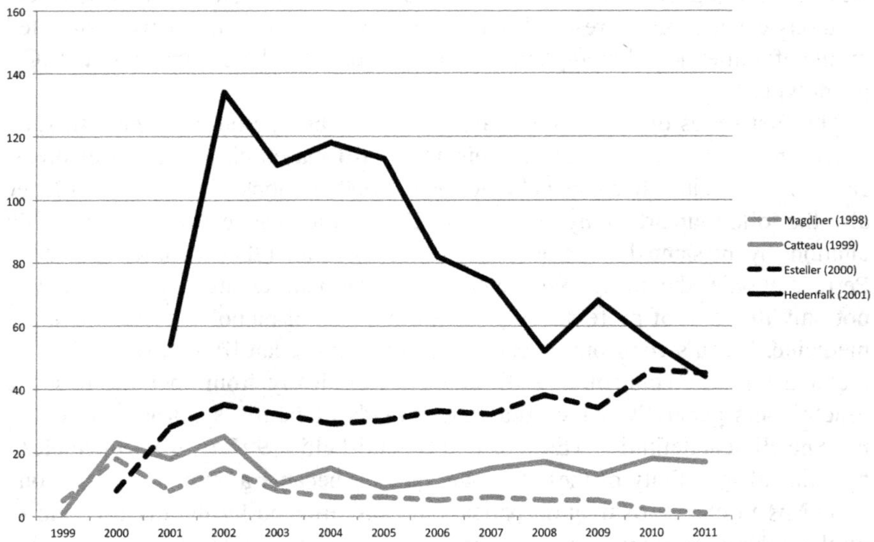

Figure 9.1 Number of citations received by the Magdiner *et al.* (1998), Catteau *et al.* (1999), Esteller *et al.* (2000) and Hedenfalk *et al.* (2001) articles.

Source: Thomson Reuters Web of Science.

(1999), which reached the opposite conclusion, and both attracted less attention than the paper by Esteller *et al.* (2000), which hypothesized methylation's role of inactivating BRCA. However, among these four early papers, the prize for most citations clearly goes to Hedenfalk *et al.* (2001), the paper that postulated the existence of a phenotypic, rather than genotypic, connection between hereditary and sporadic breast tumours. These findings immediately attracted the attention of researchers in the field, as the quick rise in citations makes clear.

Pathologists had not been passively waiting for molecular biologists to reclassify diseases. Since GEP is a 'grind and bind' approach whereby cells are destroyed to extract RNA, pathologists opted for immunohistochemical (IHC) technologies that display the presence or absence of receptors *in situ* (thus preserving tissue and cellular structures for histopathological examination) and as such are consistent with their traditional *modus operandi.* By characterizing tumours in terms of three main receptors (ER, PR and HER2), pathologists developed a system whose clinical utility, unlike the more experimental GEP molecular subtypes, was hard to dispute, since it had been evolved in constant interaction with clinical activities. While this bifurcation created a further puzzle – namely, how to align the two approaches – for our present purposes, the relevant issue is that pathologists defined a breast cancer category characterized by the absence of the three main receptors (ER, PR and HER2), which they then called, somewhat unimaginatively, triple-negative breast cancers. It soon appeared that BRCA mutant tumours were often triple-negative while, vice-versa, a large proportion of triple-negative tumours harboured BRCA defects.

The origins of triple-negative breast cancer (TNBC) as a nosological category cannot, however, be ascribed to the mechanical application of IHC tests. Many uncertainties surround the determination of IHC status, and several national and international standardization initiatives have been launched during the last decade in an attempt to increase the reliability and especially the consistency of IHC measurements, which are ultimately triangulated with clinical variables.[6] Moreover, as a nosological entity, TNBC is far from robust, as evinced by articles with titles such as 'Triple negative breast cancer: disease entity or title of convenience?' (Carey *et al.* 2010) or 'Triple negative breast cancer: proposals for a pragmatic definition' (Eiermann *et al.* 2012). Indeed, TNBC is also pragmatically defined as those tumours that do not respond to existing treatments. A number of agents, such as tamoxifen, have long been used for treating hormone-positive patients, and when the trastuzumab became available for HER2-positive patients, this led to the definition of triple-negative tumours as those tumours for which no treatment existed. As noted by a UK oncologist, 'The reason why we know it [TNBC] now is just because Herceptin was developed. . . . It's definitely not a biological entity . . . it's a practical clinical entity based on practicality, which means that we need to find treatments for it' (interview, 24 June, 2011). A measure of both the uncertainties surrounding TNBC and of its increasingly strategic position in breast cancer is provided by a surprisingly specific statement from 2012 by the U.S. Senate committee overseeing funding for the National Cancer Institute. No doubt spurred by the present climate of patient activism, the committee reported that it 'remain[ed] concerned about the toll of triple negative breast cancer and urge[d] NCI to collaborate with [other agencies] to help improve treatment and survival rates' (Ong 2012).

The situation we just described is neatly summarized by a Venn diagram consisting of three overlapping circles of basal-like, triple-negative, and BRCA-associated breast cancers (see, for example, Figure 9.1 in Carey *et al.* 2010). In other words, BRCAness emerged from the timely intersection of these three lines of work. As the next section shows, however, the situation was more complex.

BRCAness, at last

Let us now return to BRCAness. The article by Turner *et al.* from 2004, which introduced this term, and the follow-up article by the same team (Farmer *et al.* 2005) carried the notion of a BRCA *phenotype* well beyond the scope covered in the paper by Hedenfalk *et al.* (2001). Comparing the citations received by these three papers, Figure 9.2 is consistent with the hypothesis that, while the article from 2001 attracted the attention of researchers, the contributions from 2004 and 2005 displaced it and became the *locus classicus* for subsequent work on this topic. Let us examine how.

The authors of the paper from 2004 explicitly refer to Perou's molecular subtypes as the starting point for their exploration of BRCAness, drawing a direct connection between familial BRCA1 tumours and basal-type sporadic tumours. Rather than assimilate the two, however, they retained and brought to the fore the distinctive

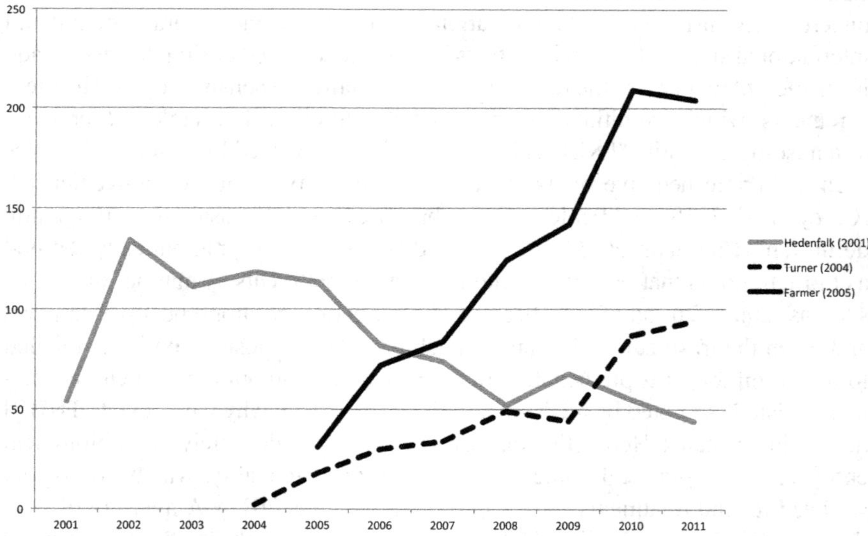

Figure 9.2 Number of citations received by the Hedenfalk *et al.* (2001), Turner *et al.* (2004) and Farmer *et al.* (2005) articles.

Source: Thomson Reuters Web of Science.

nature of the phenotype. They claimed that the inactivation of BRCA gene function might have causes other than mutations or methylation, including the 'dysfunctions of other genes acting in the same biochemical pathway'. According to the authors the elucidation of 'the many components of the pathways and numerous potential mechanisms of inactivation' was one of the main challenges of the new emerging group of 'BRCAness tumours' (Turner *et al.* 2004: p. 818). The key term here is 'pathways': it signals a shift from a narrow focus on genes and mutations to the examination of the complex chains of cellular reactions in which genes and their products are (dys)functionally involved. While we cannot go into detail here about this important transition, it should be noted that it did not take place in the contained atmosphere of laboratories, but in close connection to therapeutic investigations. The sobering clinical fact was that drugs designed to block specific pathological proteins had short-term effects, as tumours quickly developed resistance to those substances. This was ascribed to a tumour cell's capacity to develop alternative pathways to circumvent the original pathway blocked by the drug.

BRCAness did more than enshrine the existence of a BRCA phenotype; it did so by explicitly correlating BRCA phenotype with DNA repair pathways (Box 1 in Turner *et al.* 2004). The identification and characterization of BRCA genes as cancer susceptibility genes in the previous decade had led researchers to investigate their role and to conclude that their key function was to repair damaged DNA. Mutations disable this tumour-suppressing function, thus leading to an accumulation of DNA breaks and errors and, in the end, to cancer.[7] BRCAness meant that, in sporadic cancers, factors other than mutations could disable the BRCA-associated repair pathways, causing the affected cells to behave as their hereditarily mutated counterparts. But the import of the new notion did not stop there. In a remarkable argumentative turn, Turner and colleagues suggested that clinicians could, in fact, take advantage of these biopathological processes by translating them into a therapeutic strategy to fight cancer. In other words, in addition to clinically expanding the BRCA domain to sporadic cancers, the London group simultaneously opened therapeutic avenues. This is where, as detailed below, BRCAness intersected with two older lines of work: the mechanisms described by the notion of 'synthetic lethality', and pharmaceutical research on compounds known as PARP inhibitors.

Before examining these intersections, we would like to emphasize the translational nature of this line of work. As shown in Figure 9.2, the article by Farmer *et al.* (2005), which was published side-by-side with an article by a British–Swedish team (Bryant *et al.* 2005) proposing a similar approach, is the most cited of the two BRCAness articles published by the London group. This is hardly surprising, insofar as in this 'seminal article' (Domcheck 2011: p. 4224) 'a new concept' in cancer chemotherapy was detailed – namely, the therapeutic strategy outlined in the more programmatic paper from 2004. In order to get a sense of its reach, we can identify who, and in what domain, cited that article. We can do so by extracting from the citing articles a list of the journals they co-cite (two journals are co-cited when they are cited together in the same reference list). Using network analysis software, we can then map clusters of co-cited journals, thus providing an indication of the specialty areas corresponding to the citing journals. Figure 9.3

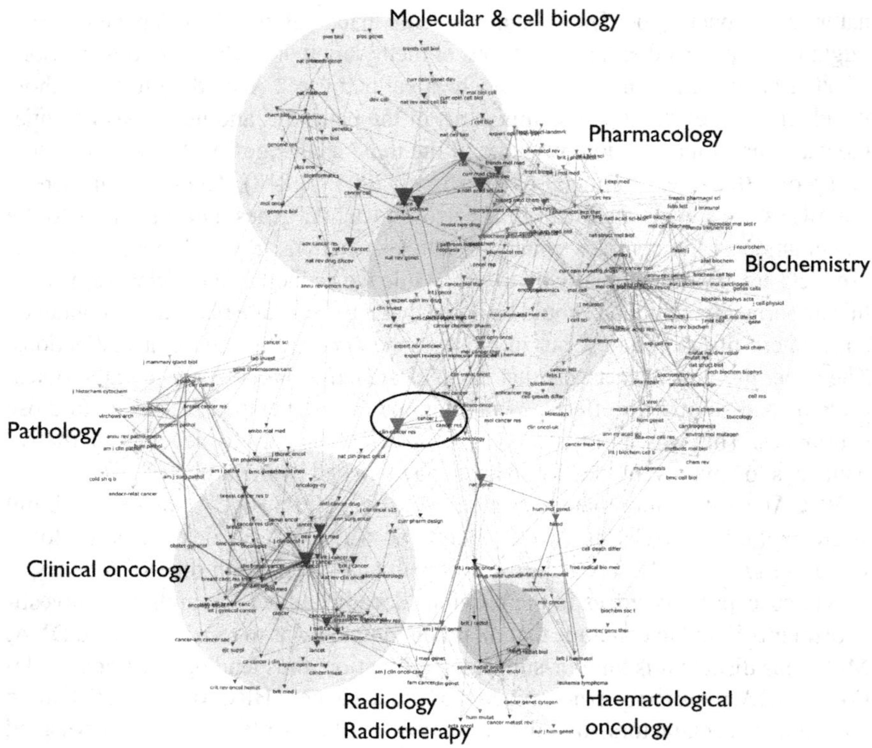

Figure 9.3 Co-citation map of the journals cited by articles citing Farmer *et al.* (2005). We processed and mapped co-citation data downloaded from Thomson Reuters Web of Science with CorTexT, a software platform for the analysis of heterogeneous and semantic networks (www.cortext.fr).

shows the resulting map with a number of clinical specialties at the bottom; at the top are fundamental research specialties. Two large nodes (the size of the nodes is proportional to the number of citations) representing the journals *Cancer Research* and *Clinical Cancer Research* connect these two poles, thus displaying once again the translational research nexus.[8] What is more, in the portrait *Nature* devoted to his work, astutely entitled 'Talking up translation' (Cressey 2010), Alan Ashworth, the last author of the BRCAness paper from 2004, openly advocated a translational approach as the necessary framework for producing clinically relevant research. Such a framework, as we endeavour to show, implies not only the intersections of separate lines of work – i.e. the establishment of a *collective,* which, as pointed out by Michel Callon (2012), should not be equated with a community (epistemic of otherwise), insofar as its members do not necessarily share a common understanding or common approaches (see also Amin and Cohendet 2004) – but also a temporal dimension, without which, as Morange (1997) maintains, such a collective would fail to assemble. This can be further exemplified by examining two additional intersections.

Synthetic lethality and PARP inhibitors: more intersections

As mentioned in the previous section, the London team proposed turning the tables on cancer and exploiting the properties of BRCA-mutated or BRCA-like cells – in other words, those at the origin of cancerous formations – in order to kill those same tumour cells via a mechanism called synthetic lethality. This somewhat complex notion is predicated on the aforementioned understanding of the plasticity of cellular processes: when a vital pathway is blocked by a chemotherapeutic drug or an antibiotic, an alternative pathway steps in to reestablish the original functions, thus creating resistance to treatment. In the present case, tumour cells with BRCA mutations have lost the capacity to use this major DNA repair pathway. When cisplatin – a key component of oncology's chemotherapeutic arsenal – plays havoc with those cells' DNA, they are killed. Cancer, however, bounces back by activating an alternative pathway known as PARP, and cisplatin-resistant tumours take over. If *both* pathways are simultaneously blocked, for instance when using a second chemotherapeutic agent from the PARP-inhibitors' family, the cells die (hence the notion of a combination that is both *synthetic* and *lethal*), or at least this is the hypothesis. Most importantly, in the present case, the London team did not confine their hypothesis to 'inherited BRCA1 or BRCA2 deficiency *per se*' but suggested that 'this approach may be more widely applicable in the treatment of sporadic cancers with "BRCAness" or other impairments of the homologous recombination pathway' (Farmer *et al.* 2005: pp. 919–20).

Where do synthetic lethality and PARP inhibitors come from? The geneticist Theodosius Dobzhansky (1900–1975) first advanced the notion of synthetic lethality in 1946, well before the advent of cisplatin, BRCA and present-day notions of pathways. Defined in simple terms as the process whereby mutations in several genes lead to cell death whereas a mutation in a single one of those genes does not lead to such an outcome, it was used in the study of model organisms (in particular the fruit fly *Drosophila* and the yeast *Saccharomyces cerevisiae*) as a tool (a 'genetic screen') to explore cellular processes and genotype–phenotype relations. Fast-forwarding to the late 1900s, an influential article by Hartwell *et al.* (1997) adopted Dobzhansky's notion in a programmatic article on the integration of genetic approaches in the discovery of anticancer drugs.[9] The London team seized this reconfigured notion in turn and translated it into the specific BRCAness domain, first by extending its definition from mutation-based transformations to phenotypic deficiencies, and second by changing it from a laboratory tool into a chemotherapeutic strategy. In order to do this, however, a second intersection was necessary – namely, a similarly long-lived line of work on PARP inhibitors.

Although the first PARP enzyme was described in the 1960s (Chambon *et al.* 1963), research on drugs that inhibit these enzymes did not begin until the 1980s. Figure 9.4 shows the increase of publications on this topic, which since 1995 has undergone marked growth (the drop between 2005 and 2008 can be accounted for through institutional factors – namely, the fusion of pharmaceutical research programmes following corporate mergers; see Ferraris 2010 and the inset in Figure 9.4). PARP-1 had been touted as a 'viable cancer target' since the 1980s, when

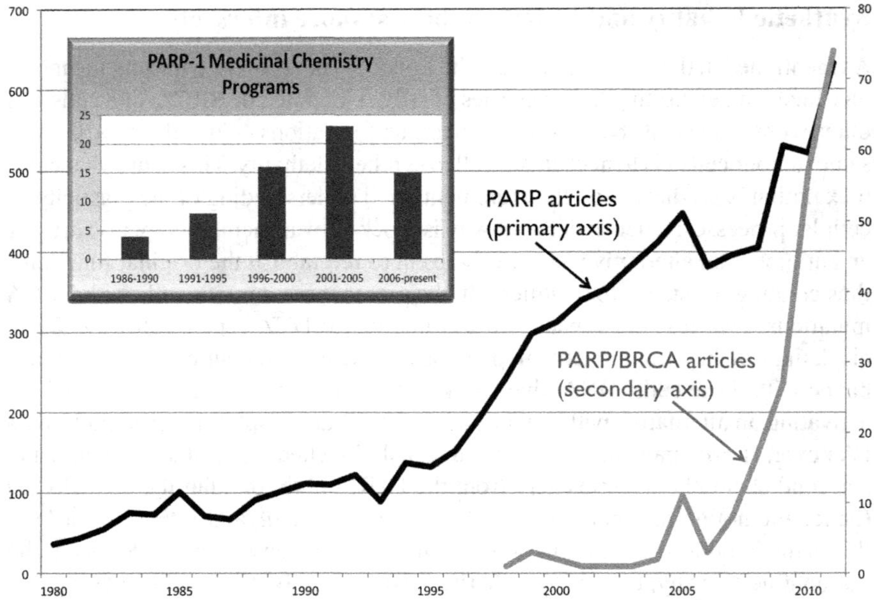

Figure 9.4 Number of articles published on PARP (primary axis) and on PARP and BRCA (secondary axis). The inset shows the number of PARP industrial programmes.

Source: PubMed. Inset reprinted with permission from Ferraris, D. V. (2010) 'Evolution of Poly(ADP-ribose) Polymerase-1 (PARP-1) inhibitors. From concept to clinic', *Journal of Medicinal Chemistry,* 53: 4561–84, © 2010, American Chemical Society.

researchers first proposed that 'dramatic synergistic potentiation of cell killing by alkylating agents and [PARP] inhibitors may be of use in the treatment of human leukaemia' (Durkacz *et al.* 1980: p. 595). This suggestion, however, came too early and thus went unheeded. In fact, the history of programmes set up to develop PARP inhibitors in the 1990s clearly resembles a case of drugs looking for a disease insofar as the medicinal chemistry programmes wandered through a series of therapeutic domains, such as cardiology, inflammation, diabetes and, of course, cancer (Ferraris 2010). PARP inhibitors did not find a disease until they crossed the path of BRCAness. Figure 9.4 also shows (on a different scale) the very rapid growth of articles on PARP and BRCA, beginning in 2006.

This was a mutually constitutive process: PARP inhibitors embarked on a new career thanks to BRCAness and, at the same time, BRCAness became a therapeutic object rather than a purely conceptual one. One of the consequences is that the clinical utility of BRCA testing may be profoundly redefined. According to the Manchester medical geneticist Gareth Evans (personal communication, August 2012), 'the recent development of drugs that target the homologous recombination repair deficiency typical of BRCA-null cancer cells [i.e. PARP inhibitors] has led to an increased referral of women who have developed TNBC to genetic services for rapid genetic testing' (see also Evans *et al.* 2011). The ripple effect of the redefinition of the therapeutic role of PARP inhibitors can also be felt beyond TNBC, as it leads clinicians to ask whether *all* women with breast cancer should be tested for mutations at the time of diagnosis (Narod 2012).

Did these intersections give rise to an unmitigated success story? Not quite. After very promising results in early-phase clinical trials, PARP inhibitors have so far produced disappointing outcomes in phase III trials in both hereditary and sporadic breast cancer (see, for example, Guha 2011). These results have not led to the rejection of the hypothesis that PARP inhibitors represent a promising therapeutic avenue. In fact, a number of authors (Domcheck *et al.* 2011, Maxwell and Domcheck 2012), while resorting to their own form of critical inquiry (Boltanski and Thévenot 1999, Lynch 1982), have complained that therapeutic research related to BRCA-associated cancers has stalled – not due to intrinsic deficiencies, but because of a number of regulatory and socio-economic issues. These include the small size of the target patient population, although targeted therapies have been approved for tumours that affect even smaller numbers of patients. Indeed, BRCAness would expand the number of patients eligible for the new treatment. Another issue is the regulatory requirement of clearly defining the target population – namely, via an approved diagnostic test. The situation here is marred by uncertainties, especially in the US, given the monopoly of Myriad Genetics on BRCA testing thanks to its controversial patents (see, for example, Kepler *et al.* 2010), the ongoing and equally controversial attempts to modify the FDA regulatory framework for diagnostic tests (Bourret *et al.* 2011), and the fact that, to date, only one experimental test has been proposed for BRCAness (Konstantinopoulos *et al.* 2010). This is clearly a case of an innovation having arrived late on the scene, as the intellectual property field has been already staked out, depending, of course, on ongoing litigation.

A third issue concerns the ethical and regulatory obstacles resulting from the availability of active therapies for breast cancer, which makes comparisons of the new agents with the existing standard of care especially difficult. One could argue, in this respect, that BRCA-associated cancers, given their often dismal prognosis and the fact that they do not respond to existing therapies, should not be conflated with the general breast cancer category. While this is another instance of the kind of problems experienced by late arrivals, it is also a telling example of genomics' potential to reshuffle established disease ontologies and the practices they support. Last but not least, we ought to mention a more 'intrinsic' issue, as illustrated by the following episode. The excitement generated by the positive results of a phase II clinical trial gave way to disappointment when iniparib, the first PARP inhibitor to reach the phase III stage, failed to show the expected benefits at that stage before turning out to be not a PARP inhibitor after all (Rios and Puhalla 2011, Roop 2011). This episode extends ontological uncertainty to include the drugs themselves, confirming the relational and thus evolving nexus of drugs and diseases (Cambrosio *et al.* 2012).

It could be objected that our account of BRCAness relates to activities that primarily concern laboratory or, at best, clinical research rather than actual clinical practices. As shown in this paper, however, and as a component of translational research initiatives, BRCAness is hardly confined to the laboratory. Moreover, in a highly protocolized domain such as oncology, any sharp distinction between clinical research and clinical routines is moot: today's experimental protocol is tomorrow's routine treatment. In the present case, the management of breast cancer patients with BRCA or BRCA-like mutations or anomalies is a topical issue in breast cancer clinical circles. A quick search in clinicaltrials.gov (a registry and results database established by the US National Health Institute, listing publicly and privately supported clinical trials) shows that, at the time of writing this article (November 2012), there were 104 clinical trials indexed with 'PARP', of which 39 were co-indexed with 'breast cancer', while of the 154 clinical trials indexed with 'BRCA', 24 were co-indexed with 'PARP' – not a negligible number.

Conclusion

We will conclude with an image: a map of the BRCA domain from 2009–2012. Figure 9.5 shows the semantic network of terms extracted from the titles and abstracts of articles published during this period. We used text-mining techniques to select relevant terms and mapped their co-occurrences with network analysis

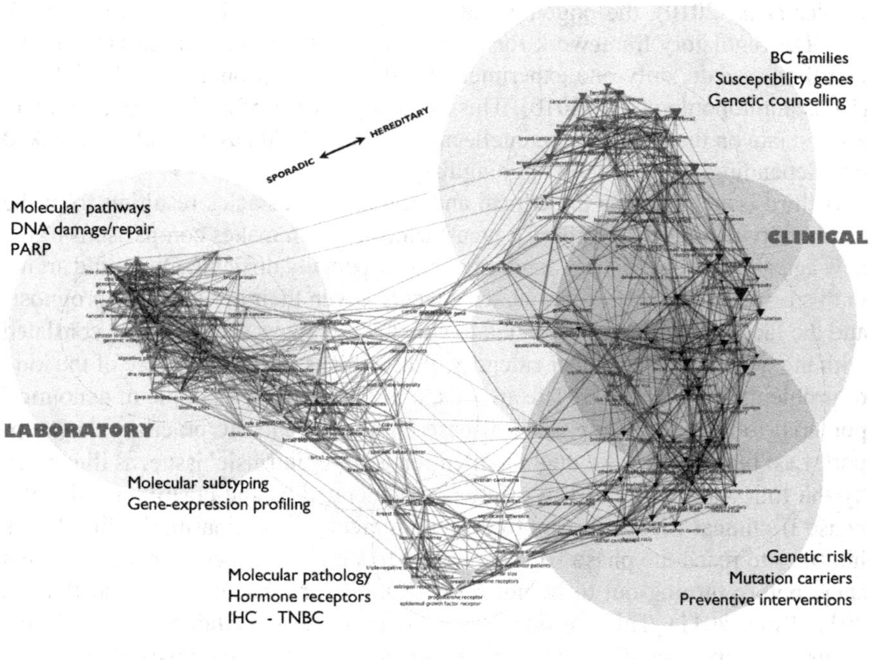

Figure 9.5 Semantic network of concepts extracted from the titles and abstracts of BRCA-related articles published from 2009–2012. We used CorTexT (see Figure 9.3) to text-mine titles and abstracts of articles downloaded from PubMed and to map the resulting concepts.

software. The map as a whole displays the thematic structure of this domain. On the right, we see the more traditional clinical pole, with a cluster on the top referring to the hereditary domain as defined by the analysis of familial forms of cancer and germline mutations. At the bottom is another large cluster focused on the assessment of risks for mutation carriers as well as preventive interventions, such as mastectomy and salpingo-oophorectomy. The left side of the map displays the laboratory pole characterized by a cluster on investigations of DNA damage, DNA repair pathways and PARP inhibitors and by a cluster on gene-expression profiling and molecular subtyping. At the bottom centre we find a cluster corresponding more closely to pathology, its immunohistochemical analysis of hormone receptors and the resultant definition of triple-negative breast cancers.

The left and right sides of the map also display a tension between the sporadic and hereditary domains. However, as described in this chapter, we should understand this tension as both creative and essential, a tension predicated on the very existence of the translational continuum. This does not mean that separate areas cannot be distinguished within the continuum, but that these areas are the components of a hybrid research collective (to use Callon's notion once again), which interact and collaborate in ways that go beyond explicit initiatives. Less a translation from one domain to another (from hereditary to sporadic cancer), these activities amount to the reconfiguration of a cancer research domain that generates novel entities, such as BRCAness, as well as related lines of therapeutic innovation. Once again, the term 'emergence' is meant to emphasize the temporal dimension of these processes. Future work exploring these processes should focus on characterizing the ongoing trajectory of BRCAness – for instance, by investigating the circulation of this notion and of the practices to which it relates, and its implementation in clinical trials and clinical settings. In parallel, one could explore how the events related in this chapter contribute to the ongoing redefinition of the notion of patient, how these refer back to existing notions of familial risk and how they do or do not contribute to the characterization of the elusive notion of 'personalized medicine'. For now, we hope we have demonstrated the heuristic interest in exploring the BRCA domain by conceiving of it as the result of multiple associations with different entities and processes, rather than reducing it to preestablished categories that do not take into account the fluidity of research practices, their capacity to shift boundaries and connect previously unconnected elements, and thus lead to novel configurations.

Notes

1. Research for this chapter was made possible by grants from the Canadian Institutes for Health Research (CIHR MOP-93553), the Fonds Québécois de la Recherche sur la Société et la Culture (FQRSC SE-124896 and SE-164195), the Social Sciences and Humanities Research Council of Canada (SSHRC 410–2011–2290) and the French National Cancer Institute (INCa 0610/3D1418/SHS08). Our special thanks go to Jean-Philippe Cointet and Andrei Mogoutov, who developed the software platform CorTexT and who contributed decisively to the production of

Figure 9.5. We would also like to thank the scientists and clinicians who kindly agreed to be interviewed, and the participants of the 'BRCA Gene Research and Medical Practices: A Comparative Transnational Social Science Workshop' (Brocher Foundation, Geneva, 5–7 December, 2011) for their comments and suggestions.

2. HBOC accounts for less than 10 per cent of all breast and ovarian cancer cases; moreover, only a subset of HBOC involves BRCA mutations. As for the alleged reasons for the focus on BRCA, critics mention biomedical 'reductionism' and the unwillingness to tackle alternative (including environmental) causes (Klawiter 2008, McCormick *et al.* 2012).
3. See also Nelson *et al.* (2013) for a discussion on the shift from risk to actionability in recent oncology.
4. The title is a clear reference to a celebrated paper (almost 10,000 citations by October 2012) published in 2000 by Hanahan and Weinberg under the title 'The hallmarks of cancer'.
5. While somatic BRCA mutations surfaced in ovarian cancer, they remained exceedingly rare.
6. See, for instance, the guidelines jointly designed by the American Society of Clinical Oncology and the College of American Pathologists for ER and PR testing (Hammond *et al.* 2010) and for HER2 testing (Wolff *et al.* 2007). For more on the debates surrounding these pronouncements, see, for example, Allison (2010) and Schmidt (2011)
7. This is an extremely simplified description, as many other factors are involved in these processes. But for our present purpose it should suffice.
8. It could be argued that Figure 9.3 shows a dichotomous rather than a translational domain, but this is due to the fact that co-citation maps display a more conservative view of the field – one based on the contributions authors consider key to their domain. An inter-citation map of the same domain (not shown), which displays a more comprehensive view of the relations between the field and its subfields, shows a densely interconnected network with no clear subdivisions. The two approaches are, in fact, complementary; nonetheless, we have opted for the co-citation map because it allows for a clearer identification of the subfields concerned in the article by Farmer *et al.* For a discussion on these methodological issues, see Jones *et al.* (2011).
9. Hartwell *et al.* (1997) did not cite the original Dobzhansky article; instead they cited a review from 1995 by Doye and Hurt, also unrelated to cancer. A recent article by Bernards (2012) has repackaged the synthetic lethality approach as a general strategy for overcoming drug resistance in the case of targeted therapies.

References

Allemani, C., Sant, M., Berrino, F. et al. (2004) 'Prognostic value of morphology and hormone receptor status in breast cancer – a population-based study', *British Journal of Cancer*, 9: 1263–68.

Allison, M. (2010) 'The HER2 testing conundrum', *Nature Biotechnology,* 28: 117–19.

Amin, A. and Cohendet, P. (2004) *Architectures of Knowledge. Firms, Capabilities, and Communities.* Oxford: Oxford University Press.

Bazell, R. (1998). *Her-2: The Making of Herceptin, a Revolutionary Treatment for Breast Cancer.* New York: Random House.

Bernards, R. (2012) 'A missing link in genotype-directed cancer therapy', *Cell,* 151: 465–68.

Boltanski, L. and Thévenot, L. (1999) 'The sociology of critical capacity', *European Journal of Social Theory,* 2: 359–77.

Bourret, P. (2005) 'BRCA patients and clinical collectives. New configurations of action in cancer genetics practices', *Social Studies of Science,* 35: 41–68.

Bourret, P., Mogoutov, A., Julian-Reynier, C., Cambrosio, A. (2006) 'A new clinical collective for French cancer genetics: a heterogeneous mapping analysis', *Science, Technology, and Human Values*, 31: 431–64.

Bourret, P., Keating, P. and Cambrosio, A. (2011) 'Regulating diagnosis in post-genomic medicine: re-aligning clinical judgment?' *Social Science and Medicine,* 73: 816–24.

Boyd, J. (1995) 'BRCA1: more than just a hereditary breast cancer gene?' *Nature Genetics,* 9: 335–36.

Brown, H. (2007) 'Translational cancer research in the USA', *Molecular Oncology,* 1: 11–13.

Bryant, H.E., Schultz, N., Thomas, H. D. et al.(2005) 'Specific killing of BRCA2-deficient tumours with inhibitors of poly(ADP-ribose) polymerase', *Nature*, 434: 913-17.

Butler, D. (2008) 'Crossing the valley of death', *Nature,* 453: 840–2.

Callon, M. (2012) 'Les sciences sociales confrontées aux nouvelles pratiques de recherche et d'innovation' (manuscript submitted for publication).

Carey, L., Winer, E., Viale, G. et al. (2010) 'Triple-negative breast cancer: disease entity or title of convenience?' *Nature Reviews Clinical Oncology*, 7: 683–92.

Cambrosio, A., Keating, P. and Mogoutov, A. (2012) 'What's in a pill? On the informational enrichment of anti-cancer drugs'. In Gaudillière, J. P. and Hess, V. (eds) *Ways of Regulating Drugs in the 19th and 20th Centuries.* Houndmills: Palgrave, 181–205.

Catteau, A., Harris, W. H., Xu, C. F. and Solomon, E. (1999) 'Methylation of the BRCA1 promoter region in sporadic breast and ovarian cancer: Correlation with disease characteristics', *Oncogene*, 18: 1957–65.

Chambon, P., Weill, J. D. and Mandel, P. (1963) 'Nicotinamide mononucleotide activation of new DNA-dependent polyadenylic acid synthesizing nuclear enzyme', *Biochemical and Biophysical Research Communications,* 11: 39–43.

Cressey, D. (2010) 'Talking up translation', *Nature,* 463: 422–3.

Dobzhansky, T. (1946) 'Genetics of natural populations: XIII. Recombination and variability in populations of Drosophila Pseudoobscura', *Genetics,* 31: 269–90.

Domchek, S. M., Mitchell, G., Lindeman, G. J. et al. (2011) 'Challenges to the development of new agents for molecularly defined patient subsets: lessons from BRCA1/2-associated breast cancer', *Journal of Clinical Oncology*, 29: 4224–6.

Doye, V. and Hurt, E. C. (1995) 'Genetic approaches to nuclear pore structure and function', *Trends in Genetics,* 11: 235–41.

Durkacz, B. W., Omidiji, O., Gray, D. A. and Shall, S. (1980) '(ADP-ribose)n participates in DNA excision repair', *Nature*, 283: 593–96.

Eiermann, W., Bergh, J., Cardoso, F. et al. (2012) 'Triple negative breast cancer: Proposals for a pragmatic definition and implications for patient management and trial design', *Breast*, 21: 20–26.

Essioux, L. and Bonaïti-Pellié, C. (1997) 'Epidémiologie des prédispositions héréditaires aux cancers et évaluation du risque héréditaire en oncologie'. In Bignon, Y. J. (ed.) Oncogénétique. Vers une médecine de présomption/prédiction. Paris: Lavoisier, 33–47.

Esteller, M., Silva, J. M., Dominguez, G. et al. (2000) 'Promoter hypermethylation and BRCA1 inactivation in sporadic breast and ovarian tumours', *Journal of the National Cancer Institute*, 92: 564–69.

Evans, D. G., Howell, A., Ward, D. et al. (2011) 'Prevalence of BRCA1 and BRCA2 mutations in triple negative breast cancer', *Journal of Medical Genetics*, 48: 520–2.

Farmer, H., McCabe N., Lord, C. J. et al. (2005) 'Targeting the DNA repair defect in BRCA mutant cells as a therapeutic strategy', *Nature*, 434: 917–21.

Ferraris, D. V. (2010) 'Evolution of Poly(ADP-ribose) Polymerase-1 (PARP-1) inhibitors. From concept to clinic', *Journal of Medicinal Chemistry*, 53: 4561–84.

Gibbon, S. (2007) *Breast Cancer Genes and the Gendering of Knowledge. Science and Citizenship in the Cultural Context of the 'New' Genetics,* Houndsmills: Palgrave.

Grushko, T. A. Dignam, J. J., Das, S. et al. (2004) '*MYC* is amplified in *BRCA1*-associated breast cancers', *Clinical Cancer Research*, 10: 499–507.

Guha, M. (2011) 'PARP inhibitors stumble in breast cancer', *Nature Biotechnology,* 29: 373–4.

Hammond, M.E.H., Hayes, D. F., Dowsett, M. et al. (2010) 'American Society of Clinical Oncology/College of American Pathologists guideline recommendations for immunohistochemical testing of estrogen and progesterone receptors in breast cancer', *Journal of Clinical Oncology*, 28: 2784–95.

Hartwell, L. H., Szankasi, P., Roberts, C. J. et al. (1997) 'Integrating genetic approaches into the discovery of anticancer drugs', *Science*, 278: 1064–68.

Hedenfalk, I. Duggan, D., Chen Y. et al. (2001) 'Gene expression profiles in hereditary breast cancer', *NEJM*, 344: 539–48.

Jazaeri, A. A., Yee, S. J., Sotiriou, C. et al. (2002) 'Gene expression profiles of BRCA1-linked, BRCA2-linked, and sporadic ovarian cancers', *Journal of the National Cancer Institute*, 94: 990–1000.

Jones, D., Cambrosio, A. and Mogoutov, A. (2011) 'Detection and characterization of translational research in cancer and cardiovascular medicine', *Journal of Translational Medicine,* 9: 57.

Keating, P. and Cambrosio, A. (2001) 'The new genetics and cancer. The contributions of clinical medicine in the era of biomedicine', *Journal of the History of Medicine and Allied Sciences,* 56: 321–52.

Kepler, T. B., Crossman, C. and Cook-Deegan, R. (2010) 'Metastazing patent claims on BRCA1', *Genomics,* 95: 312–14.

Klawiter, M. (2008) *The Biopolitics of Cancer. Changing Cultures of Disease and Activism,* Minneapolis: University of Minnesota Press.

Kohli-Laven, N., Bourret, P., Keating, P. and Cambrosio, A. (2011) 'Cancer clinical trials in the era of genomic signatures: biomedical innovation, clinical utility, and regulatory-scientific hybrids', *Social Studies of Science,* 41: 487–513.

Konstantinopoulos, P. A. Spentzos, D., Karlan, B. Y. et al. (2010) 'Gene expression profile of BRCAness that correlates with responsiveness to chemotherapy and with outcome in patients with epithelial ovarian cancer', *Journal of Clinical Oncology*, 28: 3555–61.

Löwy, I. and Gaudillière, J. P. (2008) 'Localizing the global: testing for hereditary risks of breast cancer', *Science Technology and Human Values,* 33: 299–325.

Lynch, M. (1982) 'Technical work and critical inquiry: investigations in a scientific laboratory', *Social Studies of Science,* 12: 499–533.

Magdinier, F., Ribieras, S., Lenoir, G.M. et al. (1998) 'Down-regulation of BRCA1 in human sporadic breast cancer; analysis of DNA methylation patterns of the putative promoter region', *Oncogene*, 17: 3169–76.

Maxwell, K. N. and Domcheck, S. M. (2012) 'Cancer treatment according to BRCA1 and BRCA2 mutations', *Nature Reviews Clinical Oncology,* 9: 520–8.

McCormick, S., Brown, P., Zavestoksi, S. and Cordner, A. (2012) 'The personal is scientific, the scientific is political. The public paradigm of the environmental breast cancer movement'. In P. Brown, R. Morello-Frosch and S. Zavestoksi (eds) *Contested Illnesses. Citizens, Science, and Health Social Movements*, Berkeley: University of California Press.

Morange, M. (1997) 'From the regulatory vision of cancer to the oncogene paradigm, 1975–1985', *Journal of the History of Biology*, 30: 1–29.

Narod, S.A. (2012) 'Should all women with breast cancer be tested for BRCA mutations at the time of diagnosis?' *Journal of Clinical Oncology*, 30: 2–3.

Nelson, N., Keating, P. and Cambrosio, A. (2013) 'On being "actionable": clinical sequencing and the emerging contours of a regime of genomic medicine in oncology', *New Genetics and Society*, 32: 405–28.

Ong, M.B.H. (2012) 'Senate increases NIH funding for 2013, rejects President's $200+ million increase for program evaluation activities,' *The Cancer Letter*, 38, 25: 1, 7–9.

Parthasarathy, S. (2007) *Building Genetic Medicine: Breast Cancer, Technology, and the Comparative Politics of Health Care*. Cambridge, MA: MIT Press.

Perou, C.M., Sorlie, T., Eisen, M.B. et al. (2000) 'Molecular portraits of human breast tumours', *Nature*, 406: 747–52.

Rabeharisoa, V. and Bourret, P. (2009) 'Staging and weighting evidence in biomedicine: comparing clinical practices in cancer genetics and psychiatric genetics', *Social Studies of Science*, 39: 691–715.

Reis-Filho, J. and Pusztai, L. (2011) 'Gene expression profile in breast cancer: classification, prognostication and prediction', *Lancet*, 378: 1812–23.

Rice, J.C., Massey-Brown, K.S. and Futscher, B.W. (1998) 'Aberrant methylation of the BRCA1 CpG island promoter is associated with decreased BRCA1 mRNA in sporadic breast cancer cells', *Oncogene*, 17: 1807–12.

Rios, J. and Puhalla, S. (2011) 'PARP inhibitors in breast cancer: BRCA and beyond', *Oncology*, 25: 1014–25.

Roop, R. P, Ma, C.X. and Ellis, M.J.C. (2011) 'PARP inhibitors and their evolving role in breast cancer', *Oncology*, 25: 1033–34.

Schmidt, C. (2011) 'How do you tell whether a breast cancer is HER2 positive? Ongoing studies keep debate in high gear', *Journal of the National Cancer Institute*, 103: 87–9.

Sorlie, T., Perou, C.M., Tibshirani, R. et al. (2001) 'Gene expression patterns of breast carcinomas distinguish tumor subclasses with clinical implications', *Proceedings of the National Academy of Sciences USA*, 98: 10869–74.

Turner, N., Tutt, A. and Ashworth, A. (2004). 'Hallmarks of "BRCAness" in sporadic cancers', *Nature Reviews Cancer*, 4: 814–19.

van't Veer, L.J., Dai, H., van de Vijver, M.J. et al. (2002) 'Gene expression profiling predicts clinical outcome of breast cancer', *Nature*, 415: 530–36.

Wolff, A.C., Hammond, M.E.H., Schwartz, J.N. et al. (2007) 'American Society of Clinical Oncology/College of American Pathologists guideline recommendations for human epidermal growth factor receptor 2 testing in breast cancer', *Archives of Pathology and Laboratory Medicine*, 131: 18–43.

10 Ethical analysis of PGD for BRCA

Attending to more than risks and benefits

Lisa R. Rubin and Inmaculada de Melo-Martín

Introduction

Among the supposed benefits of BRCA gene mutation testing is that individuals, particularly women, identified as carrying a BRCA mutation can then take steps to manage the risk of, and possibly even prevent, the development of breast and ovarian cancer. However, until recently, there were few options available for BRCA carriers to manage or prevent transmission of this inherited gene mutation to their biogenetically related children. BRCA mutations are autosomal dominant, and men and women who carry a BRCA1 or BRCA2 mutation confront a 50 per cent chance that their children will inherit the mutation. Although it is not clear that BRCA has shifted childbearing decisions for the majority of carriers (Van Asperen *et al.* 2002), this has nonetheless been identified as a significant concern for many carriers and their parents (Claes *et al.* 2004).

Until the clinical implementation of preimplantation genetic diagnoses (PGD), options for individuals wishing to avoid the risk of transmitting a BRCA mutation were limited to remaining child-free, or adoption. The use of PGD in combination with *in vitro* fertilization (IVF), however, currently allows determination of whether an embryo carries genetic mutations or chromosomal abnormalities that can cause disability or might increase a future child's risk of suffering from a particular disease (Geraedts and De Wert 2009, Simpson 2010). With that information, prospective parents can make decisions about whether to prevent certain embryos from being implanted.

As is the case with most technological developments, these new abilities raise important ethical challenges. In general, these challenges tend to be evaluated within the framework of risks and benefits (Noble *et al.* 2008). The use of PGD for BRCA, as well as for other gene mutations associated with inherited risk of adult-onset cancer, is not an exception. This risk–benefit framework has been used to inform policy making, and even outside of policy making, it has the potential to influence medical practice. However, much of the literature about the ethics of using PGD for BRCA focuses on a limited range of questions about the risks and benefits of the use of this technology. Although, of course, risk assessments are an important component of an ethical evaluation, an ethical analysis packaged entirely within a traditional risk–benefit framework may provide too narrow a lens through which to locate the ethical issues at stake in the use of PGD for BRCA1/2. In this chapter, we call attention to several ethical concerns regarding the use of PGD for BRCA that extend beyond risk–benefit considerations.

The benefits of PGD seem clear to most people: it allows the identification and elimination of a variety of diseases and impairments, thus promoting the goal of having healthy children (Bredenoord *et al.* 2008, Esplen *et al.* 2007, Harper and SenGupta, 2012, Malek and Daar 2012, Mansour 2004, Savulescu 2001, SenGupta *et al.* 2012). The potential harm most often discussed has centred on matters of eugenics, which is particularly relevant in light of recent and cross-national histories of eugenic practices (Baum 2006; King, D. S. 1999; McCabe and McCabe 2011, Parens and Asch 1999). Ethical assessments of PGD thus usually attempt to determine how to balance the potential benefits of this technology with a variety of harms, including the eugenic harms that it might cause. Such balance is thought to be attained by providing parameters and criterion that presumably help minimize the risks of using PGD and maximize its possible benefits, thus demarcating ethically appropriate from inappropriate uses of PGD. For example, the 'seriousness of the genetic condition' is supposed to provide us with such a criterion. However, what counts as 'serious' when evaluating diseases and impairments has turned out to be – unsurprisingly – not an easy matter. Indeed, when attending to factors such as the impact of the condition on health, the severity of symptoms, degree of penetrance of the genetic mutation, the existence of a cure or treatment, the rate of progression and the age of onset, all make determinations of seriousness fraught with challenges. A significant amount of debate has thus centred on trying to examine, probe, refine and dispute this criterion as a guide for the moral acceptability of PGD (Camporesi 2010, Clancy 2010, Krahn 2009, Mansour 2004, Oster *et al.* 2008, Robertson 2003, Scott *et al.* 2007, SenGupta *et al.* 2012, Snelling 2008).

Dilemmas of line-drawing around seriousness have taken centre stage in critiques using a risk–benefit framework of ethical evaluation, foreclosing the examination of other limitations of this framework. Because evaluations of risks and benefits are not value-neutral, focusing ethical concerns exclusively on identifying and balancing risks and benefits can draw attention away from the need to consider the values underlying risk–benefit analysis. For example, values are implicated in evaluations of what counts as a risk or a benefit, when is a risk considered too risky (or not risky enough) and what is an acceptable level of risk. Determination of the relevant time frame for investigating risks, the manageability of the proposed risks or the standards with which to judge whether unmanageable risks are not present are all value-laden judgments, as are evaluations of how compelling the benefits are. The value-laden nature of risk–benefit analyses is underscored by the considerable cross-national variability in the regulation of PGD across the globe – from all out bans on this technology in countries such as Germany, Austria, and Italy, to regulatory systems in the UK and Canada, and the use of professional guidelines within the US and Japan (King 2008). To the extent that this is the case, it seems important to evaluate the value judgments that play a role in determinations about the risks and benefits.

Another related drawback of the risk-benefit framework is that it conceals other concerns that are morally relevant when evaluating technologies in general and PGD in particular. Indeed, general questions such as (1) how the practices and values of knowledge production influence the types of technologies that we choose to develop, (2) how these affect the technologies that are found desirable or even feasible and (3) how new technologies that promote or challenge particular values fail to find a place in these types of evaluations. However, even more specific questions about the desirability of the goals that PGD presumably helps us achieve, or the appropriateness of PGD as a means to such goals, also become clouded when limiting the evaluation of PGD to an assessment of risks and benefits. The purpose of this chapter is to uncover some of those aspects. In particular, we focus here on relevant concerns, such as the constraints that the availability of PGD for BRCA puts on prospective parent's choices, the emphasis on PGD as a solution to breast and ovarian cancer risks at the expense of other possible solutions, the construction of health and disease in reductionist ways and the value assumptions about good parenting that are presupposed by the use of PGD. Although these concerns fit uneasily within a risk–benefit framework and thus tend to be ignored in bioethical evaluations within academic medicine and by those involved in direct clinical care, they are nonetheless essential to a robust ethical analysis of this technology.

This chapter is the product of an ongoing collaboration between a philosopher (de Melo-Martín) and a psychologist (Rubin). We explore ways of integrating normative ethical analysis with qualitative research to deepen our understanding of ethical, social and psychological issues involved in repro-genetic technologies (Rubin and de Melo-Martín 2012). For de Melo-Martín, this includes a programme of research that examines the often neglected and unacknowledged role of values within scientific and bioethical evaluations. Within the field of philosophy, the empirical investigation of patient stakeholders' attitudes and values may not always be relevant to a normative ethical analysis (i.e. analysis of what 'ought to be'), but they certainly can be. This became apparent to Rubin when she noticed how de Melo-Martín's work of drawing out the unspoken values at stake in the practice of PGD often mapped the concerns of women and men she interviewed who carried a BRCA1/2 mutation as they weighed the option of PGD. To this end, this chapter draws on interviews conducted as part of a larger study exploring attitudes toward using PGD to prevent the transmission of inherited breast and ovarian cancer risk associated with BRCA1 and BRCA2 mutations among reproductive-age mutation carriers living in the US. The normative conclusions about the failures of the risk–benefit analysis of PGD for BRCA made here are illustrated by the experiences of BRCA1/2 mutation carriers as they contemplated the possibility of PGD. Our aim here is not to advocate for or against the use of PGD for BRCA1/2, or for any other condition. Instead, by drawing from interviews with BRCA1/2 mutation carriers considering the possibility of PGD, we illuminate some of ethical issues that are not readily locatable within a traditional risk–benefit framework but are deeply relevant to the experiences of individuals navigating these technologies in their everyday lives.

Methods

As part of the aforementioned study led by Rubin and colleagues (Rubin 2008–2011), thirty-three reproductive-age women and men who had undergone genetic screening for a BRCA mutation and tested positive for a BRCA1 or BRCA2 mutation were recruited from the Clinical Genetic Service (CGS) of a private, comprehensive cancer centre in New York City to participate in an interview study about their views regarding PGD for BRCA. Inclusion criteria required that participants (1) were identified as carriers of a deleterious BRCA mutation documented by CGS, (2) were of 'reproductive age' defined as under the age of 43 for women and under the age of 50 for men and (3) had not undergone hysterectomy or risk-reducing oophorectomy. In addition, a second sample comprised of six individuals seeking consultation for PGD to screen embryos for a BRCA gene mutation were recruited through the Center for Reproductive Medicine (CRM) in New York City. Eligibility criteria were the same, with the exception that female partners of male BRCA carriers were also eligible to participate.

A total of 39 interviews were conducted, with 34 female and 5 male participants. The majority were white (92 per cent), married (76.9 per cent), working full-time (59 per cent) and affluent (nearly 70 per cent reported annual incomes greater than $100,000). Just over half of the sample had children (56.4 per cent), and nearly 80 per cent reported they were not finished (or not sure they were finished) with plans for having children. In addition, 61.5 per cent identified as Jewish with a range of identifications from secular to Orthodox. All participants were BRCA mutation positive except one female participant who was undergoing PGD to identify and screen out a BRCA gene mutation carried by her husband.

After providing informed consent and completing a brief survey of background demographics as well as prior knowledge of and experience with repro-genetic technologies, participants viewed a brief, standardized educational tutorial, developed in collaboration with a doctoral-level genetic counsellor and CGS genetic counsellors, reviewing risk and inheritance patterns associated with BRCA gene mutations, defining preimplantation genetic diagnosis and prenatal genetic diagnosis and describing the procedures and associated features (including cost) for each. This ensured that all participants were exposed to the same basic knowledge regarding patterns of cancer risk and inheritance associated with a BRCA gene mutation, the procedures involved with PGD as well as the costs and alternatives. Following the educational presentation, participants completed a brief knowledge assessment to ensure comprehension of the key points of the educational presentation.

Participants then took part in an in-depth, semi-structured interview with a clinical psychologist or social worker, both of whom were experienced in qualitative interviewing and were knowledgeable about hereditary cancer risk. Interviews lasted approximately one hour and explored experiences of familial cancer and genetic testing, screening and/or surveillance options for BRCA mutation carriers, the impact of a BRCA mutation on family planning, attitudes toward the use of PGD as well as prenatal diagnosis to screen for BRCA. Concerns relating to religion, family views and costs were also explored.

All interviews were audio-recorded and transcribed verbatim by a professional transcription service. As part of the larger study, data were analysed using a grounded theory approach (Charmaz 2000), which identified key tensions expressed between and among participants in relation to their attitude toward and interest in PGD for BRCA. With an *a priori* framework of thinking beyond risk–benefit analysis in mind, we reviewed interviews and coded data to examine ways in which participants' interviews expanded our understanding of the ethical issues involved in PGD for BRCA beyond the risk–benefit framework.

The limits of risk–benefit evaluations of PGD for BRCA

Interview findings shed light on several ethical concerns raised by participants that go beyond a risk–benefit framework. We believe that these deserve consideration when providing ethical analysis of PGD for BRCA. Our goal is not to ascertain how ethical concerns of PGD for BRCA *ought* to be evaluated. We simply aim to reveal some ethical factors that are typically neglected when the main focus of an evaluation of PGD is the determination and assessment of the risks and potential benefits of PGD for BRCA. We illustrate such concerns by presenting the voices of individuals who are confronted with the use of this technology.

Constraints on choice

The introduction of new technological developments is normally hailed as a way to increase people's choices. The use of PGD for BRCA is no exception. Prospective parents at risk of transmitting BRCA mutations to their biogenetic offspring now have the choice to use the technology, so as not to pass on such mutations. Expanded choices are usually seen as benefiting people, as more choices usually increase the chances that people will be able to satisfy their own particular desires or address their own concerns. And yet this increase in choices often comes at a cost, and such a cost is rarely acknowledged. For instance, because PGD requires the use of IVF, the existence of this choice can constrain BRCA carriers' desires to become pregnant without the help of technologies. In the words of one participant, a 30-year-old woman who originally heard about PGD from her uncle and tried to become pregnant several times using PGD but failed:

> I had heard about it, my uncle is a doctor . . . and he had heard about it. He had mentioned it to me. And initially I was very upset about it. Like, I was very upset that I *had to,* like, go through this process. I was twenty-seven years old and I wanted to just have kids! I wanted to, like, be normal! Like all my friends who were getting pregnant. And I really didn't, I really thought pregnancy was, like, oh, you tried and you got pregnant.
>
> (emphasis added)

Of course, BRCA carriers are not prevented from choosing to become pregnant without the use of IVF and PGD. The concern is that the existence of this choice might decrease the likelihood that one can exercise previous choices that one would have preferred, such as trying to conceive naturally. Once this participant learned about PGD, she felt she no longer had the choice to become pregnant naturally. Rather, she felt that after hearing about it, she *had to* use PGD.

The concern expressed by this participant – that being presented with the choice of using PGD actually constrained the possibility of choosing alternate options – was also experienced by other participants in various ways that illustrate the often neglected costs of introducing technological choices. For instance, one 36-year-old male participant, who had a daughter before learning about PGD for BRCA and was trying to decide whether to use PGD as he and his wife planned for their next pregnancy, was conflicted about this choice. He wished that he had never been presented with what Kenen (1996) has described as the 'diagnostic invitation and the "gift" of knowing' about PGD for BRCA, while he reluctantly acknowledged that the invitation now could not be ignored.

> [The doctor] probably also almost certainly regarded it as giving me a choice, you know, giving me an opportunity . . . I'm sure I take it for granted and have the childish approach to it, complaining about having the opportunity. It is an opportunity, and – you know, no one would really in the end rather be ignorant, I don't think . . . it's nobody's fault that we were then presented with all the information.

This cost of increased technological choice – that the availability of PGD necessitated its use (Dumit and Davis-Floyd 1998) – was raised by several participants, a few of whom also discussed the consequent constraints on other previously available choices. Others experienced the 'invitation' as a burden of responsibility. Indeed, having a choice, and being aware of it, raised the issue of responsibility. A failure to choose could now be used to hold someone, and oneself, responsible and to judge them, and oneself, blameworthy. Indeed, some participants who opted for not using PGD expressed trepidation that the decision not to do so could be construed as being irresponsible. As one participant, a 38-year-old woman who was pregnant at the time of the interview put it:

> It's a little irresponsible. I think my husband feels differently. He's like, you know, you could just, you could get rid of this thing and you know, instead of having her live a life of, you know like you might have to, I don't know.

With responsibility also comes the need to justify that one has made responsible choices. For instance, another participant – a 34-year-old woman who unexpectedly became pregnant naturally after several failed IVF attempts – regarded the fact that she used IVF and PGD, even if unsuccessfully, as sufficient to fulfil her responsibilities of not transmitting the BRCA mutation to her child, and therefore saw herself as not blameworthy:

> I've done my part, right. I've been responsible, I've done my part and now I just have to leave it up to whatever's going to happen. And I'm okay with letting go, as long as I've done my part.

Limiting solutions to BRCA risks

An aspect of technological innovation that risk–benefit analyses often fail to consider is the way that they frame solutions to a particular problem. In this respect, the use of PGD for BRCA is certainly a blunt solution to the problem of reducing the transmission of cancer risks associated with BRCA mutations. After all, this technology allows for such reduction by selecting against embryos that carry such mutations. The elimination of the increased cancer risks is thus inseparable from the elimination of the embryo.

However, an emphasis on PGD as a solution to increased cancer risk associated with BRCA mutations might also limit the solutions offered to address such risk by directing research efforts in particular ways at the expense of others. Thus, if a technology is available that limits the chances of having offspring with BRCA mutations, efforts directed at understanding the ways in which such mutations contribute to cancer, or addressing the environmental contributors to breast and ovarian cancer in this population, might be reduced. As a 35-year-old participant who was undecided about having children but confident that she would not use PGD for BRCA if she did, emphatically put it:

> We're the sickest country. We have disease rates that are climbing astronomically. And, you know, even with BRCA1 and BRCA2 it's not 100% of the people that come down with a cancer. Genetics plays a part, but I think that if more effort could be – what is the secret of the people that don't get it? . . . . And that's where I focus . . . good genetics can take you pretty far, and it can compensate for a lot of problems. . . . But I don't think – it doesn't concern me as much as it used to.

Moreover, the emphasis that underlies the use of PGD for reducing the risk of passing on BRCA mutations also obscures the ways in which such cancer risks might be managed in other ways. For instance, one 30-year-old cancer survivor, who also lost her mother to cancer, called attention to this concern in a poignant way:

> You know, if my mom were alive, would she be blaming herself for giving me breast cancer? Maybe, but do you think that would've stopped her from having me? I don't think so. You know, so it's almost like, yeah, I think I might feel guilty if I did pass that down . . ., but I also think I might be knowledgeable enough, and I feel like in the times that we're living in now, like there's so much care that's available, and it's – you know, it could be cured at that point in time. . . . I don't think that [BRCA] would ever stop me from having kids.

Indeed, most participants felt optimistic that better options than PGD would develop by the time their children would begin to face an increased cancer risk, assuming they had inherited their parents' mutation. For example, a 40-year-old breast cancer survivor who was diagnosed in the middle of IVF treatment and who was not interested in PGD, stated: 'They're doing a lot of research in this area so eventually they're going to find what to do to correct the mutation. So I felt that in my child's lifetime, that correction would be done.'

Health and values

The main goal of PGD is to produce healthy children. The risk–benefit analyses of PGD take for granted the ethical appropriateness of such a goal. However, health and disease are not simply descriptive concepts; they involve normative considerations. Because of such normative considerations, health and disease states are not always easy to determine, at least in part. Moreover, health is one among many other goods that human beings value dearly, and at times, those goods can conflict. Conflicts between goods and the value-laden nature of the concepts of health and disease are also aspects that fit uneasily within the risk–benefit framework normally used to evaluate PGD. Indeed, one of the ethical concerns obscured by risk–benefit analysis is the fact that the use of PGD solves these conflicts between goods in a particular way. Thus, because PGD is aimed exclusively at limiting the possibility that prospective parents will pass on their BRCA mutations to their offspring, this technology in fact prioritizes concerns about health, and in particular a future child's health, over other aspects of human existence. This concern was expressed over and over by participants who were forced to face the existential question (Ormondroyd *et al.* 2012): Would I have been born if my parents had had the option of using PGD?

For instance, one 35-year-old woman who was using PGD for another condition but did not feel it was necessary for BRCA, wondered:

> Why would I? If my mother had this opportunity I wouldn't be here maybe. I don't know. I mean, that's just the way I was thinking. . . . I'm fine, I'm here. . . . When I look at my daughter, who could have the BRCA gene. . . . It doesn't make – it's not – I mean, would I not want her? That's what it comes down to.

Similarly, another participant who was 41 years old at the time of the interview had cancer a few years earlier and had frozen eggs just before her cancer treatment. However, despite the fact that she would need to undergo IVF to have biogenetically related children, she was nonetheless uninterested in PGD. She explained:

> . . . now that I have eggs frozen on First Avenue waiting for me – I've thought about it a lot and I don't think I would do the PGD because [pause]. Believe me this sucks – would I say my life hasn't been worth living because of it? No. Would my mother say, 'I wish I never had kids?' No.

Or, as another 38-year-old woman who participated simply stated: 'Would I have chosen never to be born? No, obviously.'

The emphasis on health at the expense of other aspects of human existence is also voiced by a 35-year-old cancer survivor with seven children, all daughters, who notes:

> I think most people walking around, I think if they tested corpses you would find that most people walking around are predisposed to many things. It's not a reason not to live. And it's not a reason not to have kids. This is not – I don't know. It's not guaranteed to be a terminal – you know, this isn't, you know, I don't know, maybe if it was a worse cancer.

Risk–benefit analyses fail to attend to the fact that the use of PGD presents a particular solution to the conflicts between goods, and they thus ignore the ethical consequences of the weighing of such goods. Moreover, such analyses also neglect considerations about how the use of PGD actually alters the boundaries between health and disease and encourages a particular construction of health, one that reduces health to the absence of genetic risks. Indeed, to the extent that PGD is thought of as an appropriate means to achieve the goal of having healthy children, its use for BRCA implies that people with such mutations are not healthy. This concern was clearly expressed by some of our participants, who challenged this view of health and disease. For instance, as one 35-year-old participant, whose mother and grandmother were both breast cancer survivors, explained: 'I just, I look at somebody with BRCA as healthy.' Another participant, a 30-year-old breast cancer survivor quoted earlier, explained that 'just because you have the gene doesn't mean you're gonna get cancer. It's not a sure thing. And I mean I'm healthy, I'm fine.'

She thus echoed the previous participant's challenge to equating risk with disease. However, as a cancer survivor, she takes this statement further to say that, even after having been through a cancer diagnosis and cancer treatment, she still views herself as healthy – a statement that was not uncommon among participants who had been diagnosed with early-stage breast cancer. Still another participant, a 34-year-old woman who had already undergone a prophylactic mastectomy and viewed this decision not as a signifier of illness but as a way to preserve her status as a healthy individual, explained: 'I'm still a healthy person and I'm still able to make decisions that preserve my health, so it feels different from having something where you're just not healthy.'

The boundaries between health and disease are often contested and unstable (Greene 2007). To the extent that PGD involves value-laden understandings of health and disease, such values must be open to scrutiny and critical evaluation. However, in taking such values for granted, risk–benefit analysis prevents just such an evaluation.

Conceptions of good parenting

PGD for BRCA is aimed at the selection of particular children – i.e. children who are not carriers of BRCA mutations. It is thus important that its use is grounded in particular assumptions about what it means to be a good parent. One such assumption is that good parenting is compatible with making decisions about a child's characteristics, even when such characteristics are unlikely to make the life of the child not worth living. However, such a conception conflicts with other widely accepted notions of good parenting that call for parents to love whatever child comes along (Herissone-Kelly 2007a, Herissone-Kelly 2007b, McDougall 2005). Indeed, some participants regard the use of PGD for BRCA as being at odds with this understanding of parenting. For instance, a 29-year-old Orthodox Jewish woman hoping to have children in the near future says about the likelihood of her using PGD:

> Probably not because in general I really do feel you get the lot that you get and you make the most of what you have. And if you start playing with – and again, let's say, I'll just have to teach my child how to deal with it. Medicine in general is going to help you deal with what you're genetically predisposed to.

Similarly, a 27-year-old participant – Catholic, Latina, and a cancer survivor – challenged the use of PGD for BRCA, which she viewed as conflicting with her own understanding of good parenting. In her words:

> Me personally – and this is coming from a girl who's never had a kid. I mean I don't know, I can theoretically think about the responsibility and the awesome, you know, burden on a parent's shoulder when they have a child with any condition, whether it's cancer or Down Syndrome. I would like to think that I would welcome any child, you know? And that when I become a parent I'm accepting to become a parent no matter what that child has, whether it's an emotional condition or psychological or – you know, I'd like to – I would hope that that would be my case. But I know that I haven't been a parent. I don't know what it is to walk into a doctor's office and have a doctor tell you your child is almost certain to have cancer one day, or that your child will have Down Syndrome, or . . .

This is not to say that the conception of good parenting that calls for parents to love whatever child comes along is a better conception than the one underlying the defence of PGD for BRCA. It is to say that such a defence actually presupposes a particular conception of good parents. Thus, while the use of PGD might have an important effect on our understanding of what it means to be a good parent, such considerations are ignored when we use a risk–benefit framework as a sufficient way to provide ourselves with a robust ethical analysis of PGD for BRCA mutations.

Conclusion

There is little doubt that, when evaluating medical technologies such as PGD for BRCA, paying attention to risks and benefits is often necessary and helpful. Although it is not emphasized in this chapter, participants in the study from which our data were derived certainly discussed matters that fall within a traditional risk–benefit analysis, including matters of eugenics and concerns about 'drawing lines', as well as the potential medical risks of IVF for women and children. However, as our paper illustrates, they raised further issues that are generally not recognized within this traditional analytic framework. While acknowledging the importance of the risk–benefit analysis, we contend that its use as the primary and exclusive strategy for engaging with an ethical analysis of PGD can direct and delimit how we understand the value and limitations of this technology. For example, if the central and primary concern is eugenics, debates will centre on whether PGD for hereditary cancer risk is a eugenic practice and on how to mitigate potential eugenic harms by establishing limitations and parameters on its use. However, while a variety of other ethical concerns are also relevant, these are disregarded by a risk–benefit framework as traditionally understood. These include questions about the cost of increased choices, the limitations that an emphasis on PGD as a solution to breast and ovarian cancer risks can introduce when considering solutions to such risks, the meaning of the goal of creating healthy children, and with it, the construction of health and disease in reductionist ways as well as the value assumptions about good parenting that are presupposed by the use of PGD.

Moving beyond a risk–benefit framework engages many issues that are raised throughout this volume, including matters of temporality, subjectivity, empowerment and prevention. When considering PGD, interview participants often engaged with the past – particularly their mother's, aunts' or grandmothers' experiences of cancer – to weigh concerns about their (future) children's lives. PGD gives BRCA mutation carriers hope that they can halt devastating intergenerational legacies of cancer. However, the discourse of empowerment that supported their decision to undergo BRCA testing already made BRCA feel less devastating. Thus, participants could be observed weighing decisions about PGD in a context in which the meaning of BRCA itself is continually shifting and 'mutating' (Gibbon 2007: 74). Indeed, some participants resisted the geneticization of identity that has accompanied predictive genetic testing (Novas and Rose 2000), refusing ways of reformulating risk as disease (Fosket 2010) and reconceptualizing the category 'at risk' as 'chronically ill'.

As we noted earlier, when considering disease prevention, PGD – while halting a particular BRCA mutation within a family line – is a 'blunt instrument' that is a limited strategy for cancer prevention. Several participants felt that the option of PGD (as well as the other preventive measures available, such as preventive surgery and chemoprevention) was an overly individualized and unsatisfactory strategy for prevention. It is noteworthy that our data were collected within the US health care context. Indeed, a risk–benefit framework sits comfortably within the US neoliberal health care context, which emphasizes such individualized solutions. However, as a handful of participants highlighted, it also limits our imagination regarding the kind of solutions that are sought in relation to cancer prevention.

Through the voices of people who are carriers of BRCA mutations – people living in the US who were invited to discuss the use of PGD – we have illustrated several important ethical considerations here that fit uneasily within the risk–benefit framework. To the extent that attention to these concerns is arguably relevant to be able to adequately evaluate PGD, exclusively focusing on the assessment of the risks and benefits of PGD – which is the primary approach taken within academic medicine and which informs everyday practice – will fall short of providing a compelling ethical evaluation of this technique.

References

Baum, M. (2006) 'Pre-implantation genetic diagnosis (PGD): the spectre of eugenics or a "no brainer"', *International Journal of Surgery,* 4: 144–5.

Bredenoord, A. L., Dondorp, W., Pennings, G., De Die-Smulders, C. E. and De Wert, G. (2008) 'PGD to reduce reproductive risk: the case of mitochondrial DNA disorders', *Human Reproduction,* 23: 2392–401.

Camporesi, S. (2010) 'Choosing deafness with preimplantation genetic diagnosis: an ethical way to carry on a cultural bloodline?' *Cambridge Quarterly of Healthcare Ethics,* 19: 86–96.

Charmaz, K. (2000) 'Grounded theory: objectivist and constructivist methods'. In Denzin, N. K. and Lincoln, Y. S. (eds) *Handbook of Qualitative Research,* 2nd ed. Thousand Oaks, CA: Sage Publications.

Claes, E., Evers-Kiebooms, G., Boogaerts, A., Decruyenaere, M., Denayer, L. and Legius, E. (2004) 'Diagnostic genetic testing for hereditary breast and ovarian cancer in cancer patients: women's looking back on the pre-test period and a psychological evaluation', *Genetic Testing,* 8: 13–21.

Clancy, T. (2010) 'A clinical perspective on ethical arguments around prenatal diagnosis and preimplantation genetic diagnosis for later onset inherited cancer predispositions', *Familial Cancer,* 9: 9–14.

Dumit, J. and Davis-Floyd, R. (1998) 'Cyborg babies: children of the third millennium'. In J. Dumit and R. Davis-Floyd (eds) *Cyborg Babies: From Techno-Sex to Techno-Tots.* New York, NY: Routledge.

Esplen, M. J., Madlensky, L., Aronson, M. et al. (2007) 'Colorectal cancer survivors undergoing genetic testing for hereditary non-polyposis colorectal cancer: motivational factors and psychosocial functioning', *Clinical Genetics,* 72: 394–401.

Fosket, J. R. (2010) 'Breast cancer risk as disease: biomedicalizing risk'. In Clarke, A. E., Mamo, L., Fosket, J. R., Fishman, J. F. and Shim, J. K. (eds) *Biomedicalization: Technoscience, Health, and the Illness in the U.S.* Durham, NC: Duke University Press.

Geraedts, J. P. and De Wert, G. M. (2009) 'Preimplantation genetic diagnosis', *Clinical Genetics,* 76: 315–25.

Gibbon, S. (2007) *Breast Cancer Genes and the Gendering of Knowledge: Science and Citizenship in the Cultural Context of the 'New' Genetics.* New York: Palgrave MacMillan.

Greene, J. A. (2007) *Prescribing by Numbers: Drugs and the Definition of Disease.* Baltimore: Johns Hopkins University Press.

Harper, J. C. and SenGupta, S. B. (2012) 'Preimplantation genetic diagnosis: state of the art 2011', *Human Genetics,* 131: 175–86.

Herissone-Kelly, P. (2007a) 'Parental love and the ethics of sex selection', *Cambridge Quarterly of Healthcare Ethics,* 16: 326–35.

——. (2007b) 'The "parental love" objection to nonmedical sex selection: deepening the argument', *Cambridge Quarterly of Healthcare Ethics,* 16: 446–55.

Kenen, R. H. (1996) 'The at-risk health status and technology: a diagnostic invitation and the "gift" of knowing.' *Social Science and Medicine,* 42: 1545–53.

King, D. S. (1999) 'Preimplantation genetic diagnosis and the "new" eugenics', *Journal of Medical Ethics,* 25: 176–82.

King, J. (2008) 'Predicting probability: regulating the future of preimplantation genetic screening', *Yale Journal of Health Policy, Law, and Ethics,* 8: 283–358.

Krahn, T. (2009) 'Preimplantation genetic diagnosis: does age of onset matter (anymore)?' *Medicine, Health Care and Philosophy,* 12: 187–202.

Malek, J. and Daar, J. (2012) 'The case for a parental duty to use preimplantation genetic diagnosis for medical benefit', *American Journal of Bioethics,* 12: 3–11.

Mansour, R. (2004) 'Preimplantation genetic diagnosis for Y-linked diseases: why not?' *Reproductive Biomedicine Online,* 8: 144–5.

McCabe, L. L. and McCabe, E. R. (2011) Down syndrome: coercion and eugenics', *Genetics in Medicine,* 13: 708–10.

Mcdougall, R. (2005) 'Acting parentally: an argument against sex selection', *Journal of Medical Ethics,* 31: 601–5.

Noble, R., Bahadur, G., Iqbal, M. and Sanyal, A. (2008) 'Pandora's box: ethics of PGD for inherited risk of late-onset disorders', *Reproductive Biomedicine Online,* 17 Suppl. 3: 55–60.

Novas, C. and Rose, N. (2000) 'Genetic risk and the birth of the somatic individual', *Economy and Society,* 29: 485–513.

Ormondroyd, E., Donnelly, L., Moynihan, C. et al. (2012) 'Attitudes to reproductive genetic testing in women who had a positive BRCA test before having children: a qualitative analysis', *European Journal of Human Genetics,* 20: 4–10.

Oster, E., Dorsey, E. R., Bausch, J. et al. and Huntington Study Group PHAROS Investigators (2008) 'Fear of health insurance loss among individuals at risk for Huntington disease', *American Journal of Medical Genetics Part A,* 146A: 2070–7.

Parens, E. and Asch, A. (1999) 'The disability rights critique of prenatal genetic testing: reflections and recommendations', *The Hastings Center Report,* 29: 40–47.

Robertson, J. A. (2003) 'Extending preimplantation genetic diagnosis: the ethical debate. Ethical issues in new uses of preimplantation genetic diagnosis', *Human Reproduction,* 18: 465–71.

Rubin, L. (2008–2011) 'Awareness and attitudes regarding prenatal and preimplantation genetic diagnosis for inherited breast-ovarian cancer risk'. Online. http://projectreporter.nih.gov/project_info_description.cfm?aid=7533877&icde=18536649&ddparam=&ddvalue=&ddsub=&cr=2&csb=default&cs=ASC

Rubin, L. and de Melo-Martín, I. (2012) '"Dilemmas of choice": exploring how oocyte recipients manage information about prospective donors', paper presented at the conference Selective Reproductive Technologies – Routes of Routinisation and Globalisation, University of Copenhagen, Denmark, 13–15 December.

Savulescu, J. (2001) 'Procreative beneficence: why we should select the best children', *Bioethics,* 15: 413–26.

Scott, R., Williams, C., Ehrich, K. and Farsides, B. (2007) 'The appropriate extent of pre-implantation genetic diagnosis: health professionals' and scientists' views on the requirement for a "significant risk of a serious genetic condition"', *Medical Law Review,* 15: 320–56.

SenGupta, S. B., Vadaparampil, S. T. and Menon, U. (2012) 'Preimplantation genetic diagnosis for hereditary cancers', *Advances in Experimental Medicine and Biology,* 732: 103–13.

Simpson, J.L. (2010) 'Preimplantation genetic diagnosis at 20 years', *Prenatal Diagnostics,* 30: 682–95.

Snelling, J. (2008) 'Preimplantation genetic diagnosis for susceptibility conditions: a new frontier or a logical extension?' *Journal of Law and Medicine,* 16: 263–78.

Van Asperen, C.J., Van Dijk, S., Zoeteweij, M.W. et al. (2002) 'What do women really want to know? Motives for attending familial breast cancer clinics', *Journal of Medical Genetics,* 39: 410–414.

Afterword

Studying BRCA performativity: re-calibrations by and of the social sciences

Susanne Bauer

It was in the heyday of a new genetic determinism when the two breast cancer genes BRCA 1 and BRCA 2 were postulated in the early 1990s. At the time, the new genetics epitomized what Mike Fortun analyzed as 'futural, promissory economy' (Fortun 2008: 20). Biomedical scientists prepared the public for the revolution of biological knowledge that they envisioned with the sequencing of the human genome, including radical changes in the understandings of disease and new therapeutic avenues. The health sciences also prepared for the new technologies and data that emerged from human genome research. In epidemiology, for example, there was widespread optimism that strong associations between genetic polymorphisms and disease were about to be discovered and confirmed at the population level. This held especially for cancer, which was already conceived of as a mostly genetic disease, not only in terms of hereditary components, but also at the molecular level, with DNA mutation understood as the first step in the development of a tumour. Tackling these mechanisms of carcinogenesis at their molecular origin – DNA mutations – epidemiologists expected that genetics would open what they called the 'black box' between exposure and disease. Earlier biomedical models described tumour development as initiated by DNA mutation causing 'uncontrolled cell proliferation', followed by 'cancer promotion' depending on further carcinogenic agents. Scientists envisioned that variation in genetic sequence, such as single nucleotide polymorphisms (SNPs) might even prove to be the main epidemiological determinants of cancer at the population level.

What kind of thing is BRCA today, two decades after it entered the world? To what extent have developments in biomedical research altered understandings of health and disease, modes of knowing the body and medical practices? How does the related scientific apparatus of observation work and what are the socialities that have emerged with BRCA?

With expression profiling and the study of gene-environment interaction, other variables have moved to centre stage, and a shift toward epigenetics seems to have dissolved much of the earlier determinisms. As genes are, with a few exceptions, no longer conceived of as deterministic, knowledge of gene sequences and mutations, including those in BRCA, has largely lost its promissory potential. As a result of the epidemiological search for genes and gene patterns that would be associated with cancer, no single genes could be stabilized as major causal determinants; what emerged were but a few new clinical markers. Despite these developments, however, as any search in databases such as PubMed will confirm, there is a huge biomedical research industry that continues to test associations of BRCA mutations, related expression profiles and postgenomic markers with different cancers as well as other diseases in various population subgroups in many regions and countries. The new genetics has had effects beyond the discursive level, in that genomics now provides the technological and institutional infrastructures of future research in the biosciences. Indeed, to use a term from actor-network theory,[1] BRCA has emerged as an important 'nonhuman actant' in the biomedical research landscape and in clinical practice. Health and disease continue to be reshuffled through genomic infrastructures and its refined technologies, in which BRCA features as one involuted actant.

Debates within biomedicine over further breast cancer genes in addition to BRCA 1 and BRCA 2 also point to a host of gene–gene interactions and epigenetic mechanisms in the process of carcinogenesis. Epidemiological attempts to test for these genes enrol histories of previous databases and surveillance practices that are recombined into novel quasi-experimental configurations (Bauer 2008). In contrast to commercial testing, clinical researchers—as Bourret *et al.* describe—no longer sharply divide between hereditary and sporadic breast cancer nor between genotype and phenotype. Instead, somatic mutations of tumour tissue have moved to centre stage. BRCA also has become 'BRCAness' (Bourret *et al.*, this volume), denoting a set of phenotypic characteristics. Bourret *et al.* show how BRCA and PARP inhibitors helped each other into new career paths, bringing about 'BRCAness' as a therapeutic object and stabilizing the conditions for translational research by increasing the target population. The biomedical understanding has moved to a concept of markers in sporadic cancers, rather than understanding genes as hereditary component. BRCA is done as a biomarker and, for example, 'triple negative' is understood as a tumour characteristic. While powerfully resonating with earlier expectations, what BRCA is has been subject to change from a causal claim to a clinically applicable tumour characteristic.

In addition to its role in debates concerning disease causation and its entry into clinical practice, BRCA has also been taken up in preventive risk reduction. At the time of writing this chapter, the case of Angelina Jolie's preventive breast surgery featured on the first pages of tabloid papers and in the mainstream press (see also the Introduction, this volume).[2] The extent to which media accounts revolved around 'taking responsibility' begs witness to how much preventive risk management has become common sense. Prevention options informed by personalized genomics and brought forward to individualized 'at-risk subjects' range from the management of risk factors through enhanced screening to prophylactic surgery and recently even pre-implantation diagnostics as a 'choice not to pass on these mutations' (Rubin, this volume). Perhaps less an effect of the new genetics specifically, this is symptomatic of a more general rise of preventive governmentality, based on self-surveillance and active monitoring.

How can we situate these emerging practices of self-surveillance, early interventions and preemptive optimization? Information technologies and biomedical computing (November 2012) laid the ground for large-scale databases, routines of information storing and linkage, and organizations such as the Cochrane movement for evidence-based medicine. Evidence-based-medicine epitomizes the contemporary mode of technocratic acting in medicine based on guidelines grounded in clinical trials and epidemiological evidence. Guideline medicine works at the same time as a new bureaucratic regime and as a movement against hierarchies ('evidence versus eminence'), changing the organizational hierarchies of the clinic to the hierarchies of biostatistical evidence. Especially genomics can be situated in the history of Cold War research and the Human Genome Project was a direct outcome of the infrastructures established by the Atomic Energy Commission.[3]

Novel modes of securitization have joined the Cold War biomedical and information technologies in forming contemporary modes of rationalizing and handling risk. Post-9/11 securitization has generated new technologies and routines of surveillance that also extend to data-tracking in health monitoring. These configurations of surveillance techniques shape the distributed anticipatory infrastructures of what public health is today (Adams *et al.* 2009; Joseph, this volume).

How can we, from a social science perspective, understand the technoscientific actant 'BRCA' within the larger bio-technopolitics? One of the contributions the social studies of technoscience can make is to bring to the fore the situated and often black-boxed infrastructural constellations that have shaped contemporary technocratic rationalities. I take up Donna Haraway's notion of diffraction (Haraway 1997: 273) to unpack and reposition what is otherwise considered given knowledge and neutral sets of methods. Haraway introduces the strategy of diffraction as different from reflection in that diffraction focuses on heterogeneous patterns of inference and interaction rather than asking for causal origins and levels of representation. This strategy of diffraction has been elaborated by Karen Barad, to shift from word to matter, include nonhuman agency and move from representationalism to performativity (Barad 2007). Drawing on Niels Bohr's philosophical writings on quantum physics, Barad's concept of diffraction brings to the fore intra-actions within the material apparatus of observation, thereby moving beyond the division of subject and object in observation and conceptualizing them as entangled. What does it mean to diffract the bio-technopolitics of BRCA in this sense? How can we examine the technoscientific apparatus in which BRCA remains elusive but at the same time is enabled to travel further, enter the clinic and materialize in BRCA socialities?

The apparatus of observation

Zooming in on the apparatus of observation from which BRCA emerges leads to several interconnected sites, including the laboratory of molecular biology, the clinic, information technology and corporatized research in genomics. Together these are linked through cross-disciplinary 'biomedical platforms', to use a term Keating and Cambrosio (2003) introduced in their study of immunophenotyping. One of the connecting platforms between these sites is epidemiology.[4] As a mode of relating multiple potential influences to disease within sets of population data, epidemiology draws together otherwise disparate contexts. Its techniques of deriving statistical inferences with large-scale data have been enabled by information technologies and record linkage. To examine the connections between BRCA mutations and disease statistically on this epidemiological platform, genetic epidemiologists collect and link together data in particular ways. They transform these data from different contexts into quasi-experimental constellations, in which they calculate quantitative estimates of the effects of a genetic mutation on disease frequencies by comparing groups with and without the mutation under study. The resulting risk estimates are the technical core of evidence-based medicine; its formalized decision-making draws on the strength and statistical significance of the association as read through the risk estimates.

These concepts – the epidemiological platform and the specific apparatus of observation that makes this platform – help analyze what I call the BRCA assemblage, a notion that accounts for heterogeneous knowledge configurations and situated ways of doing BRCA or, in other words, both epistemological issues and situated ontologies. The notion of platform points to the flexibility, the traffic and intersection of the data that make up the flow through this platform as a hub for variables that come in from many directions. The apparatus, in turn, can be thought of as a specific material constellation of measurement devices with a long, contingent history of stabilization, with certain fixed technological components, shaping the methodological infrastructure of scientific knowledge production.

Genetic epidemiology works as an engine of difference production that generates blendings and slippages between genetic and nongenetic categories. It results in a heterogeneous collation of interrelated probabilistic risk estimates. A whole spectrum of mutations enters epidemiological risk modelling, each with different characteristics and largely unknown effects. Genetic epidemiologists deal with this complexity by introducing additional coefficients for variable 'gene penetrance' and gene–gene interactions as well as 'molecular environments'. In this way, the epidemiological model containing BRCA as one actant reshuffles large bodies of medical knowledge, data, samples – and, with it, the contexts in which these were generated or collected. We can think of epidemiological modelling as a generative simulacrum (in the Deleuzian sense) that produces difference and, rather than remaining merely virtual, constantly feeds novel variables into scientific debates. It is the scientific modelling that enacts new proximities and distances, connections and disconnections, shortcuts and convergences. As several contributions in this volume show, modelling endeavours constantly transform the particular pasts generated in now genomics-informed sciences of human origins, migration histories and disease aetiologies as well as the particular futures in their predictive twist.

How the results of a genetic test for a mutation are interpreted is informed by epidemiological results – risk estimates, the results of risk modelling. In risk estimation, BRCA status is formalized as exposure and subjected to the hypothesis test for association with breast cancer. Interpreted as measures of genetic susceptibility or tumour characteristic, they take on clinical relevance. As chapters in this volume make clear, these have implications even in the absence of a genetic test. Patient profiling by sets of proxy categories are used as a pre-diagnostic tool and as a proxy for genetic susceptibility and a proxy of the test itself; these often include the category ethnicity or, more recently, 'biogeograhical ancestry'. Yet, as one might ask, what happens when ancestry and belonging are calculated as a matter of statistics and proportions and when individual study participants are categorized as 'between 20 to 80 per cent European' in Latin American countries?[5]

These estimates of susceptibility can be viewed as lived simulacrum and statistics of the real at the same time. However, as they leave the realm of science, they also bring about social stratification and become performatively linked to socialities. The so-called 'Ashkenazi mutations' discussed by Mozersky and Gibbon (this volume) are one example of the ways in which biostatistical techniques recombine, align and collapse genomic markers, founder mutations, historical events and disease rates. Mozersky and Gibbon show how, in the UK, studies of 'Ashkenazi mutations' reiterate and naturalize narratives of Jewish history, with Jewish ancestry itself made into a risk factor and indication for the test. At the same time, the presence of a mutation shown by the test is often not in line with self-identified categories of belonging, thereby adding more layers to everyday negotiations of identity and difference.

Physicians and patients deal with this messiness of categories, acting within this simulacrum of probabilistic differences, a data space in which proxies and surrogate variables come to materialize and matter. In her work on HIV/Aids, Paula Treichler coined the term 'epidemics of signification' for this epidemiological practice of fixing risk groups (Treichler 1999). Surrogate variables and proxies of proxies are reshuffled and recombined with the data incessantly produced by new measurement techniques and by the travelling of these techniques into different social settings. Such effects in mundane research routines also become visible in the attempts to adapt questionnaires channelled through the same sets of variables and procedures, from a US funding context to places in the 'global south'. Focusing on the apparatus of observation helps ground the transformations of what disease and a disease marker become in the specific relations enacted through the scientific modelling practices.

The BRCA story is characteristic of the larger development of (post)genomics, in its departure from deterministic visions to multiple interactions and conditional pathways that are being modeled.[6] Recently, postgenomic exercises of co-relating have been reported under the elusive notion of 'translational medicine'. This includes a wide range of translations from sequence to protein, but also bench to bedside, epidemiology to health policy and population patterns to individual profile in evidence-based prevention and therapy as well as genomics education. Chapters in this volume give an empirical account of these renegotiations, sense-making, discriminations and appropriations of BRCA, and thereby of the scientific career and social life of BRCA.

BRCA socialities

The chapters in this volume provide empirically situated accounts of how BRCA is worked into lives, renegotiated, transformed or rejected. As BRCA entered clinical decision-making, it has brought about precarious socialities, from the stratified access to healthcare to the uncertainties and implications of a positive test.[7] BRCA has become an intersection through which breast cancer-related practices, identities and bodies are made to pass. By examining localized BRCA assemblages, lived realities and situated bodies, these case studies demonstrate how BRCA is not one entity, but many entities, to use Annemarie Mol's notion of multiplicity (Mol 2002).

The situated BRCA at-risk subjectivities enacted by genetic testing (or proxy profiling techniques) also have in common certain features. These include the specific regimes of risks brought about by stratified biomedicalization (Clarke *et al.* 2003) as well as specific entanglements of futures and past in these regimes (Adams *et al.* 2009). The apparatus of risk assessment through which BRCA socialities are coproduced are entangled in western choice-based reasoning in a market logic, leading to overemphasis of behaviour and individualized decision-making. Risk factor epidemiology had tended to make imperceptible social disparities and environmental disadvantage. More recently with the prominence of epigenetics and recognition of the complexity of environmental health, several shifts have taken place. New epigenetic accounts mobilize different, molecularized versions of the environment (Landecker 2011) – and the social – which recombine into novel experimental configurations. While these seem to open up a new space in which environmental variables can be included, we need to attend to and follow these developments closely in order to understand the specific effects of these turns to biomedical complexity.

The transnational studies collated in this volume are part of the project to situate and diffract BRCA empirically. Chapters show the dramatic disparities in relation to public health services and their gaps, where diagnostic technologies such as BRCA testing only arise as option for the most wealthy, including elite cancer aid activities, self-organized breast cancer survivors, and attempts to introduce early diagnosis. Alison Macdonald (this volume) describes landscapes of cancer activism in urban India and ways of dealing with breast cancer as a disease of modernity as opposed to traditional ways of living. She traces different articulations within activist groups in contemporary Mumbai, in which the 'absence' of BRCA is notable. Within local health care, breast cancer heredity is differently made and reworked into concerns about modernization, social change in matters of health, lifestyle and environment. Even in the absence of genetic testing, BRCA talk brings about specific gendered bodies, and constant negotiation of different cosmologies, both indigenous and biomedical.

The African American Family History Project described by Galen Joseph (this volume) as an example of biosocialization processes in the US, shows how public health genomics on the one hand produces a geneticized, biohistorical understanding of health disparities, while on the other hand, BRCA is renegotiated and linked to experiences of racism. Joseph's essay provides insight into the paradigms of anticipatory biosocialization as these communities become enrolled through public health programs aimed at identifying high-risk women in these communities. Complementary to Joseph's case of a specifically negotiated 'anticipatory habitus', Mozersky and Gibbon show how genetic tests for three specific BRCA mutations, also labelled 'Ashkenazi mutations', reconfigure the past, collapsing historically shaped identity and materiality of gene sequence in different ways in the UK and Brazil. In the Brazilian case (Mozersky and Gibbon, this volume), screenings for mutations are accomplished through links to migration history, and incorporated into public health in Brazil, where the difference categories of the risk prediction tools developed in the US fail. This prompts practitioners to improvise when working with the test in which category, in terms of the US-specific census categories, they apply when working with patients in Brazil.

Largely commercial products of personalized genomics feature as 'direct-to-consumer marketing' from endeavours in genetic epidemiology that Sarah Franklin once called a 'burgeoning translation industry' (Franklin 1995: 175). Giving an update of the status of that industry, Sandra Soo-Jin Lee (this volume) explores the relationship of patents, personalized medicine and participation in this corporate context, taking customers of companies such as 23andMe as an example. Lee focuses on the shift 'from reactive to preventive' and the rhetoric of 'P4' – 'predictive, personalized, preemptive and participatory', which comes as a corporate strategy, shifting the meaning of participatory and the right to know. These commercial options and corporate practices construct patients as mere consumers. Corporate constructions of patients as mere consumers of commercialized testing stands in contrast to the case described by Pelters of queer appropriations of at-risk-subjectivity (Pelters, this volume). She focuses on ways of handling BRCA risk and possibilities of queering the medicalized BRCA femininity reinforced in pink ribbon campaigns. Pelters reconstructs how BRCA-positive women navigate risk management to challenge gender stereotypes in breast cancer treatment.

Much of North American biomedical research is discussed in the framework of the inclusion paradigm (Epstein 2007), which is also linked to the particular North American connection between identity politics and the civil rights movement. Inclusion and difference are closely connected; inclusion can be demanded as a right *because* of difference. Different from contexts which centre on equality, American biomedical research even draws on this paradigm to market 'ethnic' drugs to African Americans (Kahn 2004). In the research routines of genetic epidemiology, gene frequencies are brought in alignment with census categories. For instance, researchers at Howard University[8] working on health disparities focus especially on African American populations with the aim to study 'minority biologies', a huge project of difference production. Attending to transnational differences in the histories and politics of equality and difference, as in the chapters by zur Nieden and Mozersky and Gibbon, helps to further decentre this US-specific bio-multiculturalism that travels with biomedical categories. For the case of Germany, zur Nieden describes how the citizenship discourse, albeit modernized and no longer exclusively based on the former *ius sanguinis,* builds on notions of integration rather than diversity. She shows how in Germany, US-centred biomedical notions of bio-multiculturalism clash in various ways with what is speakable in the German context. First, contemporary notions of biological difference described as 'ethnic' in the German context strongly resonate with the Nazi history and the role of race science in the Holocaust; therefore, such a production of difference is viewed as stigmatizing rather than anything else. Second, alternative articulations of difference used in Germany such as categories of 'migrant' or 'migration background' still work within a conservative integration paradigm, reifying differences even of the second and third generations of immigrants.

When BRCA genotyping is too expensive and researchers use proxies such as census categories or other self-identifications in the clinic as a shortcut to disease risk, racialized markers or one founder mutation become proxies for genetic susceptibility. Compared to the US, those work very differently in Brazil (Mozersky and Gibbon). Biomedical scientists problematize that US risk estimates are not transferable to the Brazil situation as a need for 'local' research. In this context, US foundations suddenly see the Brazilian mixed population as 'a unique research resource' and an experimental test site. Conceived of as laboratories of admixture, European ancestry subgroups in Latin American populations become 'unique populations', in a geographical and institutional 'outsourcing' of US research. International agencies and pharmaceutical companies identify populations as 'underserved' or 'with unmet needs' in public health genomics. In the Brazilian context especially, this stands in sharp contrast to the strong social epidemiology tradition that works with 'class' as a socio-economic variable and etiologic factor in disease causation.

Re-calibrating social studies of biomedicine

To what extent does BRCA testing work like other screening technologies such as the Pap smear or mammography? The latter could also be viewed as a product of the Cold War and the women's health movement.[9] Given the hype and hope as well as the concerns about biosurveillance and overmedicalization of women's bodies, what is at stake 20 years after BRCA was reported for the first time? What are the concerns that the social studies of science should follow up?

Social scientists have trained their attention on new biotechnologies in the tradition of risk sociology and conditions of subjectification as well as for their biopolitical effects. Technology assessment research was institutionalized since the 1980s and, in particular in the UK, many sociological research centres were organized around studies of the new genetics during the 1990s. In a funding niche within genomics, studies of ethical, legal and social implications (ELSI) took shape. These, however, often were limited to studies of effects without engaging in science in-the-making. Going beyond ELSI, this volume updates and extends studies of biosociality in Paul Rabinow's initial understanding (Rabinow 1996) as well as reflects on the question of how the social sciences can position themselves in relation to changing biomedical technologies. This project also involves a reflexive take on social science performativity when acting with biomedicine.

Even though not exactly organized around a genetic test result as in Rabinow's example, the social studies of BRCA do evolve around a genetic test technology. In a certain way, undertakings in the social studies of BRCA can be viewed as part of such biosocialities. Seen from this perspective, what are the political challenges to social science of biomedicine here, and how do social studies themselves perform in the BRCA assemblage? How are we to recalibrate the social studies of BRCA sciences when the goal is to generate more polyvocal accounts on stratified vulnerabilities in order to decenter mainstream notions of BRCA? What can an engagement in diffraction rather than subscribing to biosociality look like? The empirical studies of BRCA assemblages presented in this volume contribute to this analytical project in various ways. Following the enactments of technoscientific BRCA socialities, they begin to outline and reconstruct the ontologies as they emerge from actual BRCA-associated practices.

For an account of contemporary BRCA sociality, its ambiguity and contradictions, following BRCA objects in practice can work as a reality check. After all, BRCA may be viewed as just another biomarker consulted in technocratic clinical decision-making. As a biomarker, BRCA carries the culture of a post-Cold War technoscientific entity and a product and legacy of the late twentieth-century new genetics hype. While it proved responsible for just a proportion of hereditary breast cancer overall, BRCA has become a global actant in breast cancer genetics and reshaped the ways breast cancer is known and practised.

In order to grasp the transnational impact and consequences of BRCA, more varied stories of BRCA are needed that help lay out BRCA multiplicity. Adopting the biomedical shift from a genotypic to a phenotypic definition to include emergent BRCA socialities, one could describe the effects of this development as social 'BRCAness' to highlight the socially stratified appropriations implicated in BRCA practices. The stakes in this mode of public health genomics include issues of racism, deprivation/social disparities, good life, health, citizenship, global economies, markets, corporate structures, patents and technoscientific infrastructures. Here, social sciences can also draw from post-race debates within biomedicine (Fujimura and Rajagopalan 2011). Significantly, the term 'mestizaje' continues to appear in Brazilian BRCA population genetics. Bringing this trope in resonance with the postcolonial difference figure of the 'mestiza' (Anzaldúa 1999), are there possibilities in which such hybrid tricksters can be made to perform otherwise? Could this work in a mode similar to the queering of 'normative BRCA femininity', discussed by Pelters, this time as a means of queering and strategically countering Euro-American 'race science'? Notions of hybridity and 'mixture as a resource' evoke decolonial agendas and political tactics, too. To what extent can performative appropriations change biomedicine – despite the legacies of 'race science' and the hegemony of Euro-American risk factor epidemiology? These questions can open up new avenues that shift the focus from the coproduction and mutual reifications of the social and biological toward decentering Euro-American epistemologies and go beyond long standing Western divisions between nature and culture, whilst developing a critique of the biomedical body politic and of health technologies. Societies of control have refined the technological apparatus of public health through far-reaching monitoring and surveillance. At the same time, social networks, commercial ancestry and health testing have changed the ways in which genomics-based risk estimates are consumed and circulate in various publics. Diffracting BRCA and examining how BRCA is actually done in the assemblages of biomedicine can develop these analyses further and beyond biosociality.

Notes

1. See for example Latour, *Reassembling the Social. An Introduction to Actor-Network-Theory* (Oxford: Oxford University Press, 2005). Actor-network-theory does not limit agency to human actors but conceives of agency as chains of agency that are distributed among human and non-human actors, also termed 'actants'.
2. Jonathan Haynes and Denis Campbell, 'Angelina Jolie praised for revelation over double mastectomy. Health campaigners praise actor's decision to go public to encourage other women to check for defective gene BRCA1'. guardian.co.uk, 15 May, 2013.
3. See Schlünder (this volume) for more details on the history of biomedical sciences.
4. 'Modern epidemiology' has been defined as the study of 'statistical distributions and determinants of health and disease in populations' (Last 2001), a definition also adopted by the World Health Organization.
5. See Ana Egana, 'Genetic ancestry and breast cancer risk in an admixed Latin American population from Uruguay'. Conference presentation, Hermance, 5 December, 2011.
6. The term modeling integrates several more specific practices – from statistical testing via regression modeling, an optimization that fits the explanatory models to empirical datasets and systematic models that work with certain assumptions about pathogenic mechanisms.
7. I introduce the concept of socialities here to broaden concepts of 'biosociality' (Rabinow 1996) and to account for the multiplicity and range of renegotiations taking place in the transnational configurations of BRCA.
8. Howard University is a prominent historically Black US college.
9. See Murphy (2012) for a detailed account of the history of the Pap smear.

References

Adams, V., Murphy, M. and Clarke, A. (2009) 'Anticipation: technoscience, life, affect, temporality', *Subjectivity* 28: 246–65.

Anzaldúa, G. (1999) *Borderlands/La Frontera: The New Mestiza.* San Francisco: Aunt Lute Books.

Barad, K. (2007) *Meeting the Universe Halfway: Quantum Physics and the Entanglement of Matter and Meaning.* Durham and London: Duke University Press.

Bauer, S. (2008) 'Mining data, gathering variables and recombining information: the flexible architecture of epidemiological studies', *Studies in History and Philosophy of Biological and Biomedical Sciences* 39: 415–26.

Clarke, A.E., Mamo, L., Fishman, J.R., Shim, J.K. and Fosket, J.R. (2003) 'Biomedicalization: technoscientific transformations of health, illness, and U.S. biomedicine', *American Sociological Review* 68: 161–94.

Epstein, S. (2007) *Inclusion. The Politics of Difference in Medical Research.* Chicago: University of Chicago Press.

Fortun, M. (2008) *Promising Genomics. Iceland and deCODE Genetics in a World of Speculation.* Berkeley: University of California Press.

Franklin, S. (1995) 'Science as culture, cultures of science', *Annual Review of Anthropology* 24: 163–84.

Fujimura, J.H. and Rajagopalan, R. (2011) 'Different differences: the use of "genetic ancestry" versus race in human genetic research', *Social Studies of Science* 41 (1): 5–30.

Haraway, D.J. (1997) *Modest_witness@Second_Millennium.FemaleMan©_Meets_OncoMouse ™: Feminism and Technoscience.* New York: Routledge.

Kahn, J. (2004) 'How a drug becomes "ethnic": law, commerce, and the production of racial categories in medicine', *Yale Journal of Health Policy, Law, and Ethics* 4: 1–46.

Keating, P. and Cambrosio, A. (2003) *Biomedical Platforms. Realigning the Normal and the Pathological in Late-Twentieth-Century Medicine*, Cambridge MA: MIT Press.

Landecker, H. (2011) 'Food as exposure: nutritional epigenetics and the new metabolism', *BioSocieties* 6: 167–94.

Last, J.M. (2001) *A Dictionary of Epidemiology.* Oxford and New York: Oxford University Press.

Latour, B. (2005) *Reassembling the Social: An Introduction to Actor-Network-Theory.* Oxford: Oxford University Press.

Mol, A. (2002) *The Body Multiple. Ontology in Medical Practice.* Durham, NC and London: Duke University Press

Murphy, M. (2012) *Seizing the Means of Reproduction: Entanglements of Feminism, Health, and Technoscience.* Durham, NC and London: Duke University Press.

November, J. (2012) *Biomedical Computing. Digitizing Life in the United States.* Baltimore: John Hopkins University Press.

Rabinow, P. (1996) 'Artificiality and enlightenment: from sociobiology to biosociality'. In P. Rabinow (ed.), *Essays on the Anthropology of Reason,* 91–112. Princeton: Princeton University Press.

Treichler, P.A. (1999) *How to Have a Theory in an Epidemic. Cultural Chronicles of Aids*, Durham: Duke University Press.

Index

Page numbers in italic format indicate figures and tables.

9780415824064